W9-AFK-910

FOURTH EDITION

THE NURSE EDUCATOR'S
Guide to Assessing Learning Outcomes

Mary E. McDonald, MA, RN

Educational Assessment Consultant

Brooklyn, New York

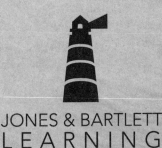

JONES & BARTLETT
LEARNING

World Headquarters
Jones & Bartlett Learning
5 Wall Street
Burlington, MA 01803
978-443-5000
info@jblearning.com
www.jblearning.com

Jones & Bartlett Learning books and products are available through most bookstores and online booksellers. To contact Jones & Bartlett Learning directly, call 800-832-0034, fax 978-443-8000, or visit our website, www.jblearning.com.

Substantial discounts on bulk quantities of Jones & Bartlett Learning publications are available to corporations, professional associations, and other qualified organizations. For details and specific discount information, contact the special sales department at Jones & Bartlett Learning via the above contact information or send an email to specialsales@jblearning.com.

Copyright © 2018 by Jones & Bartlett Learning, LLC, an Ascend Learning Company

All figures, tables, and exhibits in this book are copyrighted to Mary E. McDonald and have been used with permission. All rights reserved. No part of the material protected by this copyright may be reproduced or utilized in any form, electronic or mechanical, including photocopying, recording, or by any information storage and retrieval system, without written permission from the copyright owner.

The content, statements, views, and opinions herein are the sole expression of the respective authors and not that of Jones & Bartlett Learning, LLC. Reference herein to any specific commercial product, process, or service by trade name, trademark, manufacturer, or otherwise does not constitute or imply its endorsement or recommendation by Jones & Bartlett Learning, LLC and such reference shall not be used for advertising or product endorsement purposes. All trademarks displayed are the trademarks of the parties noted herein. *The Nurse Educator's Guide to Assessing Learning Outcomes, Fourth Edition* is an independent publication and has not been authorized, sponsored, or otherwise approved by the owners of the trademarks or service marks referenced in this product.

There may be images in this book that feature models; these models do not necessarily endorse, represent, or participate in the activities represented in the images. Any screenshots in this product are for educational and instructive purposes only. Any individuals and scenarios featured in the case studies throughout this product may be real or fictitious, but are used for instructional purposes only.

The authors, editor, and publisher have made every effort to provide accurate information. However, they are not responsible for errors, omissions, or for any outcomes related to the use of the contents of this book and take no responsibility for the use of the products and procedures described. Treatments and side effects described in this book may not be applicable to all people; likewise, some people may require a dose or experience a side effect that is not described herein. Drugs and medical devices are discussed that may have limited availability controlled by the Food and Drug Administration (FDA) for use only in a research study or clinical trial. Research, clinical practice, and government regulations often change the accepted standard in this field. When consideration is being given to use of any drug in the clinical setting, the health care provider or reader is responsible for determining FDA status of the drug, reading the package insert, and reviewing prescribing information for the most up-to-date recommendations on dose, precautions, and contraindications, and determining the appropriate usage for the product. This is especially important in the case of drugs that are new or seldom used.

Production Credits

VP, Executive Publisher: David D. Cella
Executive Editor: Amanda Martin
Associate Acquisitions Editor: Rebecca Stephenson
Editorial Assistant: Christina Freitas
Production Manager: Carolyn Rogers Pershouse
Production Assistant: Molly Hogue
Senior Marketing Manager: Jennifer Scherzay
Product Fulfillment Manager: Wendy Kilborn
Composition: S4Carlisle Publishing Services

Project Management: S4Carlisle Publishing Services
Cover Design: Michael O'Donnell
Rights & Media Specialist: Wes DeShano
Media Development Editor: Shannon Sheehan
Cover Image (Title Page): © Jonathan Knowles/Stone/Getty
Chapter Openers: © Anteromite/Shutterstock
Printing and Binding: Edwards Brothers Malloy
Cover Printing: Edwards Brothers Malloy

Library of Congress Cataloging-in-Publication Data

Names: McDonald, Mary, author.
Title: The nurse educator's guide to assessing learning outcomes / Mary E.
    McDonald.
Description: Fourth edition. | Burlington, Massachusetts : Jones & Bartlett
    Learning, [2018] | Includes bibliographical references and index.
Identifiers: LCCN 2017010375 | ISBN 9781284113365 (pbk. : alk. paper)
Subjects: | MESH: Education, Nursing | Educational Measurement--methods |
    Program Development
Classification: LCC RT81.5 | NLM WY 18 | DDC 610.73--dc23 LC record available at https://lccn.loc.gov/2017010375

6048

Printed in the United States of America
21 20 19 18 17   10 9 8 7 6 5 4 3 2 1

Dedication

This book is dedicated to the nursing educators across the country who continue to express their desire to improve their assessment skills. Special thanks go to the nurse educators who shared their assessment experiences with me; took the time to review the third edition; and offered many helpful suggestions, which I incorporated in this new edition.

I also want to acknowledge the continuous encouragement of my family, friends, colleagues, and editors throughout the process of revising this book. I especially want to thank my husband, Ed, for his continued support of all of my personal and professional endeavors.

Contents

Preface

"Nursing faculty at our school have a part-time schedule. They only work 12 hours each day."

—ANONYMOUS NURSING FACULTY MEMBER

This fourth edition of *The Nurse Educator's Guide to Assessing Learning Outcomes* expands, updates, and reorganizes the concepts and strategies presented in the third edition. The goal of this edition continues to focus on assisting nurse educators to increase their level of confidence in the decisions they have to make about students based on the results of their classroom exams. The premise of this edition continues: To create trustworthy exams, nurse educators must acquire competency in both developing and analyzing assessment instruments. This book is meant to be a resource for nurse educators, a text to be read through and then used as an ongoing reference for test development and analysis.

Since the publication of the third edition, I have continued to work with nurse educators who are committed to improving their assessment skills. I have consistently found that nurse educators want to ensure that their methods are fair to the students whose lives are affected by their decisions. This fourth edition refines the approach of the text based on the feedback of readers and incorporates the ideas and insights of numerous nurse educators who continue to share their experiences with me. In the interest of clarity, some of the subject matter has been revised and rearranged. Tables and exhibits are updated, and dozens of new exhibits have been added. The improvements in this edition increase its usefulness as a resource for developing valid and reliable assessment plans for nurse educators in both the education and practice settings.

This edition of *The Nurse Educator's Guide to Assessing Learning Outcomes* has a dual focus. It is a textbook for the continuing professional development of nurse educators and for prospective nurse educators in graduate school programs. It is also useful as a text and a reference for experienced nurse educators. In fact, educators in all fields will find that this book includes extensive and detailed practical information about classroom test development, although the examples are all related to nursing. This edition has also expanded the features introduced in the third edition at the end of each chapter: the "Web Links" and "Learning Activities" at the end of each chapter have been revised and updated. These features provide educators with an opportunity to test their knowledge and provide an impetus for further investigation of the topics presented in each chapter.

A new appendix also has also been added to this edition. Appendix F, "Sample Item Stems for Client Needs Using the Nursing Process Format," is designed to assist faculty to write items in the nursing process format that address the NCLEX client needs. These stems can be used as a starting point for developing items that address your course content while incorporating the NCLEX client needs.

Chapter Synopses

There is considerable overlap in the components of the assessment process; therefore, there are numerous possibilities for arranging the sequence of the topics in this book. The order selected here reflects my attempt to organize the process of assessment logically for the reader. Because several of the topics apply to a variety of assessment situations, they are referred to in several chapters. Therefore, you will note that the reader is frequently referred to discussion on a topic in a previous chapter or advised that a topic is further developed in a subsequent chapter. This approach is designed to assist the reader in accessing discussion on topics that are unfamiliar while providing a reference that is organized for ease of access during the process of test development.

Chapter 1, "The Role of Assessment in Instruction," updates the discussion related to the critical role of assessment in the educational process. The rationale for developing a systematic plan for assessing educational outcomes is presented, and the ethical responsibilities associated with classroom testing, the implications of assessment decisions on the lives of students, and assessment competency standards of educators are discussed. The mounting effects of the nursing faculty shortage on nursing education and resources designed to enhance the educational expertise of nursing faculty are reviewed.

Chapter 2, "The Language of Assessment," is a review of fundamental assessment concepts and terminology to enhance the reader's understanding of the discussion in the chapters that follow. An overview of the principles of assessment is presented, and the common language associated with educational assessment is defined. Discussion of the terminology related to establishing learning outcomes, objectives, and competencies is included, as is an explanation of the difference between norm- and criterion-referenced test score interpretation. The essential nature of reliability and validity in the process of test development is reviewed, and a discussion of the revised guidelines for establishing validity evidence as a basis for establishing trustworthy assessment instruments is presented.

The role of objectives and outcomes as the foundation for the instructional process is presented in Chapter 3, "Developing Instructional Objectives." Criteria for developing objectives and learning outcomes are proposed. The chapter also identifies the characteristics of mastery- and developmental-level objectives and addresses the application of strategies to assess those objectives. A comparison of Bloom's original and Krathwohl's revised taxonomies is presented. A detailed example for developing learning outcomes that illustrate progression toward program objectives is included, as is a discussion of applying the levels of the cognitive domain to classroom test development.

Chapter 4, "Implementing Systematic Test Development," examines the process of developing tests in a variety of formats. A systematic approach for outlining content or concepts and developing a test blueprint is discussed in detail. Several sample blueprint formats are provided. Particular attention is paid to selecting the appropriate format for assessing course objectives, and detailed discussion related to determining how difficult a test should be and issues associated with preparing students for a test is included.

Chapter 5, "Selected-Response Format: Developing Multiple-Choice Items," continues the discussion of test development by examining the advantages and disadvantages of multiple-choice exams. Item-writing logistics are presented, and the characteristics of effective multiple-choice items are analyzed in great detail. Specific guidelines are proposed for both developing and revising items. This edition includes 63-item examples that illustrate the presented guidelines. An exhibit reference list (Box 5.3) is included to expedite the process for finding a particular item example. Strategies for framing questions in the National Council Licensure Examination (NCLEX) Alternate Item Format are suggested, with several new illustrative examples included.

Chapter 6, "Writing Critical Thinking Multiple-Choice Items," builds on the previous chapter to present the issues associated with the creation multiple-choice items that require the students to use critical thinking. The unique characteristics of these test items are discussed, and a proposal for introducing critical thinking items in the course sequence is presented. Strategies for using sequential reasoning to craft and revise multiple-choice items that assess critical thinking are proposed. Forty item examples are presented, including several examples that elaborate on the item development approaches used on the NCLEX exams that were presented in the previous chapter. An exhibit reference list (Box 6.1) is included to expedite the process for finding a particular item example.

Detailed guidelines for writing true–false and matching items are provided in Chapter 7, "Selected-Response Format: Developing True–False and Matching Items." The advantages and disadvantages of these item types are discussed, and detailed item-writing guidelines are updated, with numerous specific examples provided. The value of using these item types is explained.

The constructed-response format is often the best choice for accurately assessing an objective. Chapter 8, "Constructed-Response Format: Developing Short-Answer and Essay Items," is focused on discussing the advantages and disadvantages and providing updated guidelines for developing and scoring items in this format. Sample scoring rubrics are presented and discussed, and suggestions are offered for developing essay exams that assess critical thinking. As in the previous chapters, numerous examples are offered to illustrate the guidelines that are presented.

Issues related to assembling, administering, and scoring tests are addressed in Chapter 9, "Assembling, Administering, and Scoring a Test." Concerns such as cheating and maintaining test security throughout the testing process are discussed. Updated guidelines for deterring cheating on both paper-and-pencil and online exams are included, along with methods for identifying plagiarism. The chapter also deals with the considerations for qualitative peer review, student posttest review, and student challenges to exam questions. Discussion related to computer administration of exams is addressed in this edition. Chapter 10, "Establishing Evidence of Reliability and Validity," examines the issue of documenting the reliability and validity of test results. Measures of reliability and the effects of measurement error are discussed. Validity is also examined as a crucial ingredient for teacher confidence in assessment decisions. Statistical formulas are presented for those who appreciate a mathematical explanation of the concepts of reliability.

A careful test analysis is a prerequisite for assigning objective scores to a multiple-choice exam. Both qualitative and quantitative analyses contribute to fair evaluation of a measurement instrument. Chapter 11, "Interpreting Test Results," explains the meaning of the statistics included in a test data report as the basis for translating raw test scores into fair grade assignments. Individual item analysis is also carefully examined, both as a test analysis tool and for its value in guiding the improvement of existing items. This chapter also includes a careful examination of how to deal with test items that are flawed.

Chapter 12, "Laboratory and Clinical Evaluation," which was contributed by Veronica Arikian for the second edition, is updated again in this edition. It establishes the importance of the course objectives when designing both clinical experiences and evaluation tools. The process of clinical teaching and evaluation is closely examined, from the perspectives of both mastery- and developmental-level learning. Valuable suggestions are offered for both designing and using clinical evaluation tools as well as for incorporating portfolio assessments in the evaluation plan. Sample evaluative tools that incorporate the course objectives and are based on scoring rubrics are included.

One of the most difficult aspects of the teacher's role is grading. Chapter 13 "Assigning Grades," examines how a grading plan evolves from the principles of grading and a teacher's personal grading philosophy. Practical suggestions for implementing a grading plan, including issues such as criterion- versus norm-referenced grading, are explored and updated in this edition.

Chapter 14, "Instituting Item Banking and Test Development Software," offers practical suggestions and examples for improving items based on item analysis, establishing an item bank, and implementing test development software. This chapter discusses the requirements for utilizing a system to streamline the development and improvement of multiple-choice items. The objective of this chapter is to consolidate the important information that will help you expedite the process of implementing these programs. Several websites that offer valuable information for investigating test development software are referenced.

The primary focus of Chapter 15, "Preparing Students for the Licensure Exam: The Importance of NCLEX," is to update and explain the details of the most recent NCLEX exams. This chapter offers valuable information to familiarize nursing faculty members with the current NCLEX development process. It also examines in detail the concerns among nurse educators associated with preparing students for the NCLEX, including curriculum focus, predictor exams, progression policies, and NCLEX prep courses. Valuable suggestions for facilitating student success are presented.

All of the appendices have been updated. Appendix E, "Sample Item Stems for Phases of the Nursing Process," has been updated to present stems that incorporate the alternative item formats include in the NCLEX examinations. Appendix F,

"Sample Item Stems for Client Needs Using the Nursing Process Format," has been added to this edition. This appendix offers more than 200 suggestions for item stems that facilitate the development of items that address course content/concepts and incorporate the client needs and the nursing process.

This edition expands and updates the discussions in the third edition and provides guidelines that incorporate the principles and practices of assessment to assist you in developing a plan for systematic assessment of learning outcomes. While the best use of this book is to read it cover to cover, it should not be read once and put on your bookshelf. As with the previous editions, it is a significant resource as both an introductory textbook and a working reference for educators who are seriously interested in developing trustworthy assessment instruments. Remember, there are no hard and fast assessment rules. However, you should seriously consider adopting the guidelines suggested in this book because they are based on generally agreed on opinions of measurement experts. The guidelines presented in this edition are essential for developing measurement instruments on which you can confidently base your assessment decisions.

The Role of Assessment in Instruction

CHAPTER 1

"Every student can learn, just not on the same day, or the same way."

—GEORGE EVANS

Teachers make decisions about students—decisions that have serious effects on students' lives. For teachers to have confidence that the decisions they make are fair, they must base those decisions on information that is valid and reliable.

Assessment is the systematic process of collecting and interpreting information to make decisions about students. High-quality assessments not only provide valid and reliable information about student achievement, they also assist educators to determine the effectiveness of their instructional strategies. The higher the quality of the information you collect, the higher your confidence level will be when you are making important decisions about students, and the better you will sleep at night!

The Process of Assessment

All assessments begin with a purpose. Classroom assessment is a formal process that involves a deliberate effort to gain information about a student's status in relation to course content and objectives. This process includes a wide range of procedures and has the ultimate goal of obtaining valid and reliable information on which to base educational decisions.

In 1999, Brookhart identified planning, teaching, and assessment as the three interactive components of educational instruction. Planning involves the establishment of instructional objectives and learning outcomes, which leads to decisions about the types of learning activities that will provide students with appropriate opportunities to achieve the required outcomes . The desired learning outcomes and instructional activities then guide the assessment techniques. Finally, the assessment results direct, and even modify, the teaching approach. **Figure 1.1** illustrates this relationship, which Brookhart (1999) describes as effective when the assessment instruments provide accurate, meaningful, and appropriate information.

While the main goal of classroom assessment is to obtain valid and reliable information about student achievement, assessment procedures also assist in appraising the effectiveness of the instruction. A well-designed assessment plan helps you to optimize your teaching by identifying your own strengths and weaknesses. The results of a classroom test based on such a plan provide answers to the following questions:

- What is the level of the students' achievement?
- Are the course objectives realistic?
- Is the difficulty level of the content appropriate?
- Are the instructional methods effective?
- How well are the learning experiences sequenced?

In addition to being the primary indicator of student achievement and the effectiveness of an educational program, student assessment is also an integral part of the learning process. Effective assessment is a continuous process that provides valuable feedback for students and thus reinforces successful learning and offers information about additional learning needs. While a poorly designed assessment interferes with learning, an assessment that is well designed not only promotes learning but also enhances teaching by assisting both the student in learning and the teacher in teaching (Miller, Linn, & Gronlund, 2009). Well-developed classroom assessments contribute to effective student learning by helping students identify their strengths and weaknesses to guide their future study.

You probably have heard a student say, "There is no way I can pass this test." If students believe that they will not be able to pass their classroom exams no matter

Figure 1.1	Interaction of planning, teaching, and assessment in educational instruction

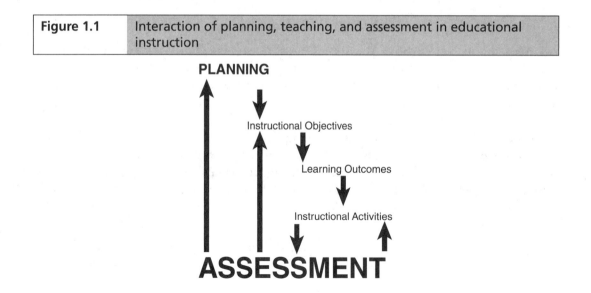

what they do, their self-confidence is undermined. When tests are perceived as unfair or too difficult, many students protect their self-esteem by giving up rather than failing repeatedly. Educators can counteract this syndrome by ensuring that students have a clear understanding of what is expected of them to demonstrate success, offering them learning opportunities to achieve the expectations, informing them about how their learning will be assessed, and providing them with feedback to guide future learning.

Ethical Responsibilities

Educators have an ethical responsibility every time they assess students. Nurse educators also have a responsibility to the healthcare consumers whose care will be entrusted to the students who graduate and enter nursing practice. It is therefore imperative that your assessments be trustworthy so that you obtain high-quality information. While you may not be happy about some of the decisions you have to make, you will be comfortable with those decisions if they are based on trustworthy assessment instruments.

Teacher-made tests play a central role in student assessment. In light of the influence that decisions based on these tests have on the lives of students, elaborate care must be taken when testing and grading. Fundamental to the development of valid assessments is the recognition that classroom test preparation deserves the same priority as the preparation of classroom instruction. Consider the amount of group effort invested in the development of a course in a nursing program. Endless meetings and discussions are held to develop objectives, outcomes, and content outlines and to plan learning activities that afford students the opportunity to attain success in the course. Yet test development is often a solitary process: Individual faculty members contribute pieces to the final product without seeing the whole picture until the test is completed.

What Clements and MacDonald identified in 1966 stills holds true today: Ethical responsibility for student assessment requires teachers to ensure that each assessment tool:

- is appropriately designed, and
- actually measures what it claims to measure

In addition, Clements and MacDonald pointed out that, when interpreting the results of assessment instruments, teachers must seriously consider the following:

- The emotional and social impact on students
- The consequences of the evaluation on a student's academic life

Assessment and Self-Efficacy

One of the most important responsibilities of a teacher is to promote every student's self-efficacy. To promote self-efficacy, which can be described as the "I can do it" attitude, teachers need to believe that every student can be successful. Admission to a nursing program is certainly a selective process, and every admitted student has the potential for success. It is the obligation of the program's faculty to assist every student to become successful.

In the process of promoting student self-efficacy, it is essential to recognize that a student's sense of accomplishment is diminished if a task is too easy and is defeated if a task is too hard. When tests are perceived as trivial, students perceive schoolwork as trivial and can adopt the attitude that the process of learning is one of passive recall. We cannot expect students to be successful, to have the "I can do it" attitude on high-stakes examinations such as the National Council Licensure Examination (NCLEX), if they are accustomed to taking poorly constructed classroom exams that are perceived as too easy or too difficult.

It is unrealistic to believe that a postprogram review course can teach students to be successful on a national examination. The best approach for fostering a realistic sense of self-efficacy is to expose students throughout their entire nursing program to well-constructed tests that require them to think critically and to apply their acquired knowledge.

How many exams do students take over the course of a nursing program—20, 30, 40? It is certainly not unusual for students to answer more than 2,000 multiple-choice items during a nursing program. By presenting them with well-written exams that assess higher-order thinking, nursing programs can challenge students' critical thinking ability and provide them with the best preparation for passing NCLEX. Chapter 15, "Preparing Students for the Licensure Exam: The Importance of NCLEX," offers suggestions for increasing your students' self-confidence.

Assessment Inadequacy

Although most teachers recognize and strive to fulfill their assessment role, many experience conflict originating from feelings of inadequacy. These feelings of assessment inadequacy are understandable. While assessment is integral to instruction and learning, classroom assessment and grading are generally acknowledged as the weak links in modern education. Despite the widespread use of classroom achievement tests and the important role they play in the instructional process, teachers of all disciplines, at every level of education, lack the understanding of assessment methods. Surveys of teacher preparation (National Council of State Boards of Nursing [NCSBN], 2008; Penn, Wilson, & Rosseter, 2008; Schoening, 2009; VanBever, 2010; Worrell et al., 2014) report that teachers often lack the educational preparation essential for the educator role, which includes the development and use of classroom assessments. Schoening (2009) points out that, despite the fact that classroom assessment is an integral part of a teacher's responsibility, many nurse educators have not received the basic instruction in the process of assessment and grading that is necessary for fair student evaluation.

Nursing education is facing a particular dilemma with the assessment competency of faculty. In 1980, Fitzpatrick and Heller identified that the number of nurse educators with the necessary preparation in education was dwindling. That trend has continued for more than 35 years.

The National League for Nursing (NLN, 2013b), the American Association of Colleges of Nursing (AACN, 2015), and the National Advisory Council for Nursing Education and Practice (NACNEP, 2010) have all identified the need for increased enrollment in schools of nursing to address the growing shortage of nurses in the United States. The AACN, the NLN, and the NACNEP all documented that, while we need to increase enrollment, the inverse is occurring. Substantial numbers of qualified applicants are being denied admission to nursing programs. The critical factor identified for limited student enrollment is the shortage of faculty at nursing schools across the country.

Both the NLN (2013a) and the AACN (2015) support the doctoral degree as the preferred preparation for nurse educators. The NLN (2013a) recommends several strategies to increase the number of nurse educators prepared at the doctoral level (pp. 4–5). However, because of the growing shortage of qualified nurse educators, expert clinicians, rather than educators, are increasingly filling nurse faculty positions. Although these faculty members have valuable clinical expertise, the role of nurse educator requires specialized knowledge and preparation.

A variety of proposals have been advanced to promote the interest and expertise of Master's prepared nurses in the educator role (Benner, Sulphen, Leonard, & Day, 2009; Bond, 2017; Ganley & Sheets, 2009; Penn et al., 2008). An NLN recommendation from its 2002 Position Statement that is particularly pertinent to the discussions in this book is the following:

> Schools of nursing should support lifelong learning activities that help educators maintain and expand their expertise in teaching and education as well as their clinical competence and their scholarly skills. (p. 4)

The NLN, taking action on its own recommendation, has developed a variety of resources to enhance the educational expertise of nursing faculty. A number of continuing education offerings are available through the NLN website. The NLN also encourages continuous quality improvement by recognizing nursing programs that are committed to improving the educational environment. Each year the NLN Centers of Excellence in Nursing Education Program publicly acknowledge programs that excel in one of three areas:

1. Enhancing student learning and professional development
2. Promoting the pedagogical expertise of faculty
3. Advancing the science of nursing education

Recognizing the need for expertise in the nurse educator role, the NLN also sponsors a certification program for nurse educators. The certified nurse educator (CNE) examination is based on the Core Competencies of Nurse Educators (NLN, 2012) and is administered as a prerequisite for CNE certification. The NLN provides a range of opportunities to help nursing faculty continuously improve their proficiency in the role of educator. Visit their website (http://www.nln.org) frequently to keep up to date on what is being offered.

The AACN is also taking a proactive approach to promote excellence in academic nursing. The mission of the AACN, as stated on their website (http://www.aacn.nche .edu), is to "serve as the catalyst for excellence and innovation in nursing education, research, and practice." The AACN website includes a faculty tab that provides a variety of resources, including links to webinars, conferences, curriculum guidelines, and funding opportunities.

Assessment Competency Standards

As public and professional awareness of the need for assessment competence increases, several professional organizations have developed standards to provide guidelines for the assessment skills that educators should possess. The 2014 edition of the *Standards for Educational and Psychological Testing* was developed jointly by the American Educational Research Association (AERA), the American Psychological Association (APA), and the National Council on Measurement in Education (NCME). The intent of this document is to "promote sound testing practices and to provide a basis for evaluating the quality of those practices" (p. 1). These standards represent a consensus on the skills required of teachers that enable them to use educational and psychological tests appropriately. An ad hoc committee of the NCME published the *Code of Professional Responsibilities in Educational Measurement* in 1995 to "promote professionally responsible practice in educational measurement" (p. 2). Both documents provide valuable guidelines for fair and ethical assessment in higher education.

The *Standards for Teacher Competence in Educational Assessment of Students* was developed jointly by the American Federation of Teachers (AFT), the NCME, and the National Education Association (NEA, 1990). This collaboration between teaching and measurement specialists defined seven assessment competencies that are critical to the role of educator (**Box 1.1**). Although these standards were specifically written for K–12 classroom teachers, they provide a discussion model for professional competence and fairness in assessment in higher education (Brookhart, 1999).

Unfortunately, the assessment abilities of many teachers are often inconsistent with the standards adopted by professional organizations. The assessment content presented in *The Nurse Educator's Guide to Assessing Learning Outcomes* is consistent with the most current professional standards and provides you with a foundation for achieving competence, or improving your abilities, in student assessment.

Box 1.1   Teacher competence standards

Teachers should be skilled in:

1. Choosing assessment methods appropriate for instructional decisions.
2. Developing assessment methods appropriate for instructional decisions.
3. Administering, scoring, and interpreting the results of both externally produced and teacher-produced assessment methods.
4. Using assessment results when making decisions about individual students, planning teaching, developing curriculum, and school improvement.
5. Developing valid pupil grading procedures that use pupil assessments.
6. Communicating assessment results to students, parents, other lay audiences, and other educators.
7. Recognizing unethical, illegal, and otherwise inappropriate assessment methods and uses of assessment information.

Reproduced from American Federation of Teachers, National Council on Measurement in Education, & National Education Association. (1990). *Standards for teacher competence in educational assessment of students*. Washington, DC: National Council on Measurement in Education.

Need for a Systematic Approach to Assessment

A systematic plan is defined as a procedure that is based on a coordinated approach. It ensures that no steps are omitted from a process. The only way to ensure that all steps are completed in a complicated process is to follow a system. The nursing process provides an example of a systematic method applied to a complex process. Certainly, there is no process more complex than the practice of nursing. Widely adopted by the profession, particularly in nursing education, the nursing process provides a systematic approach that ensures the comprehensive application of nursing care.

A comprehensive assessment plan involves several interacting processes. To maintain the plan's integrity, a methodical procedure, which is based on the principles of assessment, must be designed and adhered to. In fact, having a defined methodology not only ensures that all steps are followed; it also ensures that objectivity is maintained throughout the assessment process. In fact, following a systematic procedure for each component of the overall plan ensures that your assessment plan is both comprehensive and objective. The *Nurse Educator's Guide to Assessing Learning Outcomes* is designed to help you develop a system that will streamline every aspect of your assessment plan. The guidelines ensure that your plan is practical, comprehensive, and grounded in the principles of sound assessment.

Assessment Instruments

As defined in Standard One of the *Standards for Teacher Competence in Educational Assessment of Students* (1990), when planning assessment strategies, it is important that you choose the assessment technique appropriate for the particular behavior being assessed. Brookhart (1999) describes the following four categories of assessment instruments:

1. Paper and pencil (or computer administered)
2. Performance assessments
3. Oral presentations
4. Portfolio assessment

A multidimensional approach is essential to assess all aspects of a behavior. This is especially true when assessing psychomotor skills, affective behavior, or higher-level cognitive ability such as critical thinking. For a variety of reasons, teacher-made, multiple-choice, paper-and-pencil classroom tests are widely used in all educational settings, particularly in nursing education. This edition of *The Nurse Educator's Guide to Assessing Learning Outcomes* evolved from the first three editions, and so it focuses on the role of the multiple-choice format for classroom tests and elaborates on suggestions for constructing measurement instruments in several formats that were introduced in the previous editions. This edition of *The Nurse Educator's Guide to Assessing Learning Outcomes* provides you with strategies for developing well-constructed classroom exams in a variety of formats that provide valid and reliable results.

Summary

Assessment is fundamental to the instructional process. However, the assessment part of the instructional process often does not receive the attention it warrants for several reasons. The most important one is the need for faculty to recognize the integral role of assessment in the instructional process.

This edition of *The Nurse Educator's Guide to Assessing Learning Outcomes* is designed to help you develop a systematic plan for assessment of learning outcomes in the classroom. It provides a review of the theories and principles of assessment. Assessment issues are addressed and practical guidelines are presented to assist you in developing classroom exams that reflect the standards of assessment competence. The information presented in the following chapters will help you improve your overall assessment program, whatever assessment format you choose to implement.

Learning Activities

1. Consider an assessment program that you have experience with and describe an actual or potential ethical conflict associated with that program.

2. How does the "I can do it" attitude influence a student's success on both classroom and standardized exams? Identify two approaches you can use to promote the "I can do it" attitude in the classroom or clinical setting.

3. Discuss the impact of the nursing faculty shortage on the shortage of nurses in the healthcare settings across the country.

4. What suggestion would you propose to increase the number of nursing faculty prepared at the doctoral level?

5. Review the *Standards for Teacher Competence in the Educational Assessment of Students* (refer again to Box 1.1). How do standards 1 and 2 apply to classroom and clinical assessment in nursing education?

6. What do you consider to be your assessment weaknesses? What approach will you take to improve your expertise in this area?

Web Links

American Association of Colleges of Nursing
http://www.aacn.nche.edu
American Educational Research Association
http://www.aera.net
American Federation of Teachers
http://www.aft.org
American Psychological Association
http://www.apa.org
Association for the Assessment of Learning in Higher Education
http://aalhe.org/
Carnegie Mellon: Enhancing Education—Assessment
http://www.cmu.edu/teaching/assessment/index.html

Educational Resources Information Center
http://www.eric.ed.gov
Internet Resources for Assessment in Higher Education
http://www2.acs.ncsu.edu/upa/assmt/resource.htm
National Council of State Boards of Nursing
http://www.ncsbn.org
National Council on Measurement in Education
http://www.ncme.org
National League for Nursing
http://www.nln.org

References

American Association of Colleges of Nursing. (2015). *Nursing faculty shortage fact sheet.* Retrieved from http:// www.aacn.nche.edu/media-relations/FacultyShortageFS.pdf

American Educational Research Association, American Psychological Association, & National Council on Measurement in Education. (2014). *Standards for educational and psychological testing.* Washington, DC: American Educational Research Association.

American Federation of Teachers, National Council on Measurement in Education, & National Education Association. (1990). *Standards for teacher competence in educational assessment of students.* Washington, DC: National Council on Measurement in Education.

Benner, P., Sulphen, M., Leonard, V., & Day, L. (2009). *Educating nurses: A call for radical transformation.* San Francisco, CA: Jossey-Bass.

Bond, D. K. (2017). Will BSN students consider a future nursing faculty role? *Nursing Education Perspectives, 38*(1), 9–17.

Brookhart, S. M. (1999). *The art and science of classroom assessment: The missing part of pedagogy.* Washington, DC: The George Washington University Graduate School of Education and Human Development. Retrieved from http://www.eric.ed.gov/ERICDocs/data/ericdocs2/content_storage_01/0000000b/80/2a/2e/2f.pdf

Clements, H., & MacDonald, J. (1966). Moral concerns in assessing pupil growth. *The National Elementary School Principal, 45,* 29–33.

Fitzpatrick, M. L., & Heller, B. R. (1980). Teaching the teachers to teach. *Nursing Outlook, 26,* 372–373.

Ganley, B., & Sheets, I. (2009). A strategy to address the nursing faculty shortage. *Educational Innovations, 48*(7), 401–405.

Miller, M. D., Linn, R. L., & Gronlund, N. E. (2009). *Measurement and assessment in teaching* (10th ed.). Upper Saddle River, NJ: Pearson Education, Inc.

National Advisory Council for Nursing Education and Practice. (2010). *The impact of the nursing faculty shortage on nurse education and practice.* Washington, DC: U.S. Department of Health and Human Services, Health Resources and Services Administration. Retrieved from http://www.hrsa.gov/advisorycommittees/bhpradvisory/nacnep/Reports/ninthreport.pdf

National Council of State Boards of Nursing. (2008). *Nursing faculty qualifications and roles.* Chicago, IL: Author. Retrieved from https://www.ncsbn.org/Final_08_Faculty_Qual_Report.pdf

National League for Nursing. (2002). *Position statement: The preparation of nurse educators.* Retrieved from http://www.nln.org/aboutnln/positionStatements /prepofnursed02.htm

National League for Nursing. (2012). *Core competencies of nurse educators.* Retrieved from http://www.nln.org/professional-development-programs /competencies-for-nursing-education/nurse-educator-core-competency

National League for Nursing. (2013a). *A vision for doctoral preparation for nurse educators.* Retrieved from http:// www.nln.org/docs/default-source/about/nln -vision-series-(position-statements)/nlnvision_6.pdf

National League for Nursing. (2013b). *NLN nurse educator shortage fact sheet.* Retrieved from http://www.nln.org/docs/default-source/advocacy-public-policy /nurse-faculty-shortage-fact-sheet-pdf.pdf?sfvrsn=0

Penn, B. K., Wilson, L., & Rosseter, R. (2008). Transitioning from nursing practice to a teaching role. *Online Journal of Issues in Nursing, 13*(3). Retrieved from http:// nursingworld.org/MainMenuCategories/ANAMarketplace/ANAPeriodicals/OJIN /TableofContents/vol132008/No3Sept08/NursingPracticetoNursingEducation.html

Schoening, A. M. (2009). *The journey from bedside to classroom: Making the transition.* Unpublished doctoral dissertation, University of Nebraska, Lincoln.

VanBever, R. R. (2010). *Examining the effects of a National League for Nursing core competencies workshop as an intervention to improve faculty practice.* Unpublished doctoral dissertation, Liberty University, Lynchburg, Virginia.

Worrell, F., Brabeck, M., Dwyer, C., Geisinger, K., Marx, R., Noell, G., & Pianta, R. (2014). *Assessing and evaluating teacher preparation programs.* Washington, DC: American Psychological Association.

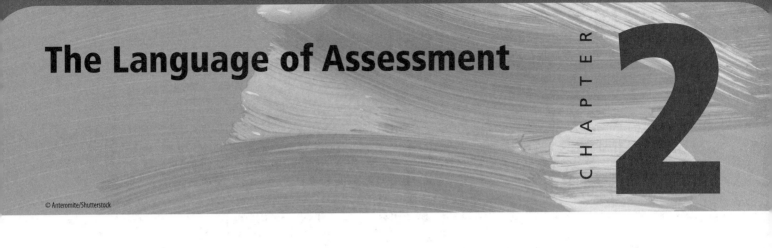

The Language of Assessment

© Anteromite/Shutterstock

CHAPTER 2

"There are three sides to every story—your side, my side, and the truth."

—JOHN ADAMS

The goal of assessment is to collect objective evidence that represents the truth about student performance. To ensure objectivity, the assessment plan must be grounded in the principles of assessment. The first step in developing an objective assessment plan is to become familiar with the terminology of assessment to facilitate your understanding of the bigger picture. The purpose of this chapter is to review the principles of assessment and the terminology as it is defined in this text. This review will provide a basic understanding of the framework on which to base an objective, comprehensive, systematic assessment plan. These concepts are elaborated on in subsequent chapters.

Many of you are familiar with these terms. However, as Frisbie (2005) points out, the terms used in assessment can be confused. This confusion can lead to misinterpretation of assessment results. The review in this chapter is intended to clarify the meaning of assessment terminology as it is referred to in this text and enhance your understanding of the proposed guidelines.

Assessment

Chapter 1, "The Role of Assessment in Instruction," introduces you to the concept of assessment as the broad and comprehensive process of collecting quantitative and qualitative data to make informed educational decisions about students. The terms *assessment*, *test*, and *measurement* are often confused because they are all involved in the same process.

Assessment involves collecting information. It is a comprehensive process that involves a wide range of strategies used to gain information to make decisions about student achievement. Assessment data also inform decisions about teaching and learning strategies and the efficacy of the individual courses and the overall curriculum. Data collection for assessment should be directed by clearly defined learning targets or objectives (Brookhart & Nitko, 2008). In nursing education, assessment answers the question, "How well has the student achieved the instructional objectives?"

Brookhart and Nitko (2008) propose five guidelines to help teachers select and use classroom assessments. These principles provide the basis for developing a plan for systematic assessment of learning outcomes:

1. Identify the desired learning targets (instructional objectives) and select the behaviors that represent achievement of the objectives (the learning outcomes).

2. Ensure that the selected assessment techniques match the learning outcomes. While assessment techniques should be practical and efficient, it is more important that they are derived from the intellectual challenge posed by the learning outcomes.

3. Provide assessment opportunities that meet a learner's needs. Students should be given concrete examples of what is expected of them and the assessment techniques should provide meaningful feedback.

4. Employ multiple measurement techniques to assess each learning outcome. The validity of assessment is enhanced by using multiple assessment modalities. A variety of measurements may be required to evaluate whether a student has attained a particular learning outcome, especially if the outcome involves higher-order thinking.

5. Consider the limitations of assessment techniques when interpreting their results. It is important to remember that the information obtained, even when multiple assessment techniques are used, is only a sample of a student's behavior and that the interpretation of all assessments is subject to measurement error. (pp. 7–8)

Measurement

Measurement is the process of assigning a score that represents the degree to which an individual possesses a characteristic or behavior according to a specific plan (Miller, Linn, & Gronlund, 2012). It encompasses a variety of techniques, including tests, ratings, and observations, which are designed to assign a score that represents the degree of a predefined trait an individual possesses. Thus, measurements provide the information that guides decision making. While valid measurements contribute to valid decisions, erroneous measures can lead to inappropriate decisions. Therefore, it is crucial for educators to ensure that their measurement instruments are trustworthy.

Objectivity is an essential element of a trustworthy measurement. If a measurement instrument is not objective, the measurement's results depend more on the subjective opinion of the person who is conducting the measurement rather than on the ability of the person who is being measured. A measurement instrument is objective only if it is confined to assigning a number or a rating to a student characteristic based on predefined objective evidence of the characteristic.

Box 2.1 **Steps for developing effective measurement instruments**

1. Develop the instructional objectives and learning outcomes.
2. Construct a test blueprint based on course content and objectives.
3. Write items to measure mastery of content and objectives.
4. Use the items to generate a test that addresses the blueprint.
5. Quantify the results of the measurement.

One common measurement error is to equate quantification with objective measurement. Numbers have a systematic quality that can be confused with objectivity. Just because a measurement instrument produces a numerical score does not mean the score is an objective one. A score of 90% on a test is meaningless and arbitrary if the score is based on a test that was poorly constructed in the first place. After all, 90% of nothing is nothing.

Measurement instruments that provide qualitative information are sometimes chosen as the most desirable instruments for classroom measurement. When a measurement instrument involves a procedure that describes student achievement in qualitative terms, extreme care must be taken to ensure objectivity when assigning a number or category as a score. Whatever technique you choose, it is essential that your measurement instruments are never based on subjective judgments.

In addition, it is very important to acknowledge that measurement skills are not intuitive. The ability to produce measurements that provide valid and reliable results is acquired; it develops with practice. Following the four steps for developing effective classroom measurement instruments, as identified in **Box 2.1**, will give you a head start. Each of these steps is incorporated when discussing assessment development throughout this text.

Note that step 1 in Box 2.1 reflects the first of Brookhart and Nitko's (2008) assessment guidelines: Identify the desired learning targets and the instructional objectives. This is also the first step in the development of a systematic plan for assessment. As you read this text, you will recognize that the steps for developing an assessment plan overlap and that each reflects Brookhart and Nitko's assessment guidelines.

Evaluation

Assessment, measurement, and evaluation are not equivalent. Evaluation is defined as the process of making a value judgment that attaches meaning to the data obtained by measurement and gathered through assessment (Brookhart & Nitko, 2014). It is guided by professional judgment and involves interpreting what the accumulated information means and how it can be used.

Evaluation compares student performance with a standard and makes a decision based on that comparison. The standard or outcomes that students are expected to achieve must be established at the beginning of the instructional process. Establishing the behavior standards and clearly communicating them to the students facilitates the evaluation of students' achievement of the learning outcomes. **Box 2.2** illustrates the difference between measurement and evaluation.

Box 2.2   **Difference between measurement and evaluation**
Measurement: The student correctly answered 85 of 100 items on the multiple-choice exam.
Evaluation: The student performed at an above average level.

While evaluation involves a judgment about the merit of an individual's performance, it also involves a judgment about the value of the measurement. Although fair evaluation should be objective, classroom evaluation is at risk for being subjective because human judgment is subjective. Therefore, it is a teacher's responsibility to verify that evaluation is based on objective measurement instruments. The more judgments are based on carefully constructed and administered classroom measurement instruments, the greater the likelihood that they are objectively sound. Furthermore, the more familiarity you have with the principles of assessment, the greater confidence you will have in the objectivity and ultimate fairness of your student evaluations.

Formative Evaluation

Formative evaluation monitors learning progress during instruction. It directs future learning by appraising the quality of student achievement while the student is still in the process of learning. It judges student progress toward meeting instructional objectives with the intent of improving teaching and learning. Formative evaluation is diagnostic evaluation; it identifies students' strengths and weaknesses to provide constructive feedback. Formative evaluation provides guidance to both students and teachers. It involves judgments about the quality of instruction and learning as they occur (Miller et al., 2012). These judgments allow the teacher to revise instructional materials, clarify objectives, update learning outcomes, and revise measurement instruments during a course of instruction. Because formative evaluation is a method that shapes the process of teaching and learning while it is in progress, it should not be used for assigning class grades.

Summative Evaluation

The focus of summative evaluation is to describe the quality of student achievement after an instructional process is completed. While a formative evaluation asks, "How are you doing?," a summative evaluation asks, "How did you do?" (Slavin, 1997, p. 491). A summative evaluation is given at the conclusion of a unit or a course of instruction, and it focuses on determining whether learning has occurred and if the objectives have been achieved. The main purpose of summative evaluation is to assign a course grade.

Summative and formative evaluation should be consistent. This consistency is achieved when both are based on the instructional objectives established at the beginning of the course. In addition, it is imperative that students know whether an evaluation is formative or summative so they understand if the evaluation is for practice or if grades will be assigned. **Table 2.1** compares formative and summative evaluation.

Table 2.1   Comparison of Formative and Summative Evaluation

Formative evaluation How are you doing?	Summative evaluation How did you do?
• Occurs during the process of learning • Assesses progress in a course • Directs learning to achieve objectives • Grades not assigned • Provides feedback	• Occurs at the completion of instruction • Summarizes achievement in a course • Assesses objective achievement • Assigns grades • Provides feedback

Instructional Objectives

The first step in the development of an assessment plan is to identify what is expected as a result of a student's course and program experience (Gronlund & Brookhart, 2009). A variety of terminology is used to describe the statement of learning intent. In fact, the use of that terminology is widely debated, and too often the debate becomes more important than the logical development of the assessment plan (Fitzpatrick, 2002; Glennon, 2006). Whatever term you use (objectives, outcomes, competencies, etc.), what is important is that the statements are consistent and clearly communicate the teacher's expectations for what is required to pass the course to the students.

A very effective method for developing instructional objectives is described by Gronlund and Brookhart (2009). They recommend stating the objectives as a broad statement and then defining them in terms of the intended student learning. The definition of *learning outcomes* used in this text follows the suggestion of Gronlund and Brookhart. Learning outcomes specify behaviors and clarify what performance you are willing to accept as evidence that the student has achieved the course objectives.

Objectives are sometimes criticized as limiting the students' learning experience. In fact, while objectives identify the end point, they do not specify the route that must be taken. Objectives are also criticized as focusing on minimal learning. While well-designed objectives do identify the minimum acceptable achievement, they also guide students to attain their own personal best. Educators must clearly communicate what minimum acceptable behaviors that students must achieve to demonstrate success or students will not know what is expected of them. When students are involved in learning experiences that inspire them to achieve their own personal best, they are most likely to develop a love of learning, which will compel them to strive for personal excellence throughout life.

As Robert Mager (1997) stated, "When clearly defined goals are lacking, it is impossible to evaluate a course or program efficiently, and there is no sound basis for selecting appropriate materials, content, or instructional methods" (p. 3). The development of instructional objectives and learning outcomes is elaborated in Chapter 3, "Developing Instructional Objectives."

Learning Outcomes

The most effective way to define an instructional objective is to establish the behaviors that you expect students to achieve by the end of a course. Gronlund and

Brookhart (2009) maintain that defining objectives in terms of desired student learning outcomes shifts the focus from the learning process to the learning outcomes and also provides a basis for the assessment of student learning. Stating the general objective first and then listing a representational sample of learning outcomes clarifies to the student what is deemed to be acceptable by the teacher as evidence that the student has attained the objective (2009). Chapter 3, "Developing Instructional Objectives," expands on this approach for student assessment.

Blueprint

To decide whether a student passes or fails a course based on the results of a test, the teacher must have evidence that the test actually represents the course. The blueprint, or table of specifications, is the foundation for validity evidence because it is the framework for the test. To establish validity evidence, the blueprint must incorporate only the objectives and content that are included in the course.

A blueprint is most effective when it is represented as a two-dimensional table that relates the objectives to the course content. A two-dimensional table requires that every item on the test be classified in terms of both objectives and content (Gronlund & Brookhart, 2009). A blueprint that is set up as a two-dimensional table is the foundation for establishing validity evidence that a test represents the content, as well as the objectives, of the course. When the blueprint guides the selection of test questions that reflect achievement of both the content and course objectives, evidence of validity is established.

A test cannot include the entire instructional domain of a course, but, it must include a sample of that domain that is a true representation of the course in order to provide validity evidence for decisions that are made based on the results of the test. A blueprint is the mechanism that guides the systematic selection of a representative sample of the content and objectives of a course. A test based on a carefully planned blueprint enables you to project that a student who receives a score of 90% on a 50-item test would receive a score of 90% on a 500-item test.

A blueprint answers the question, "What is being measured?" Although a blueprint directs the selection of test items, it is still the teacher's responsibility to plan carefully and develop test items to ensure that they actually measure student ability in the areas specified by the blueprint.

Test development is a time-consuming process. However, using a blueprint as a guide expedites this process and provides the structure for obtaining valid and reliable test results. The effort required for blueprint development is time well spent. In the long run, it facilitates test development and increases your confidence in the decisions you make based on your measurement instruments. Chapter 4, "Implementing Systematic Test Development," provides detailed guidelines for blueprint development.

Item Bank

An item bank is defined as an organized collection of items that can be accessed for test development. Testing experts often distinguish between item pools and item banks. This distinction defines a bank as a set of items whose difficulty levels have been calibrated on a common scale, while a pool simply consists of a collection of items. Because the term *item bank* is commonly used when referring to collections of items for classroom use, it is used throughout this text. Although a classroom item bank can be used to accumulate item data, the difficulty levels of the items in the classroom item banks referred to in this text are not calibrated.

The most efficient way to develop an item bank is to create and store items electronically. Several commercially produced software programs are available that facilitate item banking and test development. Educators can also organize test items electronically with a word processing or spreadsheet program. The implementation of an item banking program is closely examined in Chapter 14, "Instituting Item Banking and Test Development Software."

Test

A test is a type of assessment that consists of a group of questions that is administered during a fixed time period to a group of students who participated in a class. Tests are measurement instruments: formal events where individuals are asked to demonstrate their achievement of some knowledge or skill in a specific domain. The purpose of an achievement test is to obtain relevant and accurate data needed to make important decisions with a minimum amount of error. Gronlund and Brookhart (2009) describe a test as a tool for measuring a sample of student performance. It can be assumed that students have achieved the course learning objectives in the entire content domain when a designated score is obtained on a test that is designed to sample the content appropriately. A test measures how well a student performs either in comparison with a domain of content and objective or in comparison with others (Miller et al., 2012).

Using a single test or type of measurement instrument is not a satisfactory assessment strategy. Most course objectives require a variety of measurement and evaluation strategies to determine student competency. The selection of measurement instruments depends on the outcomes to be measured. It is important to select the most appropriate strategies for measuring each learning outcome. One premise of *The Nurse Educator's Guide to Assessing Learning Outcomes* is that multiple-choice exams can be developed to contribute to the assessment of objectives that require higher-level cognitive ability, including the construct of critical thinking.

An achievement test should consist of a sampling of tasks that represents the larger domain of behavior included in the course. The number of questions on a test is limited, so the questions you include have to be a representative sample of all the possible questions you could ask. The sample must be relevant and represent the total domain of what was included in the course (Gronlund & Brookhart, 2009). When students complain that an exam did not relate to the course content, it may indicate a mismatch between the test items and the larger domain of course content or objectives, or it may indicate that the items did not address the designated content or objectives. It is not possible to measure a student's achievement of objectives with items that do not match those particular objectives. You are most likely to obtain a representative sample of test items by following a systematic procedure for developing a test blueprint. The challenge is to develop a blueprint for the test and to write items to match the objectives and content being assessed. Chapter 4, "Implementing Systematic Test Development," provides guidelines for implementing a procedure for blueprint development.

Interpreting Test Scores

A raw test score is meaningless without a framework for interpretation. A raw score represents the number of correct responses on a test before any review or analysis of the items is done. The raw test score is only given meaning within the instructional content domain it represents. Criterion-referenced tests (CRTs) assess an individual's performance based on the percentage of the content mastered, while norm-referenced tests (NRTs) define an individual's performance by comparing it with others. Although both types of interpretation can be applied to the same test, the interpretation is most meaningful when the test is specifically designed for a desired interpretation (Miller et al., 2012).

Criterion-Referenced Tests (CRTs)

A criterion is a measurable behavior, attitude, or bit of knowledge, so CRTs assess a student's mastery of a criterion. A criterion reference approach interprets a student's raw score using a preset standard established by the faculty. Thus, each student's competency in relation to the preset standard is measured without reference to any other student. Student scores are then reported as the percentage correct, with each student's performance level determined by the preset, or absolute, standard. **Exhibit 2.1** presents an example of a criterion-referenced score.

Exhibit 2.1   Example of a criterion-referenced score

The student demonstrated mastery by correctly identifying 90% of the terms.

Because CRTs measure a student's attainment of a set of learning outcomes, no attempt should be made to eliminate easy items. The content chosen for a CRT depends only on how well it matches the instructional objectives of the course (Brookhart & Nitko, 2008). If most students in a group meet the standard, the group scores will obviously cluster at the high end of the grading scale.

CRTs are often teacher made and are closely tied to the objectives and curriculum. They are most meaningful when they are specifically designed to measure student ability in a particular area (Gronlund & Brookhart, 2009).

Gronlund (1973) describes the relationship of criterion-referenced testing to the two levels of learning: mastery and developmental. Designing tests for these two different levels of learning poses different challenges.

Mastery Learning   At the mastery level, CRTs are concerned with measuring the minimum essential skills that indicate mastery of an objective. The scope of learning tasks is limited, which simplifies the process of assessment. A score of the percentage correct is usually used to identify how closely a student's score demonstrates a complete mastery of the objective.

One challenge for the faculty is to identify (1) which specific objectives the students are expected to master and (2) which objectives represent learning beyond the mastery level, or developmental learning (Gronlund, 1973). Chapter 3, "Developing Instructional Objectives," offers a more in-depth discussion and also provides examples of objectives at the mastery and developmental levels of learning.

Developmental Learning   The concept of developmental learning applies to constructs that represent complex higher-order thinking, such as critical thinking. The abilities associated with this level are continuously developing throughout life. Objectives for developmental learning represent goals to work toward, with emphasis focused on continuous development rather than a complete mastery of a set of predetermined skills (Gronlund, 1973).

Learning outcomes at the developmental level represent degrees of progress toward an objective. Because it is impossible to identify all the behaviors that represent a complex construct, only a sample of the behaviors associated with instructional objectives at this level can be identified as learning outcomes. These behaviors should define the construct and provide a representational sample of student performance that will be accepted as evidence of the appropriate progress toward the attainment of the ultimate objective.

Students are not expected to attain full mastery of objectives at the developmental level. However, they are required to demonstrate the behaviors described by the learning outcomes, and they are also encouraged to strive for their personal level of maximum achievement toward the ultimate objective—their personal best. At this level, instructional objectives can be designed to show the development of students as they progress through an instructional program. For example, the same general instructional objectives can be used in every course in a nursing program, with the learning outcomes becoming more complex as the students progress through the program. Developing objectives for mastery and developmental learning is reviewed in Chapter 3, "Developing Instructional Objectives."

Gronlund (1973) asserts that the use of CRTs is restricted with the assessment of developmental learning. While test preparation should follow mastery level procedures, he suggests that adequate assessment of student performance beyond minimal essentials, require tests at the developmental level to include items of varying difficulty and allow for both criterion- and norm-referenced interpretations. Robinson Kurpius and Stafford (2006) suggest that teachers can designate multiple cutoff scores with CRTs. The syllabus would explain, for example, that a student who demonstrates mastery of 95% of the course content and objectives would receive a grade of "A" for the course. Students who achieve 85% would earn a "B;" 75%, a "C;" and below 75%, a "D." In this case, 75% is the minimum for passing, and students are rewarded for achieving beyond the minimum.

Norm-Referenced Tests (NRT)

While CRTs measure a student's achievement of a program's objectives without reference to other students, the aim of an NRT is to compare a student's achievement with the achievement of the student's peer group. NRTs focus on a student's performance in relation to other students rather than in relation to the attainment of a course's objectives. Norms themselves do not represent levels of performance; they provide a frame of reference to use when comparing the performances of a group of individuals. NRTs interpret a student's raw score as a percentile rank in a group and do not indicate what a student has achieved; the tests indicate only how the student compares with other students in his or her group. An example of a norm-referenced score is shown in **Exhibit 2.2**.

Exhibit 2.2   Example of a norm-referenced score

The student's performance equaled or exceeded 82% of the students in the group.

NRTs are designed to discriminate between strong and weak students. The tests are developed to provide a wide range of scores so that the identification of students at different achievement levels is possible. Therefore, items that all students are likely to answer correctly are eliminated.

The content selected for an NRT is based on how well it ranks students from high to low achievers (Brookhart & Nitko, 2008). The NRT format is commonly used on national standardized tests. These tests have a generalized content that is commonly taught in many schools. The norms established by a standardized achievement test are based on nationally accepted educational goals, which enable educators to compare a student's test score with the scores of other students in similar programs in the United States. These scores provide a general indication of the strengths and weaknesses of the students in a particular school and afford faculty members an external reference point for comparing their curriculum with a composite national curriculum.

Norm-referenced tests in the classroom setting identify how students compare with each other. Because strict NRTs are not concerned with the level of individual student achievement, they are usually not appropriate for classroom use. Chapter 4, "Implementing Systematic Test Development," elaborates on the use of NRTs and CRTs when determining how difficult a test should be. **Table 2.2** compares CRTs and NRTs.

Table 2.2   Comparison of Criterion- and Norm-Referenced Tests

Criterion-referenced test	Norm-referenced test
• Compares student performance to pre-established criteria	• Compares student performance to reference group
• Describes the performance	• Rates the performance
• Mastery reference	• Relative performance reference
• Narrowly defined content domain	• Diverse content domain
• Larger number of items for each objective	• Smaller number of items for each objective
• Includes easy items	• Eliminates easy items
• Focuses on student competency	• Focuses on student ranking
• Provides percent-correct score	• Provides percentile rank

High-Stakes Test

The term *high stakes* is commonly used among test developers when referring to a test whose results are the basis for making life-altering decisions about people. For example, a licensure examination is a high-stakes test because the examinees' scores on the test determine whether or not they will be allowed to practice their profession. When the results of one test are used to determine whether an individual will be licensed, the test results must have very high evidence of reliability and validity.

Classroom exams in nursing meet the criteria for being designated as high-stakes examinations. Life-altering decisions are certainly made based on the results of these exams. Classroom exams do differ from licensure examinations because decisions are not based on the results of one exam but rather on the accumulation of scores over a semester's worth of exams. However, because decisions that are made based on the results of classroom exams can have a profound impact on students' lives, it is obvious that faculty must pay careful attention to develop classroom exams that produce trustworthy results.

Grade

While a test score is a numerical indication of what is observed from a single measurement instrument, a grade is a label representing a composite evaluation. A course grade should be derived from the accumulation of scores obtained from several measurement instruments. Because life-altering decisions are associated with student grades, the utmost care must be used when assigning test scores and grades. Chapters 11, "Interpreting Test Results," and 13, "Assigning Grades," both discuss test analysis and grading procedures.

A cutoff score is the lowest grade a student can achieve to demonstrate proficiency in a course. Every course syllabus in a nursing program should spell out what cutoff score is required to pass the course. Suppose the pass score, or cutoff score, in a nursing program is 75%. The students would have to demonstrate an average of 75% across all the assessments in a course to pass. Every course syllabus should describe what scores correlate to each grade. If a passing grade of "C" requires an average of 75%, then an "A" might require a grade of 95%, a "B" an average of 85%, and a failing grade of "D" would be an average below 75%. The important issue is to make the grade requirements clear to the students.

Test Bias

A biased test is one that discriminates against a certain group based on socioeconomic status, disability, race, ethnicity, and/or gender (Slavin, 1997). When a measurement is biased, students who have the same ability perform differently on the same task because of their affiliation with a particular ethnic, sexual, cultural, or religious group (Hambleton & Rodgers, 1995). Hambleton and Rodgers define stereotyping as another undesirable characteristic of a test that introduces bias. Stereotyping refers to the representation of a group in a way that may be offensive to the group members. They also note that test language that is offensive can obstruct the purpose of a test when it produces negative feelings, which affect the students' attitudes toward the test and thus influence their test scores (Hambleton & Rodgers, 1995). Test bias in a nursing exam refers to the difference in a group's mean performance based on nonnursing elements in the exam, which are elements not familiar to the group.

An assessment is not fair if some students have an advantage because of factors unrelated to the purpose of the assessment. The aim of a nursing test is to measure knowledge that is essential to safe nursing practice in the United States. Reading speed, vocabulary ability, or familiarity with cultural practices that are unrelated to health should not influence a student's score (Miller et al., 2012). Therefore, it is important for teachers to collaborate with each other when developing a nursing exam. Every test should be carefully reviewed by at least two faculty members for items containing language that could offend or be misunderstood. Items with overt cultural or gender bias should be rejected. Items referring to events that are common to one culture but not to another should also be eliminated. All tests should be edited to remove stereotypical language. In fact, even the most innocent vocabulary can introduce bias into a test, as **Exhibit 2.3** illustrates. Although offensive, demeaning, or emotionally charged material may not make an item more difficult, it can cause students to become distracted, thus lowering their overall performance (Miller et al.,2012).

Exhibit 2.3   Example of a culturally biased stem

Biased Question:
A client who is taking a medication that is a sedative says to a nurse, "I am responsible for the *carpool* tomorrow." Which of these directions should the nurse give to the client?

The term carpool *could be unfamiliar to individuals for whom English is a second language or for those who live in urban areas and depend on public transportation.*

Bosher (2002) defines linguistic bias as resulting from students' inability to understand an item because the language is so complex. Students who are English language learners (ELLs) are particularly susceptible to linguistic bias. Poorly written test items can introduce structural bias into a test. Items that are grammatically incorrect, ambiguous, or vaguely worded confuse all students, but they particularly confuse ELLs and learning disabled students (Klisch, 1994). Each question should be written succinctly so that all students have a clear understanding of its meaning the first time it is read.

Although humor can be a useful tool in the classroom, it can be a distraction in an exam. Students are not inclined to get the joke during an exam, particularly ELL students. In fact, test anxiety can increase when students do not understand why others are laughing. Haladyna (2004) points out that humorous items reduce the number of plausible options and therefore make the items easier for those students who understand the joke. The detailed item development guidelines presented in Chapter 6, "Writing Critical Thinking Multiple-Choice Items," provides guidelines to assist you in eliminating bias from your test items.

Reliability

Test reliability is very important to test developers and users. You would have little confidence in a standardized nursing achievement test that ranked a student in the top

5% last week but places the same student near the mean this week. Reliability refers to the degree of consistency with which an instrument measures an attribute for a particular group. Reliability is not a property of the test itself; the test is not reliable. Reliability refers to the reproducibility of a set of scores obtained from a particular group, on a particular day, under particular circumstances (Frisbie, 2005). Achievement test results that are reliable are consistent, reproducible, and generalizable—that is, a second measurement with the same test on the same individual would obtain the same result. However, because every measurement contains error, you should expect some variation in test performance. It is highly unlikely that your efforts at obtaining a second measurement would produce precisely the same scores as the first measurement.

Reliability can be quantified by several statistical formulas. These estimates provide a reliability coefficient, or a measure of the amount of variation in test performance. While there are several procedures for obtaining a test's reliability estimate, the procedures that are most frequently reported by test analysis software estimate a test's reliability based on the internal consistency of the test. These reliability estimates range from zero to one, with zero indicating no reliability and one indicating perfect reliability. Reliability is discussed at length in Chapter 10, "Establishing Evidence of Reliability and Validity."

Validity

Although a test must be reliable to be valid, a reliable test is not always valid. A test can have high reliability and yet not really measure anything of importance or it can fail to be an appropriate measure for a particular use (Burns & Grove, 1997). Therefore, we can have reliable measures that provide the wrong information (see **Exhibit 2.4**).

Exhibit 2.4   Reliability requirement for validity
A test can be reliable without being valid.
HOWEVER
A test cannot be valid unless it is reliable.

Frisbie (2005) notes that the term *validity* is one of the most misused and misunderstood concepts in educational measurement. The American Educational Research Association (AERA), American Psychological Association (APA), and the National Council on Measurement in Education (NCME) (1999) agree that "Validity is the most fundamental consideration in developing and evaluating tests" (p. 9). Validity is not a property of the test itself. It refers to the appropriateness of the interpretation and use of the test scores—the extent of the evidence that exists to justify the inferences we make based on the results of the test. A test can have substantial evidence of validity for one interpretation and not for another. For example, an exam can have considerable evidence of validity for interpretations related to acceptance into a city's police department, whereas the same exam can be of no use for admission to the same city's fire department. This is a perfect example of why you cannot use an exam with validity evidence that supports its use to assess theoretical nursing knowledge to also assess a construct such as critical thinking unless you can collect validity evidence to justify the test's use to measure critical thinking.

Validity does not exist on an all-or-none basis. A test is always valid to some degree—high, moderate, or weak—in a particular situation with a particular sample. Validity is a matter of judgment: There are no fixed rules for deciding what is meant by high, moderate, or weak validity. Skill in making these judgments is based on test validation, and it develops with experience in dealing with tests (Miller et al., 2012). Test validation is defined as the process of collecting evidence to establish that the inferences, which are based on the test results, are appropriate. The first step in the process of test validation is to have a clear understanding of the evidence that establishes validity.

The traditional approach to establishing validity identified three distinct classifications of validity: content validity, construct validity, and criterion-related validity. Today, however, validity is viewed as a unitary concept, not as three distinct types.

The 1985 edition of the *Standards for Educational and Psychological Testing* (AERA et al., 1985) identifies validity as a unitary concept that includes each of the categories as evidence of validity:

- Content-related evidence
- Construct-related evidence
- Criterion-related evidence

Content-related evidence, criterion-related evidence, and construct-related evidence are interrelated; ideal validation includes several types of evidence, spanning all three of the traditional categories (AERA et al., 1985, p. 9). This approach emphasizes that validity is not an all-or-none proposition. It is a matter of degree and involves the judgment that you make after considering all the accumulated evidence.

The most recent edition of the *Standards for Educational and Psychological Testing* (AERA et al., 2014) refers to types of validity evidence rather than categories of validity. Validity is referred to as the most fundamental consideration when interpreting a test score. It is described as a process of collecting a variety of evidence to support a proposed interpretation of a test score. The 2014 edition outlines the various sources of evidence that can be used for evaluating the proposed interpretation of a test's score for a particular purpose (p. 11). The sources of validity evidence described in the 2014 *Standards* include:

- Evidence based on test content
- Evidence based on response processes
- Evidence based on internal structure
- Evidence based on relations to other variables
- Evidence related to the consequences of testing

When reviewing the different types of validity evidence, it is essential to keep the unitary nature of validity in mind. Types of validity evidence do not exist exclusively or separately; they overlap. They are all essential to a unitary concept of validity. Evidence from each one may be needed when attempting to validate the interpretation of a test score. The importance of selecting, developing, and using tests based on adequate validity evidence for interpreting the test scores for a particular purpose cannot be overstated (Goodwin, 2002).

Evidence Based on Test Content

Evidence based on test content represents the degree to which the items on a test reflect a course's content domain. Content-related validity is nonstatistical (Lyman, 1998); it cannot be objectively quantified with a number. Rather, the documentation of content-related evidence of validity begins with test development and is established by a detailed examination of the test content. The more closely related a test is to its blueprint, the higher the content validity will be. If a test has content-related evidence of validity, then we can use the test results to make a judgment about the person's knowledge within that specific content domain.

A well-constructed test measures every important aspect of a course, including the subject matter and the course objectives. Because a test measures only a sample of a domain, the degree to which the test items represent the content of the course is the key issue in content validation. No aspect of a course should be under- or overrepresented. The validity of the inferences based on the test results depends on how well the test sample represents the domain being tested (Gronlund & Brookhart, 2009). A blueprint establishes validity evidence based on test content by ensuring that a test provides a representative sampling of the objectives and content domain of a course. Chapter 4, "Implementing Systematic Test Development," presents detailed guidelines for developing blueprints for your classroom tests.

Content-related evidence of validity is a central concern during test development (AERA et al., 1985, p. 11). Tests that provide content-valid results are produced with careful planning. When developing a test to inform decisions about student progression in a course of study, the content domain on the test must be limited to what the students have had the opportunity to learn during the course (AERA et al., 1999, p. 12).

Standardized tests use a national panel of experts in the field being measured to establish validity evidence based on test content. When you develop a classroom test, you do not have access to a panel of experts. However, you can strengthen the evidence for the validity of the decisions you make based on your tests' results by following the steps for enhancing validity evidence based on test content (see **Exhibit 2.5**).

Exhibit 2.5 Steps for enhancing validity evidence based on test content

- State objectives in performance terms.
- Identify learning outcomes.
- Define the domain to be measured.
- Prepare a detailed blueprint.
- Write items to fit the blueprint.
- Select a representative sample of items for the test.
- Ask colleagues to review your blueprint and items.
- Provide adequate time for test completion.
- Review item and test analysis.
- Use the test only for its intended purpose.

Evidence Based on Response Processes

This type of validity evidence was formerly a component of construct-related evidence. A construct is an unobservable characteristic of an individual that cannot be measured directly, such as intelligence, creativity, and critical thinking. The 2014 *Standards* (AERA et al., 2014) focus on whether the questions are in fact measuring the intended construct or are irrelevant factors inherent in the questions influencing the performance of subgroups of examinees. Evidence based on response processes involves the collection of evidence that supports the assertion that a test measures a construct by measuring the observable behaviors, which demonstrate the construct as defined by the test developer (Goodwin, 2002).

Evidence Based on Internal Structure

This type of validity evidence was also a component of construct-related evidence in the 1999 *Standards* (AERA et al., 1999). Construct validation begins with test development, and it continues until the evidence establishes a relationship between the test scores and the construct. For example, a test claiming to measure critical thinking would require construct validation. First, a detailed definition of the construct of critical thinking, which is derived from psychological theory, prior research, or systematic observation and analyses of the behavior domain, must be developed (Goodwin, 2002).

Evidence Based on Relation to Other Variables

This type of evidence examines the relationship of test score to variables that are external to the test (AERA et al., 2014). The focus of predictive evidence is to determine how valid a test is at predicting a second measure of performance—the criteria. A study of concurrent evidence, however, is concerned with estimating present performance when compared to the criterion. The key question with criterion-related validity is, "How accurately do test scores estimate criterion performance?" (AERA et al., 2014, p. 17).

As Lyman (1998) explains, concurrent and predictive evidence differ only in their time sequence. Both test scores and criterion values are obtained at about the same time with concurrent validity. In predictive validity, however, there is a time lapse between testing and obtaining the criterion values. When criterion-related evidence is high, the test can be used to estimate performance on the criterion.

If you are using a test score to predict future performance, you must be concerned with determining the degree of the relationship between the test and the criterion (the future performance). Support of criterion validity must include empirical evidence on the comparison between test performance and performance of the criterion (Goodwin, 2002). Many tests are currently being marketed that claim to predict student success on the National Council Licensure Examination (NCLEX). When evaluating these predictor examinations, it is important for you to determine how they have established criterion-related evidence of validity. You should be able to answer this question: "How does the test predict the performance of the students on NCLEX?" The predictor test should compare an individual's test scores to NCLEX pass/fail status to provide a basis for predicting the likelihood of passing or failing NCLEX based on the score on the predictor test.

Evidence Based on the Consequences of Testing

The 2014 *Standards* focuses attention on the intended and unintended consequences of using test results to make decisions about different groups. This type of evidence answers these questions posed by Goodwin (2002):

- To what extent are the anticipated benefits of testing being realized?
- To what extent do unanticipated benefits (positive and negative) occur?
- To what extent are differential consequences observed for different identifiable subgroups of examinees? (p. 104)

The 2014 *Standards* call for the test validation process to provide evidence that the intended benefits of testing are being realized (AERA et al., 2014, p. 19). Test developers must support the claims they make for the benefits of using a particular test score as the basis for making decisions that affect peoples' lives.

Face Validity

Face validity is not validity in the technical sense; it refers to what a test appears to measure, not what it actually measures. Face validity means that the appearance of the test coincides with its use (Miller et al., 2012). While actual validity is far more important than face validity, face validity is still desirable. A test needs face validity so that it appears to be valid to the test consumer. Face validity also helps to keep the motivation of the test takers high because students seem to try harder when a test appears to be reasonable and fair (Lyman, 1998). Students respond positively to tests that represent the content and objectives of the course. Tests that students perceive as being unrelated to course content can be distracting and therefore decrease the reliability of the test's results.

Face validity by itself never provides sufficient basis on which to establish validity; the mere appearance of validity is not adequate to establish evidence of validity. We must still establish evidence that enables us to be confident in the decisions we make based on the test's scores.

Usually, when you establish evidence of validity for the interpretation of test scores, face validity is also established. Poor test item construction is a primary cause of inadequate face validity. Thus, nursing exams should refer to nursing situations. Developing an exam blueprint and including a nurse and a client in the questions add to the face validity of your nursing exams. Sharing the blueprint with the students before the test alerts them about what to expect on the test and also increases their perception of the test as a valid measurement instrument. Chapter 10, "Establishing Evidence of Reliability and Validity," offers additional discussion related to validity.

Basic Test Statistics

Test analysis is a powerful tool that you can use to increase the quality of your classroom exams and your confidence in the decisions you make based on the test results. In addition, item analysis is an invaluable guide for improving the reliability and validity of the results of future tests by directing the improvement of the individual test items. Before you can analyze test and item data and correctly interpret their meanings, it is important that you understand the basic concepts of test statistics. Appendix B, "Basic Test Statistics," provides a brief reference guide to help familiarize you with the terms related to test and item analysis, which are used throughout this book. Each of these definitions is examined in greater detail in Chapters 11, "Interpreting Test Results," and 14, "Instituting Item Banking and Test Development Software."

Summary

Assessment procedures do not make decisions about students; teachers make decisions about students. To develop procedures that ensure fair decisions, it is important to have a clear understanding of the principles of assessment. This chapter presents an overview of the terminology that is fundamental to a thorough understanding of the concepts underlying valid and reliable assessment procedures as proposed in this text. Many of these concepts are explained in greater detail in subsequent chapters. *The Nurse Educator's Guide to Assessing Learning Outcomes* explores the entire assessment process and offers guidelines for the development of instruments that provide valid and reliable results, which are an integral component of a plan for the systematic assessment of learning outcomes. Familiarity with the language of assessment is the basic requirement for establishing a comprehensive assessment plan.

Learning Activities

1. Identify one instructional objective from a course you have taught or taken. Use Brookhart and Nitko's (2008) five guidelines to outline a plan for assessing student achievement of the learning outcomes associated with the objective.
2. Compare the processes involved with assessment and measurement.
3. Explain how a blueprint establishes validity evidence for the decisions made based on the results of a test.
4. Compare norm-referenced to CRT score interpretations. Explain why norm-referenced score interpretation is inappropriate in the classroom setting.
5. Describe a situation that would result in test bias.
6. Compare reliability to validity when interpreting a test score.
7. Explain why validity is the most crucial component of trustworthy test results.

Web Links

Association for the Assessment of Learning in Higher Education
http://www.aalhe.org/
Educational Resources Information Center
http://www.eric.ed.gov/
Internet Resources for Higher Education Outcomes Assessment
http://www2.acs.ncsu.edu/upa/assmt/resource.htm

References

American Educational Research Association, American Psychological Association, & National Council on Measurement in Education. (1985). *Standards for educational and psychological testing.* Washington, DC: American Educational Research Association.

American Educational Research Association, American Psychological Association, & National Council on Measurement in Education. (1999). *Standards for educational and psychological testing.* Washington, DC: American Educational Research Association.

American Educational Research Association, American Psychological Association, & National Council on Measurement in Education. (2014). *Standards for educational and psychological testing.* Washington, DC: American Educational Research Association.

Bosher, S. (2002). Barriers to creating a more culturally diverse nursing profession: Linguistic bias in multiple-choice nursing exams. *Nursing Education Perspectives, 24,* 25–34.

Brookhart, S. M., & Nitko, A. J. (2008). *Assessment and grading in classrooms.* Upper Saddle River, NJ: Pearson Education.

Brookhart, S. M., & Nitko, A. J. (2014). *Educational assessment of students* (7th ed.). Upper Saddle River, NJ: Pearson Education, Inc.

Burns, N., & Grove, S. K. (1997). *The practice of nursing research* (3rd ed.). Philadelphia, PA: W. B. Saunders.

Fitzpatrick, J. J. (2002). Never let an objective interfere with student learning. *Nursing Education Perspectives, 23,* 5.

Frisbie, D. A. (2005). Measurement 101: Some fundamentals revisited. *Educational Measurement: Issues and Practice, 24*(3), 21–28.

Glennon, C. D. (2006). Rconceptualizing program outcomes. *Journal of Nursing Education, 45,* 55–58.

Goodwin, L. D. (2002). Changing conceptions of measurement validity: An update on the new standards. *Journal of Nursing Education, 41,* 100–106.

Gronlund, N. E. (1973). *Preparing criterion-referenced tests for classroom instruction.* New York, NY: Macmillan.

Gronlund, N. E., & Brookhart, S. M. (2009). *Gronlund's writing instructional objectives* (8th ed.). Upper Saddle River, NJ: Pearson Education.

Haladyna, T. M. (2004). *Developing and validating multiple-choice test items* (3rd ed.). Mahwah, NJ: Lawrence Erlbaum Associates.

Hambleton, R. K., & Rodgers, J. H. (1995). Item bias review. *Practical Assessment, Research & Evaluation, 4*(6). Retrieved from, http://PAREonline.net/getvn.asp?v=4&n=6

Klisch, M. L. (1994). Guidelines for reducing bias in nursing examinations. *Nurse Educator, 19,* 35–39.

Lyman, H. L. (1998). *Test scores and what they mean* (6th ed.). Boston, MA: Allyn and Bacon.

Mager, R. F. (1997). *Preparing instructional objectives* (3rd ed.). Belmont, CA: Fearon Publishers.

Miller, M. D., Linn, R. L., & Gronlund, N. E. (2012). *Measurement and assessment in teaching* (11th ed.). New York, NY: Pearson.

Robinson Kurpius, S. E., & Stafford, M. E. (2006). *Testing and measurement: A user friendly guide.* Thousand Oaks, CA: Sage.

Slavin, R. E. (1997). *Educational psychology* (5th ed.). Boston, MA: Allyn and Bacon.

Developing Instructional Objectives

3

© Anteromite/Shutterstock

"You tell me, and I forget. You teach me, and I remember. You involve me, and I learn."

—Benjamin Franklin

A systematic approach for developing an assessment plan ensures that the plan is comprehensive. Numerous educational experts (Gronlund & Brookhart, 2009; Huba & Freed, 2000; Miller, Linn, & Gronlund, 2012; Brookhart & Nitko, 2014) identify objectives as the logical foundation of the teaching–learning–assessment process and agree that the first step of an instructional plan is to identify the course objectives. Objectives set the stage for effective planning, teaching, and assessment by specifying what a student should know and be able to do at the end of an instructional course (Gronlund & Brookhart).

Educators frequently concentrate on what material to include in a course before identifying what knowledge and skills they want students to develop. This approach tends to emphasize the recall of factual information instead of focusing the students on developing higher-level learning abilities. Identifying the objectives as the initial step in planning a course guides the instructional and assessment processes and also provides the framework for developing measurement instruments that provide valid and reliable information about student achievement.

Norman Gronlund proposed a straightforward plan for preparing clearly defined instructional objectives in 1973. The most recent edition of his book (Gronlund & Brookhart, 2009) continues to refine that plan, but the basic principles remain the same: State the objectives in general terms and identify specific learning outcomes to define the objectives as behaviors that students are expected to demonstrate as evidence of attaining the objective at the conclusion of the instruction. With this approach, the objectives guide the instructional destination of an educational experience for both the teacher and the students, while the outcomes define the objectives by specifying the behaviors that represent the achievement of the objectives. When students are aware of what is required of them from the beginning of a course, they are required to assume responsibility for their own learning.

Establishing objectives and outcomes during the initial phase of course preparation compels you to identify your learning expectations in a language that explicitly communicates your intent to students. Students are much more likely to succeed if they understand what is expected of them from the outset of an educational experience and if they perceive the expectations to be realistic. When students recognize that the purpose of the instruction is relevant and useful for their educational goals, they are more likely to assume ownership of their own learning.

Clearly defined instructional objectives steer efficient course planning. In addition, they guide the selection of teaching and learning activities, direct the development of measurement instruments, and empower students to take charge of their own learning to meet the teacher's expectations, thereby increasing the validity of the assessment plan.

Role of Objectives

Objectives guide the instructional process by synchronizing the planning and implementation of teaching, learning, and assessment activities, thereby focusing on the outcomes teachers want students to achieve. Unfortunately, course preparation often involves planning for the content and teaching activities without first establishing a clear definition of desired student outcomes. This approach can lead to instructional methods and assessments that focus on knowledge acquisition rather than on higher-level learning outcomes.

If students are expected to achieve the objectives of a course, they must be provided with appropriate opportunities to learn what they need to learn (Huba & Freed, 2000). Instructional objectives require teachers to provide students with the kinds of experiences that facilitate the attainment of the objectives. When objectives are determined at the beginning of a course, they provide direction to the teacher for selecting the instructional activities that promote achievement of the desired behaviors (Gronlund & Brookhart, 2009). For example, a course objective that requires a student to demonstrate critical thinking skills necessitates that the teacher select learning experiences and assessment activities that require the ability to think critically. Refer to Chapter 12, "Laboratory and Clinical Evaluation," for a discussion related to designing clinical and laboratory experiences and assessment tools that address the course objectives.

With today's rapidly advancing computer technology, the need to develop innovative approaches to facilitate learning is paramount. The pervasive nature of the Internet and the rapid progression of distance learning mandate that teachers develop creative teaching modalities and learning opportunities to meet learner preferences. In this atmosphere of self-directed learning, instructional objectives are assuming an ever-increasing role as the basis for meeting the diverse needs of learners. Students who have the opportunity to select from a range of teacher-designed learning strategies to meet the intended objectives become active participants in the learning process. Self-direction is facilitated when an individual learner has the ability to decide how to meet a course's objectives by selecting from a variety of teaching/learning strategies designed to accommodate diverse individual learning styles.

Instructional objectives and learning outcomes also play a crucial role as the basis for valid measurement instruments by providing the framework on which a test blueprint is based. As Chapter 4, "Implementing Systematic Test Development," describes in detail, the blueprint directs the content of the test. In addition to shaping the blueprint, the objectives guide the development of the test items. Chapter 5, "Selected-Response Format: Developing Multiple-Choice Items," Chapter 6, "Writing Critical Thinking Multiple-Choice Items," and Chapter 7, "Selected-Response Format: Developing True–False and Matching Items" illustrate how selected-response items evolve from the course objectives, while Chapter 8, "Constructed-Response Format: Developing Short-Answer and Essay Items," explains how the course objectives guide the development of constructed-response items. One of the most important roles of the instructional objectives is to increase the validity of the results of assessments. When student achievement is measured with instruments that are developed from instructional objectives, fairness is ensured.

Focus of Instructional Objectives

What is the most effective way to state an instructional objective? **Exhibit 3.1** presents two different approaches for defining an objective for a hypothetical course in the foundations of nursing care.

Exhibit 3.1   Teacher-focused versus learner-focused instructional objectives

Teacher-focused: Demonstrate to students how to safely perform basic nursing procedures.
Learner-focused: The student will demonstrate safe performance of basic nursing procedures.

When an objective is teacher-focused, the attention is centered on the teaching activity. Teaching is an end in itself; learning is not a criterion. The objective, in effect, is met once the teaching takes place, regardless of whether the teaching is effective. In the traditional lecture format, the learning is teacher focused; the teacher has control of the learning. This approach focuses on transmitting information and explains the all-too-common teacher lament, "I don't understand why the students do not know that material. I covered it in class."

A learner-focused objective focuses on the learning that occurs in relation to the teaching that is taking place. Stating instructional objectives in terms of the required student achievement shifts the focus of the educational experience from transmitting volumes of information to providing learning experiences that foster attainment of the objectives. The focus changes to facilitating learner achievement. Teaching is a means to an outcome rather than an end in itself.

Learner-focused objectives require teachers to examine their teaching strategies and to develop creative methods to facilitate student learning. Because students have different learning styles, a variety of instructional methods must be integrated into a course to provide opportunities for all of the students to attain the objectives. If students do not achieve the desired outcomes with this approach, the first question that a teacher must ask is, "Were the instructional experiences appropriate?"

It is important to recognize that teachers who do not consciously identify instructional objectives are most likely operating on teacher-focused goals. When the main objective of classroom instruction is to cover the material, without concern for developing strategies to meet student needs, the goals are teacher focused and the approach usually is a didactic one. Although this instructional method can require students to think logically, it does not encourage critical thinking, and while the lecture approach to teaching is the most direct one for the teacher, it is the least beneficial for addressing individual learning styles to promote student attainment of the course objectives. That is not to say that the lecture is not important. On the contrary, a lecture can be very useful for clarifying the complicated concepts associated with nursing practice. However, with today's diverse learners, lecture cannot be the highest priority learning activity in a nursing course. Nursing education needs to focus on alternate strategies for fostering critical thinking to accommodate the wide range of students' learning styles. Refer to the websites in the "Web Links" section at the end of this chapter for a selection of teaching/learning resources.

Stating Instructional Objectives

Unless students are well informed about assessment criteria, they are placed in a no-win situation. However, by stating the instructional objectives in terms of the intended learning outcomes, you give students clear direction for the types of performance you will accept as evidence that they have demonstrated what is expected of them. A meaningful objective communicates the desired outcome behavior of the learner exactly as you understand it. In other words, if another teacher uses your objective and their student outcomes are consistent with your expectations, then you have communicated the objective in a meaningful way (Mager, 1997).

Specific Objectives

Methods for writing instructional objectives include general and specific formats. A highly specific format delineates student outcomes in very specific terms. Gronlund and Brookhart (2009) describe how specific objectives can be further defined by a list of specific tasks. These tasks can then be taught and tested sequentially. Although this process can clearly define student outcomes, it tends to overemphasize low-level skills and factual knowledge, and also stresses simple learning outcomes.

Narrowly focused specific objectives raise a concern that students will focus on the tasks as an end in themselves rather than as activities that are part of more complex learning outcomes. McMillan (2001) identifies behavior, learner, criterion, and condition as the components of highly precise objectives. **Exhibit 3.2** is an example of a highly specific objective that identifies these components. In this example, the focus is entirely on the skill. We certainly want a student to obtain a patient's apical pulse accurately, but obtaining the pulse is not an end in itself. In the real world, we want students to go beyond simply obtaining the pulse. The intended objective should be to include the ability to interpret assessment findings in unique clinical situations.

Exhibit 3.2   An example of a specific instructional objective

Within 20 minutes in the learning laboratory (condition), the student (learner) will obtain (behavior) an apical pulse on a volunteer that is accurate to within three beats per minute (criterion).

Highly specific objectives clearly indicate the behaviors that a student must demonstrate to achieve the objective. However, the degree of specificity inherent in these objectives makes them unwieldy. In a complex discipline such as nursing, faculty would have to develop extensive lists of specific objectives to address every course outcome. In addition, these objectives are very confining because they severely limit a teacher's ability to modify the instructional approach. McMillan (2001) suggests that it is better to focus your objectives on units of instruction rather than on daily lesson plans because "writing objectives that are too specific results in long lists of minutia that are too time consuming to monitor and manage" (p. 26).

Rather than having an unwieldy list of specific objectives, several general objectives can be developed to encompass the range of content in a course. This allows the teacher to address all the desired student outcomes of a course while keeping the number of course objectives manageable. A reasonable list of general objectives assists the students to demonstrate success by focusing on what is expected of them in a course.

General Objectives

A general format is a more logical approach than the specific format for developing course objectives in a complex area of study such as nursing. **Exhibit 3.3** restates the specific objective (referred to in Exhibit 3.2) as a general objective. Note that the general objective is content-free; the procedures are not identified, so you can develop a set of outcomes that are applicable with various content units in a course. This approach allows the teacher to keep the number of general objectives manageable and avoids unwieldy lists of specific objectives for each unit of study.

Exhibit 3.3   An example of a specific objective restated as general objective

The student (learner) will demonstrate (behavior) safe performance of basic nursing procedures (content).

To allow for flexibility in instructional strategies, the general objective should not include the teaching procedures for accomplishing the objective. The objective in Exhibit 3.2 prescribes a narrow skill (obtaining an apical pulse) and restricts both the setting and the teaching method. The objective requires that the learning take place in a laboratory with a volunteer, so it precludes assessment in a clinical setting. Imagine how unwieldy the list of objectives would be if they were written in this format for all the procedures in a nursing foundations course! Exhibit 3.3, in contrast, presents a general objective that can be applied for assessing a range of procedures without proscribing the setting or the instructional or assessment strategies. However, the general objectives, as stated in Exhibit 3.3, must be clarified so that the students understand what is required of them to attain the objective.

Gronlund and Brookhart (2009) propose clarifying the general objective by stating the objective first and then listing a representative sample of student behavior that is acceptable to the teacher as evidence for attaining the objective. This general objective format accommodates the development of higher-order thinking skills and leaves room for creativity in achieving and assessing the prescribed outcomes.

Learning Outcomes

One way to determine whether a person is knowledgeable about something is to observe the individual's behavior. Learning outcomes are tools for measuring mastery of information (Whittman-Price & Fasolka, 2010). They represent the behaviors that an instructor is willing to accept as evidence that the student has achieved the general objective.

Consider the general objective shown in Exhibit 3.3. The general learning objective requires that a student safely perform basic nursing procedures. However, what does "safely perform basic nursing procedures" actually mean? Although the objective is learner focused, it is very broad and does not clearly specify what behaviors a student must demonstrate to confirm attainment of the objective. To provide a basis for instruction and assessment, the behaviors acceptable as evidence of the attainment of the general objective must be identified.

Exhibit 3.4 provides an example of the learning outcomes for the student-focused general instructional objective in Exhibit 3.3. While the general objective is very broad, the learning outcomes are specific behaviors. When considered together, the learning outcomes clarify the general objective by providing an operational definition for what the teacher regards as safe performance of basic nursing procedures.

Exhibit 3.4   An example of a general objective with its learning outcomes

---

Demonstrates safe performance of basic nursing procedures:

Discusses the rationale for the procedure.
Identifies the impact of the procedure on the client.
Explains the procedure to the client.
Selects the appropriate equipment for the procedure.
Completes the procedure with a predetermined degree of accuracy.
Maintains appropriate aseptic technique during the procedure.
Interprets client responses to the procedure.
Reports and documents the results of the procedure appropriately.
Provides client follow-up based on the results of the procedure.

Note that each learning outcome begins with an action verb—a verb that denotes a behavior that can be measured. Action verbs operationalize the general objective. A student who successfully demonstrates these behaviors—at a performance level predetermined by the teacher—would meet the criteria for safe performance of basic nursing procedures.

Table 3.1   A General Objective With Learning Outcomes That Apply Across Content

1. Safely performs basic nursing procedures.

	Blood Pressure	Oral Meds	IM Injection
1.1 Discusses rationale.	X	X	X
1.2 Identifies impact.	X	X	X
1.3 Explains procedure.	X	X	X
1.4 Selects equipment.	X	X	X
1.5 Completes procedure.	X	X	X
1.6 Demonstrates aseptic technique.	X	X	X
1.7 Interprets response.	X	X	X
1.8 Reports/documents results.	X	X	X
1.9 Provides follow-up.	X	X	X

As Gronlund and Brookhart (2009) suggest, it is important to keep the objectives and learning outcomes free of specific content so they can be applied across all units of study in a course. Consider the objective in Exhibit 3.4. It does not specify which procedures the student must perform safely, and the learning outcomes are applicable to all basic nursing procedures.

When stated without specific content, learning outcomes can be applied for establishing evidence of mastery of the learning tasks required for many procedures. For example, "Discuss the rationale for the procedure" applies to all nursing procedures, while "Describe the steps of the procedure" requires that a checklist be developed for each procedure. **Table 3.1** illustrates how the general objective and learning outcomes apply to a variety of procedures.

This approach provides consistency across content for both student and teacher. It requires that a teacher carefully consider the universal requirements for safety across nursing procedures. In addition, it allows for individualization of the requirements for each procedure. It also reinforces the concept that, while principles often apply across procedures, special consideration must be made for individual situations.

Another benefit of this approach is that the focus is not solely on the skill. From the very beginning of an instructional process, students see the skill as a means to an end, as part of the procedure. Teaching, interpreting, reporting, and following up are also important considerations when performing any procedure on a patient. This approach also makes it clear that the objective is to demonstrate safe performance and not simply discussing, completing, or reporting. The learning outcomes are not ends in themselves; they describe the sample of behavior that the teacher is willing to accept as evidence of demonstrating safe performance.

Yet another benefit of developing objectives in this manner is that it focuses the instructional and assessment process on the overall objective rather than on the specific samples of behavior (Gronlund & Brookhart, 2009). For example, when teaching safe performance of a nursing procedure, you might include demonstrating the procedure or having the students read the textbook, view a video, practice the procedure, or engage in role-playing. All the learning outcomes, such as the rationale, the impact, and aseptic technique, would be included in the learning activities as part of the procedure, not as isolated activities. Then, when assessing the students, you might, for example, develop a simulation experience and have students perform a procedure on a mannequin and assess the students' ability with a checklist of all the learning outcomes. By requiring responses that were not directly taught in the classroom, you are assessing the students' ability to apply the knowledge, not to simply recall facts. You are also helping students to focus on the ultimate goal rather than concentrating on isolated tasks.

When writing objectives and learning outcomes, the goal is to communicate your objectives so they are not subject to misinterpretation. The challenge is to write your objectives at an appropriate level of generality—not so narrow that they are impossible to manage and not so general that they provide little guidance for instruction (McMillan, 2001, p. 26).

Table 3.2 provides examples of verbs to use for general objectives and verbs to use for learning outcomes to clarify the meaning of an objective. Use this list as a guide. The goal is to write broad general objectives that focus on complex learning with a list of learning outcomes that sample the observable student behaviors you are willing to accept as evidence of attainment of the objective. Decide what activities define your objective and select verbs for your learning outcomes that operationalize your general objective for the students.

A list of instructional objectives for a course usually includes objectives that address the mastery of the essentials as well as objectives that focus on development beyond the minimum level (Gronlund & Brookhart, 2009). Developing objectives and measuring these two different levels require two different sets of criteria. To ensure that the objectives form a valid basis for the assessment plan, you must have a clear understanding of the two levels.

Mastery (Performance) Objectives

Performance skills have an important role in nursing education. Nursing students are expected to master a number of performance skills. With mastery learning, the domain of learning tasks is limited and can be clearly defined. Learning outcomes, which measure mastery, are usually outcomes that we can expect all students to master. The faculty must decide which skills must be mastered and must identify the criteria for mastery.

Objectives at the mastery level are designed to establish a specified minimum acceptable performance level. Gronlund and Brookhart (2009) suggest that an objective's specific learning outcomes can be used to create a checklist to indicate satisfactory or unsatisfactory for each outcome when observing a student perform a procedure. Rating scales can also be developed by using the learning outcomes as the criteria for judging student performance on a numerical scale. The rating instrument should be easy to understand and shared with students before the instruction begins. A well-designed rating instrument facilitates providing feedback to students and offers students the opportunity to assess their own learning. The objective with learning outcomes in Table 3.1 represents an objective for mastery learning. It could be easily translated into a checklist or rating scale for measuring performance on the procedures in a nursing foundations course. The consistency across procedures helps students to recognize that skills are not an end in themselves. Chapter 12, "Laboratory and Clinical Evaluation," discusses the development of performance instruments for assessing attainment of course objectives.

Table 3.2   General and Clarifying Verbs

General Objective Verbs	Clarifying Outcome Verbs	
Analyze	Acknowledge	Identify
Apply	Adapt	Illustrate
Appreciate	Allot	Implement
Believe	Appoint	Indicate
Clarify	Arrange	Interpret
Consider	Assign	Intervene
Comprehend	Calculate	Itemize
Create	Categorize	Judge
Deduce	Choose	Label
Demonstrate	Cite	List
Distinguish	Classify	Maintain
Document	Collect	Measure
Evaluate	Combine	Name
Facilitate	Complete	Outline
Formulate	Compose	Perform
Grasp	Criticize	Predict
Infer	Defend	Prepare
Interpret	Define	Present
Know	Delegate	Provide
Observe	Denote	Question
Perform	Describe	Recite
Recognize	Develop	Rephrase
Respect	Diagram	Report
Synthesize	Differentiate	Restate
Think	Discuss	Select
Understand	Distinguish	Specify
Value	Document	State
	Employ	Stipulate
	Enumerate	Tell
	Examine	Use
	Explain	Verbalize
		Write

Gronlund (1973) notes that some objectives require a higher level of achievement to establish mastery of safe performance than others. Safety is certainly a concern that nursing faculty must consider when identifying behaviors that represent mastery for nursing procedures, such as medication administration. For example, many nursing programs require students to attain a score of 90% to 100% correct on a math calculation exam before allowing them to give medications.

No matter what level is set for mastery attainment, teachers must be ready to accept the challenge presented by Reilly and Oermann (1990): to develop strategies to meet the needs of all students in achieving mastery of learning. The best approach for defining mastery is first to establish a consensus among the nursing faculty for the minimum level of mastery for safe nursing practice and then develop the learning outcomes that define mastery. Teachers can then provide instructional activities that foster mastery and, finally, adjust the level required for evidence of mastery as needed.

Developmental Objectives

Developmental learning is learning beyond the mastery level. While mastery objectives are directed at the tasks to be performed, developmental objectives emphasize progress toward goals. The skills and abilities associated with developmental learning are continuously developing throughout life (Brookhart & Nitko, 2014). Students cannot be expected to achieve these abilities fully during a course of study; each objective represents a goal to work toward. Because each objective at this level is complex, it represents a large number of specific behaviors. It would be futile to attempt to list all possible types of behavior that represent a developmental objective. The best approach when defining a developmental objective is to list a reasonable sample of the defining behaviors as learning outcomes and share these with the students (Gronlund & Brookhart, 2009).

Gronlund (1973) explains that outcomes at the developmental level of learning represent the progress made toward attaining the objective:

> It would be impossible to identify all of the behaviors involved in such a complex pattern of response. Even if we could, the measurement of each specific behavior would not be the same as measuring the integrated response pattern. Thus, we need to focus on the types of student performance that are most indicative of progress toward the objectives at that particular level of instruction. (p. 17)

Consider the ability to apply the nursing process. This ability certainly represents developmental learning because it requires the development of skills that progress from novice to expert. An example of a specific objective designed to address the ability to apply the nursing process is shown in **Exhibit 3.5**.

Exhibit 3.5 Specific objective for the nursing process

Specific Nursing Process Objective

Given an assignment to care for an acutely ill client (condition), the student (learner) will

- Collect (behavior) data from at least two sources (criteria).
- Identify (behavior) two nursing diagnoses based on the data (criteria).
- Implement (behavior) two interventions to address each diagnosis (criteria).
- Cite (behavior) two findings that indicate success or failure for each intervention (criteria).

The drawbacks for using the specific format for developmental learning objectives are evident. This specific objective related to the nursing process is far too narrow and leaves no leeway for teaching, learning, or assessment. It also fails to represent the concept of progress toward a goal. **Exhibit 3.6** restates this objective in a general format.

Exhibit 3.6   Specific objective for the nursing process restated as a general objective

The student (learner) will apply (behavior) the nursing process in selected healthcare situations (content).

The objective in Exhibit 3.6 does not restrict the instructional process because it does not specify the number of sources, diagnoses, interventions, or evaluation findings. However, it does not provide adequate guidance for the instructional process. **Exhibit 3.7** goes further to clarify this objective by specifying the learning outcomes.

Exhibit 3.7   Nursing process general objective with learning outcomes

2. Applies the nursing process in selected healthcare situations:
   2.1 Collects assessment data.
   2.2 Identifies nursing diagnoses based on assessment.
   2.3 Develops a plan based on analysis of data.
   2.4 Maintains safety when implementing a nursing plan.
   2.5 Adapts the plan to individual situations.
   2.6 Distinguishes success or failure of the plan based on subjective and objective data.

The general objective with learning outcomes approach is clearly the most effective strategy for stating objectives related to developmental learning. The list of learning outcomes in Exhibit 3.7 serves to operationalize the general objective by specifying a sample of behaviors that demonstrate the application of the nursing process. This list of learning outcomes is also free of specific course content; achievement of the objective—applies the nursing process—can be demonstrated across the course content. In addition, the outcomes can apply to students who have different levels of expertise in their progress toward applying the nursing process.

Exhibit 3.8 is an excellent example from an introductory business communication course that clearly illustrates the advantage of using the general objective with learning outcomes approach. The two lists of behaviors are essentially the same. However, the specific approach is disorganized—the "objectives" are really activities that focus the students on tasks without an overall goal. This approach represents mastery of a narrowly defined skill set.

The general objectives approach represents developmental learning. The outcomes define the objectives at a very basic, introductory level, but the same objectives could be used in a more advanced course with learning outcomes that are more complex. The focus is on progress toward an ultimate goal while clearly defining what is expected at the introductory level.

Exhibit 3.8   Comparison of specific course objectives to general course objectives in a business communication course

Specific Course Objectives	General Course Objectives with Specific Learning Outcomes
Upon successful completion of this course, you will be able to:	*Upon successful completion of this course, you will be able to:*
1. Explain the psychology of writing effective letters and memoranda.	1. Facilitate Effective Communication in the Business Workplace
2. Examine business correspondence for effective communication of information.	• Use appropriate language in communicating ideas and information.
3. Use appropriate language in communicating ideas and information.	• Identify legal and ethical issues in communication.
4. Explain the difference between formal and informal writing styles.	• Employ effective communication techniques in an international environment.
5. Describe the process of critical thinking in business writing.	2. Create Effective Business Messages
6. Use direct, indirect, and persuasive messages appropriately.	• Compose accurate employment documents.
7. Employ effective communication techniques in an international environment.	• Explain the difference between formal and informal writing styles.
8. Prepare a formal report based on research.	• Explain the psychology of writing effective letters and memoranda.
9. Explore and present a topic to a group.	• Examine business correspondence for effective communication.
10. Identify legal and ethical issues in communication.	• Describe the process of critical thinking in business writing.
11. Write appropriate employment documents.	3. Formulate Effective Business Reports and Proposals
	• Prepare a formal report based on research.
	• Present the formal report to a group.
	• Use direct, indirect, and persuasive messages appropriately.

Refer to **Table 3.3** for a comparison between the characteristics of mastery and developmental learning objectives.

Framework for Writing Objectives

The general objectives in Exhibits 3.7 and 3.8 follow the two-step process proposed by Miller et al. (2012):

1. Each general instructional objective should encompass a readily definable domain of student responses. Each general objective should begin with a general verb (for example, *knows, understands, applies, facilitates*) and consist of only one objective.

Table 3.3 Comparison of Mastery and Developmental Learning Objectives	
Mastery Learning Objectives	**Developmental Learning Objectives**
Well-defined performance domain	Broad domain of related performances
Task oriented	Goal oriented
Focus on knowledge outcomes	Focus on complex achievements
Identify minimum skills	Identify abilities that develop continuously throughout life
Identify specific performance tasks	Identify a representative sample of performance
Measure attainable abilities	Measure the degree of achievement
Assess narrowly defined skill set	Assess progress toward an ultimate goal

2. List beneath each general instructional objective a representative sample of specific learning outcomes stated in terms of student performance. Each learning outcome should begin with an action verb (for example, *identifies, describes*), and be relevant to attaining the general instructional objective (p. 71).

This framework for developing objectives is specific enough to guide direction for teaching yet not so specific that the instruction is reduced to training. General statements provide greater freedom for the teacher in selecting instructional methods. It also provides a basis for increasing the complexity of the outcome behaviors as students progress through a course of study (Miller et al., 2012). In other words, the same general objective could be used through a sequence of courses, with the specific learning outcomes becoming more complex each semester. This framework is particularly suitable for nursing curricula, where many abilities build on each other and develop over time.

Exhibit 3.9 presents a template for the development of objectives for constructs in a nursing program. Note that the verb *applies* in the general instructional objective represents higher-order cognitive thinking. Additional aspects of higher-order thinking—analysis and evaluation—are subsumed in the learning outcomes. Lower-level thinking—knowledge and comprehension—is included in the specific learning outcomes. Application and analysis ability require ability at the lower levels of cognition. If you cannot define a concept, it is unlikely that you will be able to apply it.

Exhibit 3.9   Template for objectives for nursing constructs

---

1. Applies (nursing theory, communication skills, therapeutic nursing care, etc.) in selected healthcare setting:
   1.1 Defines
   1.2 Explains
   1.3 Interprets
   1.4 Develops
   1.5 Implements
   1.6 Adapts

The template in Exhibit 3.9 assumes that the construct being measured has been defined and that the instructional objectives and learning outcomes are derived directly from that definition. The specific verbs for the general objective and learning outcomes, listed in Table 3.2, should be selected to measure the defined construct. This example illustrates how objectives can be developed to address the levels of cognitive ability across levels and content within a nursing program.

Number of Objectives

The previous description of the process of objective development draws attention to a question that nursing professors frequently ask: "How many objectives should a course have?" While Miller et al. (2012) suggest that 8 to 12 objectives usually suffice (p. 66), there is no hard-and-fast rule. However, writing your objectives using the framework previously described will certainly enable you to keep your list manageable. If your objectives apply across content areas, you can apply the outcomes to each unit of study within your course.

You can judge the adequacy of your list of objectives by asking these questions (Miller et al., 2012):

- Does the list include all of the important objectives for the course?
- Is the list consistent with the program's general goals?
- Is the list in harmony with sound principles of learning?
- Is the list realistic in terms of student ability and the time and resources available?

It is important that you list the competencies you want students to attain at the course's end, translate those abilities into general instructional objectives, develop your learning outcomes to operationalize the instructional objectives, and keep the objectives content-free. This approach will guide you in developing a comprehensive list of general objectives while avoiding a long unmanageable list of skills.

If your objectives are written according to the framework proposed by Miller et al. (2012), the same general objectives can be used in every course, and each of its learning outcomes, instructional activities, and assessment criteria can be developed to show progress in the developmental learning associated with the required outcomes. **Exhibit 3.10** provides an example of how learning outcomes for a program objective can be developed to illustrate progression through a program's courses.

Note that the general objective represents developmental learning and that it is the same for all courses. The increasing complexity of the learning outcomes provides evidence of course progression toward achieving the desired program objective. The learning outcomes for the fourth-semester course (which would be the same as the program competencies) are much more complex than those for the first-semester course.

Also note that several of the outcomes are the same or very similar for each course, such as "Uses information technology to support patient care." In this case, the assigned activities and the setting in which technology was used would become more complex as the students progressed through the course work. Perhaps you would assign students in the first course to identify three references from an electronic

Exhibit 3.10   Learning outcomes that illustrate course progression toward program objective

---

First-Semester Communication Objective

1. Facilitates effective communication in healthcare settings:
    1.1 Defines therapeutic communication principles.
    1.2 Describes therapeutic communication techniques.
    1.3 Explains the significance of nonverbal communication.
    1.4 Discusses factors that can influence the communication process.
    1.5 Discusses cultural influences on communication.
    1.6 Describes barriers to effective communication.
    1.7 Discusses the importance of confidentiality in communication.
    1.8 Uses appropriate interviewing skills.
    1.9 Interprets the effectiveness of communication.
    1.10 Uses information technology to support patient care.

Second-Semester Communication Objective

1. Facilitates effective communication in healthcare settings:
    1.1 Uses appropriate therapeutic communication skills.
    1.2 Identifies factors that influence the communication process.
    1.3 Identifies cultural influences when communicating with patients.
    1.4 Identifies barriers to communication.
    1.5 Maintains confidentiality.
    1.6 Interprets the effectiveness of communication.
    1.7 Reports relevant information to appropriate resources.
    1.8 Documents relevant information accurately.
    1.9 Uses information technology to support patient care.

Third-Semester Communication Objective

1. Facilitates effective communication in healthcare settings:
    1.1 Uses appropriate therapeutic communication skills.
    1.2 Interprets factors that influence the communication process.
    1.3 Interprets cultural influence on communication.
    1.4 Selects techniques to minimize barriers to communication.
    1.5 Interprets the effectiveness of communication.
    1.6 Reports significant information to the appropriate resource.
    1.7 Documents relevant information accurately and appropriately.
    1.8 Identifies channels of communication.
    1.9 Maintains confidentiality.
    1.10 Uses information technology to support patient care.

Fourth-Semester Communication Objective

1. Facilitates effective communication in healthcare settings:
    1.1 Uses appropriate therapeutic communication skills.
    1.2 Adapts communication approach in culturally sensitive situations.
    1.3 Uses therapeutic techniques to minimize barriers to communication.
    1.4 Interprets effectiveness of communication.
    1.5 Reports significant information to the appropriate resource promptly.
    1.6 Documents relevant information accurately, appropriately, and concisely.
    1.7 Maintains working relationships with interdisciplinary team.
    1.8 Maintains organizational and patient confidentiality.
    1.9 Uses appropriate channels of communication.
    1.10 Uses information technology to support patient care.

library search, while the graduating students would be expected to engage in an in-depth library and web search.

Chapter 4, "Implementing Systematic Test Development," explains the development of test blueprints and elaborates on how general objectives can be applied across course content and how they guide the development of a test blueprint to establish content-related evidence of test validity.

Number of Learning Outcomes

How many learning outcomes should you identify for each objective? Obviously, there is no standard answer to this question. Gronlund and Brookhart (2009) point out that it is impossible to identify every possible behavior that is associated with developmental learning. There is no advantage to listing more than 9 or 10 outcomes for each objective. The most important concern is to make the list as representative as possible while keeping it manageable. The list of outcomes should appear reasonable to the students and also make it clear what behaviors demonstrate the achievement of the objective.

Taxonomies

A taxonomy is a classification system that describes and identifies groups. In education, taxonomies classify three domains of learning—cognitive, affective, and psychomotor. In 1956, the *Taxonomy of Educational Objectives*, edited by Benjamin Bloom, was published. Popularly referred to as Bloom's taxonomy, this well-known resource for the development of instructional objectives and test items initially covered only the cognitive domain of learning. Subsequent editions, however, deal with the affective and psychomotor learning domains as well. Bloom's taxonomy classifies three domains of learning:

1. Cognitive: Concerned with intellectual objectives. Bloom describes this domain as the central point of the work of most test development; it deals with knowledge and the development of intellectual abilities and skills (p. 7).
2. Affective: Objectives in this domain describe interests, attitudes, and values (p. 7). In nursing education, this domain relates to how these characteristics affect the practice of nursing.
3. Psychomotor: Bloom refers to this domain as the manipulative or motor skill area (p. 7). This domain is concerned with physical movements that require coordination. Oermann (1990) identifies psychomotor skills as having a cognitive aspect, which involves understanding the principles underlying each skill, and an affective dimension, which is concerned with a nurse's values and attitudes while performing a skill.

In 2001, Anderson and Krathwohl published a revision of Bloom's taxonomy. The most obvious change in the revised taxonomy is the terminology. The six categories of cognitive processes were changed from nouns to verbs. Evaluation is no longer the highest category in the new taxonomy, and a new category, creating, is now at the top of the hierarchy. See **Table 3.4** for a comparison of Bloom's original taxonomy and Anderson and Krathwohl's revision.

Table 3.4   Comparison of Bloom's and Anderson and Krathwohl's Taxonomies

Bloom's Taxonomy, 1956	Anderson and Krathwohl's Taxonomy, 2001
1. Knowledge: The ability to recall previously learned material. It refers to the simple remembrance of a fact, concept, theory, or principle.	1. Remember: Uses long-term memory to retrieve applicable information. Recognizes and recalls pertinent appropriate information.
2. Comprehension: The ability to grasp the meaning of material. Comprehension represents the lowest level of understanding and is demonstrated by translating material from one form to another.	2. Understand: Summarizes to demonstrate comprehension. Explains, summarizes, interprets meaning from oral, written, and graphic messages.
3. Application: The ability to use learned material in new and concrete situations.	3. Apply: Implements a procedure in a unique situation to solve problems. Executes a procedure in a familiar situation.
4. Analysis: The ability to break down material into its component parts so its organizational structure can be understood.	4. Analyze: Breaks down material into component parts to determine organizational structure.
5. Synthesis: The ability to combine elements to form a unique new idea, procedure, or object.	5. Evaluate: Applies qualitative and quantitative standards and criteria to make judgments.
6. Evaluation: The ability to use criteria and standards to make qualitative and quantitative judgments.	6. Create: Develops a new structure or product by reorganizing and synthesizing information.
Data from Bloom, B. S. (Ed.), Englehart, M. D., Furst, E. J., Hill, W. H., & Krathwohl, D. R. (1956). *Taxonomy of educational objectives: The classification of educational goals.* New York, NY: Longmans, Green, and Co.	Data from Anderson, L.W., & Krathwohl, D.R. (2001). *A Taxonomy for learning, teaching, and assessing.* New York, NY: Addison Wesley Longman.

In contrast to Bloom's one-dimensional taxonomy, the revised taxonomy is a two-dimensional taxonomy. The knowledge dimension identifies what has to be learned, while the cognitive process dimension represents the process used to learn. Bloom's original taxonomy, expanded and revised, is a valuable tool for educators to use when they want to move students through a learning process (Forehand, 2010).

Taxonomies relate to educational goals and are especially useful for establishing objectives and developing test items. Each domain is organized by levels of increasing complexity within the domain category. Bloom's cognitive domain, for example, includes the levels of knowledge, comprehension, application, analysis, synthesis, and evaluation. The levels build on each other, with knowledge being the lowest level. Each level in the hierarchy demands the skills and abilities of the levels that are lower in the hierarchy. For example, an objective written at the application level also requires the abilities of the knowledge and comprehension levels.

The cognitive domain is particularly applicable to classroom test development. In nursing, test items are most effective when written at the application or higher levels of cognition. In fact, most items for both the National Council Licensure Examination for registered nurses and the National Council Licensure Examination for licensed practical/vocational nurses are written at the application or higher levels of cognitive ability (National Council of State Boards of Nursing, 2016).

Taxonomies provide a useful framework for the development of objectives that accurately reflect the levels of learning. The taxonomy for each of the previous domains begins with its basic skills and progresses to its more complex abilities. Referring to a taxonomy ensures that important categories of learning are not overlooked. Miller et al. (2012) suggest that a taxonomy is useful as an aid in the development of your own unique list of objectives. Once your objectives are established, a taxonomy is also valuable in the design of test questions to accommodate your objectives.

Taxonomies can be useful guides in the development of a comprehensive list of high-quality objectives. A taxonomy assists teachers in determining if the course objectives address an adequate range of lower- and higher-order thinking skills. However, it would be counterproductive to use a taxonomy as a rigid rule book for developing objectives or test questions.

Using Instructional Objectives

Once objectives and outcomes are established, it is important to share them with students and to use them as a guide for course development. Reilly and Oermann (1990) identify the following three directions provided by instructional objectives:

1. The teaching activity best suited to meet the objective
2. The type of learning activity that enables the learner to accomplish the behavior desired in the outcome
3. Methods and criteria for evaluation of the attainment of the objective (p. 48)

Instructional objectives provide a road map for selecting teaching approaches, creating learning activities, and determining the methods for assessing outcomes. Refer to the objective presented in Exhibit 3.4. Note that it designates learning outcomes in all three learning domains: cognitive, affective, and psychomotor. Therefore, a variety of teaching/learning and assessment strategies are required to address this objective. The psychomotor component certainly suggests that the teaching activities include a demonstration of the activity, whereas the cognitive and affective components suggest activities that might include lecture, computer-assisted instruction, and/or readings. An assortment of learning activities, such as clinical or laboratory practice, process recordings, role-playing, and written assignments, should be incorporated into the plan to address each of the domains. Finally, assessment procedures should also include a variety of approaches, including written assignments, multiple-choice exams, laboratory observation, and clinical evaluation. With this design the behaviors specified as desired outcomes direct all aspects of an educational experience. **Tables 3.5** and **3.6** illustrate how teaching, learning, and assessment strategies can be planned to address all of the learning outcomes associated with the objectives identified in Exhibits 3.4 and 3.10.

Table 3.5   Worksheet for Instructional Planning Based on Learning Outcomes

Objective: Safely performs basic nursing procedures.

Learning Outcomes	Teaching Strategies				Learning Activities				Assessment Procedures			
	Readings	Computer Assisted Instruction (CAI)	Demonstration	Lecture	Written Assignments	Role Playing	Journal	Clinical/Laboratory Practice	Multiple-Choice Examinations	Journal	Clinical/Laboratory Observation	Written Assignments
Identify the rationale for the procedure.	X	X		X	X		X		X	X	X	X
Acknowledge the impact of the procedure on the client.	X	X		X	X	X	X			X		X
Describe the steps of the procedure.	X	X	X	X	X	X		X	X		X	X
Explain the procedure to the client.	X	X		X		X	X		X	X	X	
Select the appropriate equipment for the procedure.	X	X	X	X		X		X	X		X	X
Perform the procedure with a predetermined degree of accuracy.		X	X			X		X			X	
Maintain appropriate aseptic technique during the procedure.	X	X	X	X			X		X		X	
Interpret client responses to the procedure.	X	X		X	X	X	X		X	X	X	X
Communicate the results of the procedure appropriately.	X			X	X	X	X	X	X		X	
Provide client follow-up based on the results of the procedure.	X	X		X		X		X	X		X	

Table 3.6 Worksheet for Instructional Planning Based on Learning Outcomes

Objective: Facilitates effective communication in healthcare settings.

Learning Outcomes	Teaching Strategies				Learning Activities				Assessment Procedures			
	Readings	CAI	Demonstration	Lecture	Written Assignments	Role-Playing	Journal	Clinical/ Laboratory Practice	Multiple-Choice Examinations	Journal	Clinical/ Laboratory Observation	Written Assignments
Defines principles of therapeutic communication.	X	X		X	X		X		X	X	X	X
Describes therapeutic communication techniques.	X	X		X	X	X	X			X		X
Explains significance of nonverbal communication.	X	X	X	X	X	X		X	X		X	X
Discusses factors that can influence the communication process.	X	X		X		X	X		X	X	X	
Discusses cultural influences on communication.	X	X	X	X		X		X	X		X	X
Describes barriers to effective communication.		X	X	X		X		X			X	
Discusses importance of confidentiality.	X	X	X	X		X		X			X	
Uses appropriate interviewing skills.	X	X	X	X	X	X	X		X	X	X	X
Interprets effectiveness of communication.	X	X		X	X	X	X	X	X		X	
Uses information technology to support patient care.	X	X		X		X		X	X		X	

Tables 3.5 and 3.6 also demonstrate how instructional strategies can overlap. A particular strategy can address multiple outcomes during the same experience, and strategies can be applied concurrently to different areas of the instructional process. Consider written assignments. This strategy can simultaneously be a learning activity and an assessment procedure, and it addresses several outcomes. The important point is that activities are planned to address every outcome in every area of the instructional process—teaching, learning, and assessment—and that every strategy, activity, and procedure has a purpose.

Huba and Freed (2000) identify four fundamental requirements for the development of effective learner-focused assessment based on learning outcomes:

1. Formulate statements of intended learning outcomes. The first step is to describe the intentions for what students should know, understand, and be able to do with their knowledge when they graduate.

2. Develop or select assessment measures. To measure whether the intended outcomes are achieved, data-gathering measures must be used. Designing these measures forces the teacher to understand thoroughly what is really meant by the intended learning outcomes.

3. Create experiences leading to the outcomes. If students are expected to achieve the intended outcomes, they must be provided with appropriate opportunities to achieve those outcomes.

4. Discuss and use assessment results to improve learning. Discussions must take place to use assessment data for the improvement of learning. These discussions should occur between faculty and students, as well as among the faculty, to gain insights into the learning that is occurring (pp. 9–15).

Criteria for Effective Objectives

Miller et al. (2012) proposed a list of criteria to guide teachers in the development of instructional objectives. The list of criteria includes completeness, appropriateness, soundness, and feasibility. Effective objectives are also relevant, open-ended, written in terms of student behavior, and shared with students. These standards can also apply to the development of competencies or goals for an instructional course.

Complete

An objective should be included for each important aspect of a course. Knowledge objectives are easiest to include. Special attention must be paid to include objectives that focus on higher-order thinking skills as well as on the affective domain (Miller et al., 2012).

Appropriate

For the objectives to be relevant, they must be congruent with the general goals of the school, and they should be consistent with the program's mission, goals, and outcomes (Miller et al., 2012). Most objectives in a nursing program should address developmental learning and should also reflect the progress in the attainment of developmental learning.

Sound

Sound objectives are in harmony with the principles of teaching and learning. They must be appropriate to the educational and experience level of the students. Objectives that relate to the students' needs and build on prior experience appropriately motivate students. Objectives should also reflect outcomes that are permanent. Students retain knowledge that is meaningful to them, but objectives that are perceived as trivial will be dismissed by students. The nature of the learning reflected in the objectives should be permanent. Learning assumes relevance for the students when the outcomes, which are applicable to a specific situation, are transferable to other real-world situations (Miller et al., 2012).

Feasible

Clearly defined and attainable objectives are more valuable than a long list of unattainable goals. Teachers should consider whether the objectives are realistic and attainable in terms of student ability, available time, and instructional resources. Unrealistic goals discourage both students and teachers and soon become meaningless (Miller et al., 2012).

Relevant

Relevant objectives can help decrease the trivia in an educational experience by focusing teachers on what is important in a course of instruction (Reilly & Oermann, 1990). Once appropriate objectives are identified, teachers are then compelled to identify teaching, learning, and assessment strategies that address the required outcomes of the objectives. A teacher must answer the following questions: "Why am I using this strategy?" and "What purpose does it serve?"

Open-Ended

Objectives should be clear enough to define student behavior. They should provide direction without limiting the learning experience. An objective that prescribes strict methodology limits both students and teacher because it constrains the way students can demonstrate the behavior, and it requires the teacher to assess student performance only in terms of the specified method (Reilly & Oermann, 1990). Consider this example of a restricted objective: "Demonstrates safe nursing practice by accurately performing procedures." This objective suggests that only an accurate performance of the procedures demonstrates safety. In addition, it ignores the other criteria specified by the learning outcomes in Exhibit 3.4 that operationalize safe performance of nursing procedures. Writing objectives that are restricted in this manner requires that you develop an extensive and cumbersome list of objectives to address every important aspect of a course.

Open-ended objectives provide you with more flexibility. When they are content-free, it is possible to add specific learning outcomes and use the same list of objectives across units of study (Linn & Gronlund, 2000, p. 65).

Delineate Student Behavior

Outcomes for each objective should identify the student behavior that defines and signifies achievement of the objective. When objectives are written with outcomes in terms of student behavior that describes learning, they clarify your instructional intent and provide the basis for teaching methods, learning activities, and assessment strategies.

Shared with Students

This may seem too obvious to even mention, but it is very important and it must be emphasized. If you follow the criteria to develop effective objectives (**Exhibit 3.11**), implement a plan to promote learning attainment, and develop assessments based on your objectives, the objectives will be truly meaningful and students will appreciate their value. There is no point to simply giving lip service to an instructional plan. When students believe that you mean what you say and that your objectives truly reflect what is expected of them, they are provided with a framework for assessing their own progress and identifying their own strengths and weaknesses. In fact, they are encouraged to assume responsibility for their own learning. Sharing meaningful objectives with students encourages the pursuit of lifelong learning by empowering them to develop their own plan for directing their activities toward meeting objectives.

Exhibit 3.11   Criteria for effective instructional objectives
Criteria for Effective Instructional Objectives: • Complete   • Appropriate   • Sound   • Feasible   • Relevant   • Open-ended   • Delineate student behaviors   • Shared with students

Summary

Instructional objectives are the foundation for teaching, learning, and assessment in education. Not only are they the first step in establishing the validity of our instructional methods and assessments, they actually serve to expedite the process of systematic course development. The learning outcomes associated with these objectives are the common thread that is woven through all aspects of an instructional course.

Objectives provide the structure that helps educators to organize and communicate their instructional intent, they direct the development of teaching and learning strategies, and they form the basis for developing measurement instruments. Because of the critical role they play, it is imperative that you invest the effort in developing clearly written instructional objectives and learning outcomes as the initial step in the development of an instructional course.

Learning Activities

1. Develop one instructional objective with five to six learning outcomes.
2. Devise five to six learning activities that will provide students with the opportunity to achieve the each of the learning outcomes developed in Learning Activity 1.
3. Develop an assessment strategy to measure student achievement of the instructional objective developed in Learning Activity 1.
4. Use the instructional objective developed in Learning Activity 1 and refer to Exhibit 3.10 to develop learning outcomes that illustrate course progression toward program outcomes.
5. Refer to Table 3.3 to write one mastery level and one developmental level learning objective for a hypothetical nursing course or a course you have taught.

Web Links

Bloom's Taxonomy

http://www.odu.edu/educ/roverbau/Bloom/blooms_taxonomy.htm

http://projects.coe.uga.edu/epltt/index.php?title=Bloom%27s_Taxonomy

http://www.krummefamily.org/guides/bloom.html

Bloom's Revised Taxonomy

http://www.celt.iastate.edu/teaching/effective-teaching-practices/revised-blooms-taxonomy

https://tpri.wikispaces.com/file/view/05-2Bloom-16-17+Stems+for+Instruction.pdf

https://cft.vanderbilt.edu/guides-sub-pages/blooms-taxonomy/

Carnegie Mellon: Enhancing Education—Design and Teach a Course

http://www.cmu.edu/teaching/designteach/index.html

Carnegie Mellon: Enhancing Education—Technology for Education

http://www.cmu.edu/teaching/technology/index.html

MERLOT: Learning Materials for Nursing Education

http://www.merlot.org/merlot/materials.htm?category=2699&&sort.property=overallRating

Park University: Writing Quality Learning Objectives

http://www.park.edu/cetl/quicktips/writinglearningobj.html

Sloan Consortium: Committed to Quality Online Education

http://www.sloanconsortium.org/

References

Anderson, L. W., & Krathwohl, D. R. (2001). *A Taxonomy for learning, teaching, and assessing*. New York, NY: Addison Wesley Longman.

Bloom, B. S. (Ed.), Englehart, M. D., Furst, E. J., Hill, W. H., & Krathwohl, D. R. (1956). *Taxonomy of educational objectives: The classification of educational goals*. New York, NY: Longmans, Green, and Co.

Brookhart, S. M., & Nitko, A. J. (2014). *Educational assessment of students* (7th ed.). Boston, MA: Pearson Education.

Forehand, M. (2010). *Bloom's taxonomy*. Retrieved from http://epitt.coe.uga.edu /index.php?title=Bloom's_Taxonomy

Gronlund, N. E. (1973). *Preparing criterion-referenced tests for classroom instruction*. New York, NY: Macmillan.

Gronlund, N. E., & Brookhart, S. M. (2009). *Gronlund's writing instructional objectives* (8th ed.). Upper Saddle River, NJ: Pearson Education.

Huba, M. E., & Freed, J. E. (2000). *Learning-centered assessment on college campuses: Shifting the focus from teaching to learning*. Boston, MA: Allyn and Bacon.

Linn, R. L., & Gronlund, N. E. (2000). *Measurement and assessment in teaching*. Upper Saddle River, NJ: Prentice Hall.

Mager, R. F. (1997). *Preparing instructional objectives* (3rd ed.). Belmont, CA: Fearon Publishers.

McMillan, J. H. (2001). *Essential assessment concepts for teachers and administrators*. Thousand Oaks, CA: Sage.

Miller, M. D., Linn, R. L., & Gronlund, N. E. (2012). *Measurement and assessment in teaching* (11th ed.). Upper Saddle River, NJ: Pearson Education.

National Council of State Boards of Nursing (2016). *Detailed test plan for the National Council licensure examination for licensed practical/vocational nurses*. Chicago, IL: Author.

Oermann, M. H. (1990). Psychomotor skill development. *Journal of Continuing Education in Nursing, 21*, 202–204.

Reilly, D. E., & Oermann, M. H. (1990). *Behavioral objectives: Evaluation in nursing* (3rd ed.). New York, NY: National League for Nursing.

Whittman-Price, R. A., & Fasolka, B. J. (2010). Objectives and outcomes: The fundamental difference. *Nursing Education Perspective, 31*(4), 233–236.

© Anteromite/Shutterstock

Implementing Systematic Test Development

CHAPTER 4

"If you're not sure where you're going, you're liable to end up someplace else—and not even know it."

—ROBERT MAGER

Would you teach a course without developing a syllabus? Would you initiate a research project without a design? Would you compose a journal article without an outline? Certainly you would answer with a resounding no to all these questions. Yet how many of you have approached test construction without a detailed plan?

When a teacher prepares a test at the last minute, the results reflect the lack of effort. Poor planning results in grammatical and spelling errors, ambiguous questions, and clerical mistakes, all of which contribute to lack of face validity. These errors frustrate students and interfere with their ability to demonstrate mastery of the course. In a nutshell, lack of planning results in tests that fail to accurately assess student achievement.

Initiating Test Development

A good test acknowledges the knowledgeable students and identifies those who have superficial understanding about course content and objectives. Effective measurement depends on careful planning. When you develop a test you must be concerned about the validity of the inferences you make based on the scores of the test. Validity evidence based on test content refers to the degree to which the test represents the course content, or how well the test represents the domain being tested. For purposes of the discussion in this chapter, the content domain refers to health alterations or health concepts, whichever was the focus of the course. Keep this point in mind when applying the various worksheets included in this chapter to your course.

Content-related validity evidence of teacher-made classroom measurements is diminished by errors associated with the sampling of the course content and objectives. The key to ensuring that you make valid inferences about student achievement based on the results of your classroom tests lies in careful planning.

Test development refers to the process of producing a measurement by developing items and combining them to form a test according to a specified plan (American Educational Research Association [AERA], American Psychological Association [APA], & National Council on Measurement in Education [NCME], 2014, p. 75). To ensure that a test has representative content and objective sampling, development of a specified test plan should be part of course planning. Integrating test development into course planning provides the foundation for establishing evidence of validity.

In many nursing programs, several faculty members share the responsibility for teaching a course. When course responsibility is shared, it is imperative that one person be appointed to coordinate the activities of the course so that tests are produced in a timely manner. While the test coordinator has the ultimate responsibility for keeping the entire faculty group on track, all decisions related to the test should be made by consensus of the group.

Scheduling a Semester's Exams

In 1989, Victoria Schoolcraft recommended developing a master plan based on the academic calendar for all of a course's exams before generating any individual test plans. This advice continues to apply today. An efficient method for initiating test development is to base the master plan on the content to be addressed in the course; the course's objectives can be incorporated later in the blueprinting process. When developing an overall plan for a semester's tests, it is important to design the tests so that the content included in the course is represented proportionally on the tests and therefore in the final grade. Exams should be given frequently enough to allow for an adequate sampling of the content, and they should be spaced at reasonable intervals so students have adequate time for learning and are not overwhelmed.

Always consider the school's social calendar when scheduling exams. The results of a test the day after a big school event, for example, may lead to invalid inferences. Flexibility that allows appropriate postponements can enhance the reliability and validity of your test results. As with each step of test development, using a systematic plan that incorporates your professional judgment expedites the process. **Table 4.1** represents a sample master plan for a semester's exams.

Identifying the Purpose of the Test

Before you begin test development, you must decide what the purpose of the test is. Classroom tests can be used for a variety of purposes. Standard 1.0 of the *Standards for Educational and Psychological Testing* emphasizes that "no test permits interpretations that are valid for all purposes." It requires that test developers clearly describe how test scores will be interpreted and used (AERA et al., 2014, p. 23).

The items used on a test depend on the type of test you want to administer. If you are interested in determining the extent to which students have already achieved the objectives, you can administer a pretest. The goal of pretesting is to help a teacher

Table 4.1   Example of a Master Test Plan

Date	Examination	Content Area	Items	Final Grade Weight
10/12	Examination 1	Unit I Unit II	50	25%
11/20	Examination 2	Unit III Unit IV	50	25%
12/18	Comprehensive final examination	Unit I Unit II Unit IV Unit V Unit VI Unit VII	100	50%

identify the information to focus on during instruction and to assist students to identify what they need to review. Items on a pretest are designed to determine what skills the students have already mastered.

The purpose of a formative test is to assess students during instruction. Questions for a formative test are directed at monitoring student progress, detecting problems, and providing feedback to both the student and the teacher. These tests usually include a limited sample of course content and sample of objectives (Miller, Linn, & Gronlund, 2012).

Formative evaluation is more concerned with evaluating the teaching and developing appropriate instructional approaches than with assessing individual students (Miller et al., 2012). Therefore, it is usually not designed for the assignment of grades. If you use formative quizzes as graded assessments, be sure that students understand the grading implications. In any event, scores on formative quizzes should have less weight than summative evaluations in the determination of the final course grade.

Summative evaluation involves the process of assessing students in terms of the instructional objectives. Summative tests are designed to provide information about individual student achievement. A summative measurement presents questions that provide a representative sample of the objectives and content of a course. Summative tests are usually given at the end of a unit of study (unit exam) or at the end of a course (final exam) and are used to assign a grade.

When a test is being administered to assign a grade, it is important to decide whether the test will be norm- or criterion-referenced. As we discuss later in this chapter, it is beneficial to design criterion-referenced tests (CRTs) that are subject to norm-referenced interpretation when developmental learning is being measured. Most important, it is crucial that you clearly communicate the intent of a test to students so that they are aware of the implications of their test scores.

Determining the Length of the Test

How many questions will be on the test? Several factors enter into this decision, including the purpose of the measurement and the type of test items used. Most often, however, the main determinant is the amount of time allotted for the test.

For example, if 1 hour is the available time slot for an exam schedule, then you have to balance the blueprint so that it covers the desired content and objectives with a reasonable number of items that can be answered in 1 hour.

It is very important that students have enough time to finish the test. A general rule of thumb for well-constructed four-option multiple-choice questions is to allow 60 minutes for every 50 questions. Sixty minutes allows adequate time for 75 to 80 well-constructed true–false items; three-option multiple-choice items would allow you to include more than 50 items on the test in 60 minutes (Piasentin, 2010), which enables you to include a broader sample of the course. The underlying principle is to write items that are clear and unambiguous so they can be read and answered in the allotted time.

Speed influences reliability. Speed should not be a factor in a test unless the objective being measured relates to speed, such as when determining how many words per minute an individual can type. Testing situations already cause anxiety; when you add severe time constraints, anxiety increases and interferes with the student's performance. An essential requirement is to allow ample time for all students to complete all questions. Of course, ample time does not mean unlimited time. There are always stragglers who seem to engage in a tug-of-war with the proctor before giving up their answer sheets. If, after the allotted time, most of the students have finished, you can feel comfortable calling an end to the test and collecting the answer sheets from the few remaining students.

In many nursing programs, unit exams are frequently limited to 1 hour and final exams are often administered over 2 hours. If limits such as these dictate the number of questions that you can include on a test, you need to schedule several exams during the semester. It is important to present the students with a sufficient number of test questions over the course of a semester so that you adequately sample the content and objectives of your course.

The practical issues associated with timing a test are also a reminder of the need to use a variety of assessment techniques. Assessment should not be confined to class time. Providing a variety of out-of-class assignments such as care plans, journals, or a portfolio assessment increases the amount of information on which you can base your decisions. In addition, it also enables you to make informal (or formal, if you are so inclined and have adequate resources) correlations of your assessment measures. Remember this principle: The more assessment information you have, the more confidence you will have in the decisions you make based on that information.

Selecting What to Test

"The construct or constructs that the test is designed to measure should be clearly described" (AERA et al., 2014, p. 23). The content and objectives measured by a test should be a representative sample of what was included in the course during the period covered by the test. The challenge of matching what is taught to what is assessed and how it is assessed requires careful planning and professional judgment. A blueprint is the mechanism that links the course content and objectives to the questions on a test.

Clear descriptions of what is to be assessed and how it is to be assessed are the first steps in test development. Ideally, during course planning the instructional objectives are identified, the content is mapped out, and exams are scheduled. The *what* of assessment is defined by the instructional objectives and the course content. The *how* is directed by the test plan, or blueprint. The objectives and course content serve as the framework for the blueprint.

Nitko (2004, p. 125) identifies three important and fundamental principles that guide the development of classroom tests. These criteria are critical for sound assessment of students:

1. Classroom tests should focus only on objectives and important course content. Testing trivia or minor points is a waste of time. Every item should incorporate a learning outcome and focus on what is educationally important.

2. Test items should be crafted to assess mastery of the learning outcomes only. Test items should focus exclusively on eliciting the behaviors that are specified as learning outcomes. Students who have achieved the desired learning should be able to answer the item correctly, while those who have not achieved the desired learning should be unable to use test-taking skills to answer the item correctly.

3. Classroom tests should be meticulously designed. Ambiguous wording, inappropriate vocabulary, poor directions, or careless formatting, for example, can inhibit a student's ability to demonstrate attainment of the learning outcomes.

Once the instructional objectives and course content are identified, the tests for the course can be blueprinted. The tests can actually be prepared before instruction even begins. However, many teachers prefer to allow for unexpected course developments before finalizing an exam. Nevertheless, item development to meet a test plan should begin as soon as the blueprint is organized.

Selecting the Appropriate Assessment Format

Determining how well your students have achieved the instructional outcomes requires that you match each outcome with an appropriate assessment strategy. The more clearly you have stated your instructional objectives and learning outcomes, the more helpful they will be in assisting you in your decision on how to assess them. The challenge is to identify the most appropriate format for assessing the achievement of each instructional objective. You want to select the format that provides you with the best evidence of student achievement. The learning outcomes that are associated with the objectives provide the basis for determining how to assess the objectives.

The following basic types of measurement instruments provide a variety of formats that you can select from when deciding how to assess student achievement:

1. Selected-response or supply-type items are also referred to as objective items because subjective judgment is not involved in scoring them. With these questions, the correct answer is supplied and the student has to select it. Selected-response type items include the following:
   - True–false items present a statement and the student must decide whether it is true or false. These items are easy to write and score. However, if they

are poorly constructed, their use is limited to the testing of knowledge, and the potential for guessing is a concern.

- Multiple-choice items present a question or incomplete statement (stem) that is followed by two or more options. The student is required to select the correct or best choice to answer the question or complete the sentence. These items are easy to score, can test a broad content range, and lend themselves to objective analysis. Multiple-choice items can be written to assess higher-order thinking; however, well-written items can be time consuming to develop.

- Matching exercises provide two columns of options and require the student to select a choice from one column that parallels an option on the other column. These items are moderately easy to write, and a broad range of content can be assessed. However, higher-order thinking can be difficult to assess with this format.

2. Constructed-response type items are also referred to as subjective items because scoring can be open to interpretation by the scorer. These items require the student to construct a response to a statement or question. These items include the following:

- Completion or short-answer questions present the student with a question or a statement with one or more blanks. The student is required to provide a word, a phrase, or a sentence to complete the statement or to answer the question. These items are easy to write and can be administered in a short amount of time. However, verifying that the students have addressed the item's criteria can make scoring time-consuming.

- Essay questions ask a student to compose an original composition to respond to an idea or answer a question. These items can measure higher-order thinking skills and guessing is limited. Although the items are easy to write, scoring can be time-consuming and only a limited content range can be assessed.

3. Performance assessments refer to assessments in which students are asked to demonstrate mastery of the concepts beyond simply answering questions. Usually, there is no single right or wrong answer—a variety of responses can be considered correct. There are numerous examples of performance assessment, including oral presentations, experiments, journals, projects, case studies, and portfolio assessment. Although performance assessments are particularly well suited for assessing higher-order thinking, they are open to subjective interpretation and are time-consuming to administer and score.

4. Psychomotor assessment is concerned with assessing motor skill performance. Psychomotor skills are essential in nursing practice because they are fundamental to safe practice. Psychomotor assessment involves observing a student's performance of motor skills and assessing the cognitive skills that are essential for the adaptation of procedures for safe nursing practice.

Each of these assessment formats has advantages and disadvantages. Your main concern is to select the method that is most appropriate for assessing a particular instructional objective. The specific behaviors that define the learning outcomes help guide the selection of the assessment format. Chapters 5–8 provide detailed guidelines for developing measurement instruments in each of these formats.

Weighting the Content and Course Objectives

The content/objectives worksheet for a semester's exams in **Table 4.2** is a form designed to systematically assign items for each content unit and course's objectives. Note that the form enables you to weight the content areas for an entire semester. Also keep in mind that the content refers to what is taught in the course, whether the focus is on concepts or health alterations. The important fact is that the test must equally measure what was taught in the course.

The first step is to tally the total number of questions on all tests for a semester and then to identify the number of semester hours devoted to the course. Once the number of lecture hours for each content unit is identified, the percentage of the course that each content unit represents and the corresponding number of questions for each unit can be calculated.

In the hypothetical course presented in Table 4.2 there are 200 total semester exam items and 126 total semester lecture hours. By determining the percentage of the total lecture hours for each unit of content, it is easy to calculate the corresponding number of total exam items for each content area.

For example, the 24 lecture hours for Unit I represents 19% of the 126 total lecture hours; therefore, Unit I can be represented by 19% of the 200 total exam questions, or approximately 38 items. Notice that a single value is not assigned to the number of items for each unit; rather, a range is indicated. For example, instead of 38 items for Unit I, the worksheet indicates a range of 36 to 40 items. Planning a semester's exams is far from an exact science—flexibility is important with test development.

Table 4.2   Content/Objectives Worksheet

A. Number of unit examinations	2
B. Number of items per unit examination	50
C. Total unit examination items (A × B)	100
D. Number of final examination items	100
E. Total number of examination items (D + E)	200

				OBJ 1	OBJ 2	OBJ 3	OBJ 4	OBJ 5
				20%	25%	30%	10%	15%
Content	Lecture Hours	Percentage of Lecture Hours	Number of Semester Items					
Unit I	24	19%	36–40					
Unit II	20	16%	30–34					
Unit III	22	18%	34–38					
Unit IV	18	14%	26–30					
Unit V	14	11%	20–24					
Unit VI	14	11%	20–24					
Unit VII	14	11%	20–24					
Total	126 hours		200 items	38–42 items	48–52 items	58–62 items	18–22 items	28–32 items

The content is listed down the far left column in the worksheet, while the objectives are identified across the top row. Notice that the objectives are not equally weighted. Each objective is assigned a percentage. Assigning percentages to the objectives is a matter of professional judgment and reflects the relative emphasis of the objective in the course. Note that percentage weight for each objective translates into a range of items, which can be included in assessing the objective on the exams over the semester. These ranges are indicated across the bottom row of the worksheet.

Determining the relative weight of a particular content area for a semester based on the amount of instructional time devoted to that content is a practical approach to blueprinting an exam. Instructional time is an important measure of the amount of emphasis given to each topic. Because learning experiences do not occur only in the classroom, it is reasonable to include out-of-class assignment time as instructional time when weighting the content areas of a course. In the end, the percentage of instructional time (both in and outside the classroom) devoted to each content area should represent the relative emphasis of each content area in the course, and so it should also determine the number of items for the content area on the exams.

While there are no hard-and-fast rules, the most effective approach for determining how many test items should deal with each unit of content in a semester's exams is to use a systematic procedure. Completing a content worksheet, such as the one shown in **Table 4.3,** systematizes the process of identifying items for specific content

Table 4.3   Sample Content Item Worksheet

A. Number of unit examinations	2
B. Number of items per unit examination	50
C. Total unit examination items (A × B)	100
D. Number of final examination items	100
E. Total number of examination items (D + E)	200

Total Lecture Hours	126	Total Examination Items	200

Content Area	Lecture Hours	Percentage of Total Lecture Hours	Percentage of Exam Lecture Hours	Total Number of Items for Unit	Exam I Items	Exam II Items	Final Exam Items
Unit I	24	19%	55%	36–40	25–29		7–15
Unit II	20	16%	45%	30–34	21–25		5–13
Examination I					50		
Unit III	22	18%	55%	34–38		27–29	7–11
Unit IV	18	14%	45%	26–30		21–25	2–8
Examination II						50	
Unit V	14	11%		20–24			20–24
Unit VI	14	11%		20–24			0–24
Unit VII	14	11%		20–24			20–24
Total	126 hours			200 items	50 items	50 items	100 items

and simplifies the development of exam blueprints. This assignment should be a flexible one, with a range of items assigned to each content category.

The most significant criterion for establishing validity evidence based on test content is to have a representative sample of course content on your exams. To ensure that this occurs, all units of content must be represented proportionately on exams over the course of the semester. Information from the content/objectives worksheet is used to complete a semester content item form. The worksheet in Table 4.3 maps out the distribution of content across the semester exams for the course represented in Table 4.2.

Note that, in the course represented in Table 4.3, four of the content units are covered on unit exams and three are not. For example, Unit II is allocated 16% of 200 items, or 30 to 34 items for the entire semester. Because only Units I and II are included in Exam I, 21 to 25 of the 50 items on Exam I are from Unit II. This number is arrived at because Unit II represents 45% of the 44 lecture hours included on Exam I. Therefore, Unit II will have an additional 5 to 13 items for the final exam. The range in the "Total Number of Items for Unit" column determines how many items for each unit should be on the final exam after accounting for the number of items included in the unit exams.

It is important to understand the purpose of mapping out your exams in this highly specific manner. Units that are not tested during a semester should be more heavily represented on a comprehensive final exam than those units that were included on tests given during the semester. If they are not, there will not be valid representation of the course content on your exams. To weight the blueprint fairly, you need to identify how many items are devoted to each semester unit exam so the areas that were not tested at all during the semester are adequately represented on the final exam.

Although the process of deciding how to apportion items requires a time commitment in your already busy schedule, the process ensures that your tests reflect the content emphasis of your course. The content worksheet in Table 4.3 will assist you in assigning items in proportion to the course content they represent and will form the basis for establishing your test blueprints.

Developing a Test Blueprint

Once you have completed a content worksheet, you are ready to prepare a test blueprint. A blueprint is a test plan that links the test items to the content and instructional objectives of the course and provides a foundation for establishing content-related evidence of validity. Refer to Chapter 2, "The Language of Assessment," for discussion related to accumulating validity evidence. Generating a blueprint before developing the test is the essential step for establishing evidence for the validity of the inferences made based on the test scores.

A blueprint consists of a two-way chart that relates the instructional objectives to the course's content. Because the blueprint represents the validity evidence for the decisions you make based on the test results, the blueprint should *only* involve your main concern: mastery of the course objectives and content. Several authors (Fliszar, 2009; Oermann & Gaberson, 2009; Tarrant & Ware, 2012) recommend blueprinting a test to the course content or to the National Council Licensure Examination (NCLEX) blueprint, nursing process, or cognitive levels. This approach is basically flawed. You are not making a decision about the NCLEX, cognitive levels or the nursing process—you are making a decision about student accomplishment of the content and course objectives. All the test items should be written at the application and analysis cognitive levels, and the nursing process should be used as the framework for every item. The activities included in the *NCLEX Detailed Test Plan* should be incorporated into the curriculum, but the pass/fail decision in a course must be based only on what was included in the course: the content and objectives of the course. Chapter 15, "Preparing Students for the Licensure Exam: The Importance of NCLEX," explains how to cross-reference for tracking the cognitive levels, the nursing process, and the NCLEX blueprint in an exam.

The blueprint incorporates the list of course objectives that are suitable for paper-and-pencil or computer-administered testing and a content worksheet that identifies the relative emphasis of what is included in the course. The chart ensures that the content and the instructional objectives receive appropriate emphasis on the test.

The blueprint chart also verifies that the sample selected for the test is representative of what was included in the course. It would be impossible to include items on a test to measure every single concept of a course because the number of items that can be included in a test is limited. Therefore, we must select a sample that represents what was included in the course. If we select the sample appropriately, we can then generalize that our test results represent the larger achievement domain, and we can make decisions about whether the students have achieved the instructional objectives of the course. Using a blueprint to develop a test ensures that the items selected for the test represent the overall course.

Table 4.4 shows a completed blueprint worksheet for the course represented in Tables 4.2 and 4.3. The instructional objectives, which the teacher identifies as being

Table 4.4   Blueprint Worksheet

	Questions	Objective 1 20%	Objective 2 25%	Objective 3 30%	Objective 4 10%	Objective 5 15%	Total
	Range	38–42	48–52	58–62	18–22	28–32	200
Unit I	25–29	5	4	7	4	6	26
Unit II	21–25	5	8	8	1	2	24
Examination I	50	10	12	15	5	8	50
Unit III	27–29	7	10	1	2	7	27
Unit IV	21–25	4	4	10	3	2	23
Examination II	50	11	14	11	5	9	50
Unit I	10–14	5	2	3	0	2	12
Unit II	6–10	4	0	2	4	0	10
Unit III	7–11	4	1	0	0	2	7
Unit IV	3–7	0	0	3	3	0	6
Unit V	20–24	2	8	10	0	4	24
Unit VI	20–24	6	5	6	2	2	21
Unit VII	20–24	0	8	8	2	2	20
Final	100	21	24	32	11	12	100
Total	200	42	50	58	21	29	

appropriate for assessment by a paper-and-pencil or computer-administered test, are listed across the top row, and the units of content are listed down the first column of the chart. This is not a rigid process—flexibility is built in. Therefore, the items for each unit exam and the final exam are expressed as a range and are transferred from the worksheet in Table 4.3 to their corresponding content units. The number of items for each objective is also expressed as the range identified in Table 4.2.

Note that all the objectives are not included in every content area on the blueprint worksheet in Table 4.4. Some of the cells on the chart show a zero because every objective does not have to be assessed in every content area. The overall assessment of each objective and content area is in accordance with the specifications from Table 4.2. The crucial concerns are that the assessment methods reflect the emphasis of course instruction (Miller et al., 2012) and that provisions are made to assess every objective.

Although the process of preparing a blueprint as detailed as the one illustrated in Table 4.4 may initially appear very time consuming, it actually promotes efficient test development. This blueprint process is well worth the effort because it removes trivia from the tests by requiring that every item address both a content area and a course objective. This approach will assist you to write meaningful test items. Once you have your framework established, use it as a guide for item development, filling in the grid as you go. Or you could develop an electronic spreadsheet to simplify the process. Some teachers complete a detailed blueprint for the entire semester at the outset of a course. Some teachers would rather identify the ranges for the content area and objectives and then fill in the chart cells as the items are developed. Whichever approach you prefer, it is important that your blueprinting is done during course planning. As soon as the blueprint is prepared, item development and selection can be initiated.

The process of test development is becoming more streamlined with the advent of computer technology. Once you understand the techniques for blueprinting, your charts can be developed easily in a spreadsheet format. Electronic item banking programs are also available that include blueprinting in their test development process. These programs allow you to categorize every item so that you can ask to see every item that is coded for Unit I and Objective 1, for example. Then you can select items from that group to include in the corresponding cell on the blueprint. The benefits of implementing an item banking program are discussed in Chapter 14, "Instituting Item Banking and Test Development Software."

Reviewing the Blueprint

Once the blueprint is designed, it is essential to examine it to verify its relevance to the course. Professional test developers frequently use panels of recognized national experts to rate the relevancy of the blueprint to the domain being tested by an exam. Classroom teachers do not have this luxury. However, if you teach as part of a team, you can develop and review the blueprint as a group. If you are the sole instructor, you can exchange blueprints and exams with a colleague for review.

The need for blueprint review introduces another reason for early preparation of tests: You cannot expect another faculty member to review your blueprint on a moment's notice. Also, members of a teaching team will probably be unable to devote adequate time to examine the relevancy of test items on short notice. The bottom line is that the greater a time frame you allow for test development, the better the quality of your tests will be. A general rule of thumb is to have the blueprint ready for peer review during the planning phase of course preparation and to circulate each exam for final peer review 3 weeks before the scheduled exam date.

Blueprinting and item writing are the most time-consuming aspects of test development. Item banking software programs that develop blueprints, provide templates for word processing, store items with data and references, have codes for classifying and querying, and enable easy access to thousands of items for test generation and revision based on data analysis are widely available. Even if you have limited computer expertise, these programs are user-friendly tools that can provide a useful mechanism for constructing and revising tests. Chapter 14, "Instituting Item Banking and Test Development Software," discusses software programs and includes suggestions for implementation in a nursing program.

Preparing Students for a Test

Classroom achievement tests should present opportunities for students to demonstrate their maximum ability. To perform at their peak, students need to be informed about what to expect, which includes the content and abilities that will be tested, what will be emphasized on the test, and how the test will be scored and weighted in the final grade (Brookhart & Nitko, 2014).

At the same time, you must be careful not to teach to the test. Addressing the content of specific questions gives students an unfair advantage and ruins the validity of your exam results. Content review prior to a test presents a particularly risky situation. Enthusiastic faculty members who want to see students succeed must be aware of the ethical implications of teaching to a test. Although faculty members are obligated to present students with fair assessments, they also have the same obligation to ensure that students are meeting the course objectives. A test that has been shared with students, in any manner, is not a fair assessment.

Sharing the Blueprint with Students

Should you give the test blueprint to students? While using a test blueprint can inform students about how they can prepare for the test, there is a difference of opinion on whether to share the blueprint with the students. Although students should be prepared for an upcoming assessment, some educators believe that sharing the blueprint gives away the test. This concern does not consider that the blueprint is simply a guideline. It does not specify test questions; it indicates the emphasis of the units of course content and the objectives on the test. Even if you were to list specific content topics on the blueprint, items written at the application and analysis levels require students to apply higher-order thinking to answer the questions correctly, and the outline thus would not be a giveaway at all. A blueprint links the test items to the tasks required to demonstrate the mastery of a body of knowledge for the teacher, and it can serve this purpose for the students as well.

The most efficient way to share what is on a test is to share the test blueprint. Teachers share the objectives and content outline in the syllabus for every course. Sharing the test blueprints demonstrates to the students that the objectives really do matter and that teachers are not expecting rote memorization of the course content.

Having a visual guide for how the objectives enter into the assessment equation makes their attainment more meaningful to students.

The blueprint shown in Table 4.4 is not necessarily suitable for sharing with students. Students need a moderate level of detail for a study guide. A chart similar to the one shown in Table 4.2, with a range of items included in each cell, may be more appropriate. Whichever form you decide to use, it is important to share test blueprints with students to decrease their misconceptions, to help them to focus on the course objectives, and to provide them with the opportunity to demonstrate their maximum performance.

Pretest Review

Educators frequently ask if they should hold a content review for the students before an exam. While it may be beneficial for the students to have an overview of the content, a review before a test presents a problem that could compromise the validity of the exam results. The problem is that the teacher knows what is on the test, which makes it very difficult to avoid emphasizing what is known to be on the test. If the focus is only on the topics that are included on the test, the students will know exactly what to study.

A safe way to hold a review before a test is to answer any questions the students have. Conduct an out-of-class session where the students can ask any question related to the course content. This approach will ensure that the review does not focus on what is actually on the test, and it will require the students to prepare for the review.

Pop Quizzes

It is common practice to provide students with a syllabus at the outset of an instructional course. The syllabus usually includes the course objectives and content outline, the standards for grading, and the exam schedule. Providing a syllabus based on the belief that students should be informed about what to expect in the course promotes effective instruction.

Yet many of the same teachers who would never consider conducting a course without a syllabus do not hesitate to surprise their students with unannounced quizzes. These pop quizzes were described by Nunnally in 1964 as "one of the few ways of hitting back at students now that corporal punishment is going out of fashion" (p. 105). Giving unannounced quizzes is the equivalent of failing to inform students.

Some may argue that these pop quizzes keep students on their toes. However, keeping students fully informed is a much better approach. How many teachers are precisely on schedule with every one of their assignments? How many nights have you been just too exhausted to correct another paper? How would you react if a supervisor came into your class to evaluate you without notice? Sometimes we seem to forget that students have lives, too. Even the most conscientious student should be afforded the opportunity to plan course work in terms of a schedule. In order to plan, a student needs to know in advance what must be accomplished. Nitko (2004) recommends giving students at least 48 hours notice before any assessment.

Pop quizzes increase anxiety because they are associated with surprise. This anxiety is reduced when students can plan a study program. These assessments can also be patently unfair. Consider the student who is thoroughly prepared the week there is no quiz and who has a valid reason for being unprepared the week there is one. Some students will try to figure out when quizzes will be given, and once the scheduled number are given many students will believe they are off the hook. These situations take the responsibility for learning away from the students. Teachers then become the study police, lying in wait to catch students who are not following the rules.

If you are concerned about providing incentives for students to keep up with course assignments, a good approach is to schedule a brief quiz on a set day each week. Give these quizzes minimal weighting in the final course grade, and allow students to drop one or two of their lowest grades. Thus, the anxiety of wondering whether a quiz will be given is removed, and the students have the responsibility for being prepared every week.

Determining the Difficulty Level of a Test

Once you have established a blueprint, the next step is to develop the items for the test. Each item must be written to address the blueprint and the difficulty level of the exam. While the blueprint provides a guide for developing the items to address the content and objectives of the course, there is no specific formula for deciding what the difficulty level of a test should be.

You may be asking yourself, "Don't I have to wait until after I give a test to determine how difficult it is?" Although it is true that you will not know for certain how difficult a test is until after it is administered, it is important to plan ahead, or you may be surprised by the results.

Identifying how difficult a new item will be is largely a matter of experience. Experienced teachers can often predict the approximate difficulty level of a test question. However, even experienced teachers can misjudge the way a question will work on a test. You must always be willing to examine the data analysis of a test and make adjustments based on that analysis, no matter how carefully you constructed the test items. The test development software discussed in Chapter 14, "Instituting Item Banking and Test Development Software," offers teachers a valuable tool for analyzing item and test data and for making adaptations to improve both the difficulty and discrimination levels of test items for use on future tests. Once you have established a bank of items with a difficulty and discrimination history, you have a much better gauge for identifying how difficult a test will be.

The passing score on a test should reflect basic mastery of the course content and objectives. A critical step when developing test items is to decide what nursing activities demonstrate safe application of the course content and objectives in a clinical setting. Most of the items should reflect basic mastery, or passing level, for the students with a grade of "C." Some of the items should be more difficult, to identify those who have gone beyond basic mastery—those students who attain grades of "A" and "B."

Are teachers playing fair when they construct items at a predetermined difficulty level? Should items be designed so that those students who have only superficial knowledge cannot guess the correct answer? The answer to both of these questions is yes. If you want to distinguish between those who have and have not attained command of the content and objectives, the only way to construct a test question is so that it truly identifies the achievement you are measuring.

When determining how difficult a test should be, you must consider the purpose of the test. CRTs do not consider the difficulty level of items; the only criterion is a student's attainment of a set of instructional objectives. Easy items are included on CRTs as long as they assess the learning outcome. Norm-referenced tests (NRTs), on the other hand, are concerned with comparing student achievement. NRTs aim to include items of average difficulty and to exclude items that are too easy.

Standardized examinations are norm-referenced. They aim to have a mean of 0.50, with an item difficulty range of approximately 0.3 to 0.8, to ensure a normal distribution of the scores. Items written within this range also provide the best discrimination indices. This approach would certainly yield a very difficult classroom exam. Therefore, because classroom tests are not the equivalent of standardized examinations, they should not be modeled on standardized examinations. Standardized examinations are administered to large numbers of examinees of varying abilities, with the ultimate goal of identifying individual ability related to a normal distribution.

A normal curve cannot be expected on a classroom test in a nursing program. First, the number of students in a class is dramatically smaller than the sample needed for a standardized examination. In addition, students in a nursing class are a select group with similar ability, so we should expect a majority of a test's scores to be at the high end of the distribution. Although many teachers operate on the assumption that a test must yield a range of scores, it is possible for everyone to pass a classroom exam that is difficult and challenging. The success of a group on a particular test is largely determined by the composition of the group.

The bottom line is this: Classroom exams cannot be norm-referenced. It is more appropriate to develop tests that are criterion-referenced. While it is important to recognize that students in a nursing program are from a select group and have met admission requirements, we must also acknowledge that there are varying levels of ability within that select group. When assessing developmental-level learning, there is always a range of ability within a group. As Gronlund (1993) suggests, tests directed at assessing developmental learning should include items of varying difficulty.

A classroom exam that is assessing higher-order thinking should be criterion-referenced while identifying various levels of student ability, or have a norm-referenced overlay. In other words, there should be some particularly challenging questions on an exam to identify those students who excel. Only the highest achieving students in a class would pass a test that had items with an average difficulty of 50%. However, it would be appropriate to have several very difficult items on an exam to identify those students who are attaining higher achievement levels without penalizing those students who have achieved the course objectives at an acceptable level. Having items with a range of difficulty levels allows a spread of scores that identifies levels of achievement without requiring that some of the students fail the test.

The challenge you face is to write items that identify levels of achievement without tricking those who have accomplished the outcomes or giving away the correct answer to those who have only superficial knowledge. You have to decide what level of mastery you expect for the concepts tested by each question. Remember: The difficulty of the test is the average difficulty of the items on the test; the more difficult the items, the lower the mean and the median. In addition, the ability of the items to discriminate (i.e., distinguish between the high achievers and the low achievers on a test) is just as important as item difficulty.

It is important to note that items that fewer than 30% of the students answer correctly or items that more than 90% answer correctly do not contribute to the reliability of the test results. Unfortunately, multiple-choice exams are too often composed of items with a wide swing of difficulty levels. A test that has a large number of very easy items (greater than 0.90 difficulty) that is offset by several extremely difficult items (less than 0.30 difficulty) provides unreliable test results for several reasons. When most of the class answers a question correctly, it is hard to determine whether the students attained the knowledge or whether the question was simply a giveaway. When most of the class answers a question incorrectly, it is hard to determine whether the students lack knowledge or whether the question was ambiguous or too difficult for the group. Your test results will be much more reliable if they are consistently challenging and discriminating.

What mean should you expect on a test? If passing is 75%, should you aim for a 75% mean on the test? This question is tricky because the mean depends on the distribution of test scores. The mean can give the wrong impression when a distribution is skewed. Therefore, in addition to the mean, it is also important to consider the median of a group of test scores. The median tells us the midpoint score for the group on the test. A median of 0.75 means that half of the scores were below 0.75 and half were above. How many students do you expect to fail a test? If the mean of a test is 0.76 and the median is 0.75, it means that, although the average grade is 76%, half of the class scored below 75% on the test. If the passing score is 75%, is it acceptable for half of the class to fail? Was the test too difficult? Does the test reflect basic mastery of the course content and objectives? Are the test results dramatically different from prior exams given to the same or different student groups? Is it a weak or particularly strong student group? Were the teaching/learning strategies effective? These are the questions you must ask. Chapter 11, "Interpreting Test Results," continues this discussion to assist you to answer these questions.

In an attempt to increase their National Council Licensure Examination passing rate, some programs increase the grade required to pass nursing courses. This approach can cause a morale problem for the students and lead them to believe that the faculty is against them. There really is no need to take this approach. Instead if you believe you need to increase the challenge for your students, require the same passing grade but make your exams more difficult. You do not even need to announce this strategy to the students, which avoids establishing an antagonistic relationship. Remember, the passing grade is really arbitrary. A program that requires students to achieve a 70% to pass a course could be a much more difficult one than a program that requires the students to attain 80% to pass. The key to how challenging a course is lies in the quality of the items on the course exams.

Unfortunately, there is no standard answer to the question of an acceptable mean for a classroom exam. All data for a test have to be examined to determine the fairness of the scores for a test. What the test developer has to strive for is to present students with clear, unambiguous items that test their ability to demonstrate mastery of the content and objectives of the course at a difficulty level that reflects the importance of the concept being tested.

Summary

Planning for classroom assessments is fundamental to establishing the validity of the inferences made based on test scores. Validity evidence based on test content refers to how closely a test represents the content domain of the course. Evidence of validity is a matter of fairness and is closely linked to careful planning. Determining the purpose of a test, how difficult the test should be, which item format to use, and how to weight the blueprint all need to be considered. If the purpose of an assessment experience is to enable students to demonstrate their maximum ability, then teachers must take every measure possible to maximize the fairness of that experience.

The discussion presented in this chapter clarifies that developing blueprints for classroom exams is essential for establishing evidence of the validity of your exam results. However, the blueprint is only one step in the process. While a good blueprint provides the foundation for a quality test, it does not guarantee quality results. Careful attention must be focused on developing appropriate, well-crafted items that meet the specifications of the test plan and measure nursing abilities that reflect mastery of the course objectives and content. No matter how well-developed a blueprint is, if the items fail to address the objectives and content of the course as specified in the blueprint, the validity of the test results will be impaired. **Box 4.1** summarizes the test development process.

Box 4.1   Guidelines for test development

A. Preliminary considerations
  1. Who is the test coordinator?
  2. How many tests are scheduled for the semester?
  3. How much time has been provided for each test?
  4. How many items should be on each test?
  5. What is the total number of items for the semester?
  6. Which item formats are appropriate?
  7. How difficult should the tests be?
B. Steps in developing the blueprint for an objective test
  1. Determine the relative emphasis for the test.
    a. Decide the content weighting that accurately reflects the focus of the course.
    b. Identify the relative weight percentage for each objective.
  2. Determine how many items should be written for each cell.
    a. Identify the range of items for each content area.
    b. Identify the range of items for each objective.
    c. Multiply the total number of items for a content area by the percentage assigned to the objective in each row.
    d. Use this figure as a guide to estimate a range of items for each cell on the blueprint worksheet.
  3. Circulate the blueprint to faculty members for review.
C. Preparing the test
  1. Determine the faculty assignment based on the number of items required for each cell.
  2. Establish a due date for item submission.
  3. The test coordinator edits and sorts the items according to the blueprint.
  4. The test coordinator circulates the test items for review by the faculty members.
  5. The test coordinator incorporates the suggestions made by the faculty for the items and assembles a final form of the test.
  6. The test coordinator circulates the final form of the test for faculty edits.
  7. Create a cover sheet, and reproduce, number, and securely store the test until examination day.

Crafting effective test items is both an art and a science. The guidelines presented in *The Nurse Educator's Guide to Assessing Learning Outcomes*, supply the science; your creative input provides the art. Remember that constructing effective test items is a skill that develops over time. Following these guidelines will help you to attain expertise with crafting items that reflect the difficulty levels that you require for making important decisions based on the results of your classroom exams.

Learning Activities

1. Select a course you are teaching, have taught, or have taken. Develop a master test plan for a semester's exams (refer to Table 4.1). The plan should consider course content distribution, the school's calendar for the semester, and the weight of each exam in the final grade for the course.

2. Identify the type of measurement format that would be most effective for each of the objectives in a course you are teaching, have taught, or have taken.

3. Compose a content/objective worksheet (refer to Table 4.2) and a content item worksheet (refer to Table 4.3) for the course you selected in Learning Activity 1.

4. Use the content/objective and content item worksheets from Learning Activity 3 to develop a blueprint worksheet (refer to Table 4.4) for the course you selected in Learning Activity 1.

5. How would you develop a criterion-referenced exam that identifies levels of student achievement?

6. Explain the role of a blueprint for establishing validity evidence for the results of an exam.

Web Links

American Psychological Association
http://www.apa.org
Educational Resources Information Center
http://www.eric.ed.gov
National Council of State Boards of Nursing
http://www.ncsbn.org
National Council on Measurement in Education
http://www.ncme.org

References

American Educational Research Association, American Psychological Association, & National Council on Measurement in Education. (2014). *Standards for educational and psychological testing*. Washington, DC: American Educational Research Association.

Brookhart, S. M., & Nitko, A. J. (2014). *Educational assessment of students* (7th ed.). Upper Saddle River, NJ: Pearson Education.

Fliszar, R. (2009). Using assessment and evaluation strategies. In R. A. Whitman-Price & M. Godshall (Eds.), *Certified nurse educator review manual* (pp. 89–116). New York, NY: Springer.

Gronlund, N. E. (1993). *How to make achievement tests and assessments.* Needham Heights, MA: Allyn and Bacon.

Miller, M. D., Linn, R. L., & Gronlund, N. E. (2012). *Measurement and assessment in teaching* (10th ed.). Upper Saddle River, NJ: Pearson Education.

Nitko, A. J. (2004). *Educational assessment of students* (4th ed.). Englewood Cliffs, NJ: Prentice-Hall.

Nunnally, J. C. (1964). *Educational measurement and evaluation.* New York, NY: McGraw-Hill.

Oermann, M. H., & Gaberson, K. B. (2009). *Evaluation and testing in nursing education* (3rd ed.). New York, NY: Springer.

Piasentin, K. A. (2010). Exploring the optimal number of options in multiple-choice testing. *Clear Exam Review, 21*(1), 18–22.

Schoolcraft, V. (1989). *A nuts-and-bolts approach to teaching nursing.* New York, NY: Springer.

Tarrant, M., & Ware, J. (2012). A framework for improving the quality of multiple-choice assessments. *Journal of Nursing Education, 37,* 98–104.

CHAPTER 5

Selected-Response Format: Developing Multiple-Choice Items

© Anteromite/Shutterstock

"Good tests consist of good test items."

—THOMAS HALADYNA

Although a good blueprint provides the foundation for a quality test, it does not guarantee quality results. While the blueprint is a pivotal step in the test development process, careful attention must be focused on developing appropriate, well-crafted test items that meet the specifications of the blueprint. No matter how well developed the blueprint is, if the test items fail to address the objectives and content of the course as specified in the blueprint, the validity of the test results will be impaired. If poorly written items are included on the test, students will have difficulty deciphering what is being asked, and the reliability of the test results will be diminished. In either situation, inappropriate decisions could be made based on the test results.

The key to effective test development is to avoid trivia and focus instead on testing important concepts, and then select the question format that is most appropriate for measuring each concept. There is no perfect format that fits all tests; every format has advantages and disadvantages. The chapters that follow help you to capitalize on the strengths and minimize the weaknesses of each format type when you are developing test items.

The selected-response item format has several advantages. One of the most important advantages is the ability to test a wider range of material that can be tested with constructed-response type items. Selected-response items include the multiple-choice, true–false, and matching formats. These item types have many qualities in common as well as several unique characteristics. An understanding of these qualities will guide you in selecting the most appropriate format for your testing needs. This chapter and Chapter 6, "Writing Critical Thinking Multiple-Choice Items," focus on the most popular selected-response type item, the multiple-choice format. True–false and matching formats are reviewed in Chapter 7, "Selected-Response Format: Developing True–False and Matching Items."

Item Writing Logistics

There are no longer any excuses for unprofessional-looking tests. Test development software enables you to create professional-looking exams. If you do not have access to this software, the availability of current electronic word processing programs can provide you with the tools that will give your classroom tests a professional appearance. Carelessness with grammar, spelling, and punctuation reflect poorly on you, the test developer. Additionally, if educators expect to hold students to high standards on their written assignments, they must hold themselves to even higher standards. Remember, nothing you write will ever be as highly scrutinized as the questions on your classroom exams will be by the students who must answer them.

A key requirement for item development is that all faculty members use the same procedure for creating test items. The ultimate goal for every nursing program should be to establish a working item bank. Because consistency is a paramount concern for item bank development, it is beneficial for faculty members to come to a consensus on several key issues at the outset of the item-development process. Chapter 14, "Instituting Item Banking and Test Development Software," explores the use of electronic item banking and test development software.

Once the blueprint for a test is agreed on, faculty can start writing items. It is a good idea to develop more questions than you need for each area of the blueprint because these extra items can be stored in the item bank. Another practical suggestion is to write a few questions each day, particularly after a classroom or a clinical experience when the material is fresh in your mind. Just be careful not to use the same examples that you used to illustrate a point in class or you will be writing at the recall cognitive level. If a particularly interesting illustration of a concept occurs with a group of students, use the experience to write an item and bank it for next year.

Electronic Item Development

In this era of electronic word processing, you are wasting your time if you handwrite items and then type them into a test. It is essential that you create your items in an electronic file. If you are not already doing so, start composing your items with a word processing program. You will get a much better feel for the item when you see it in typeface, and with very little practice you will be electronically cutting and pasting your way to item-writing proficiency.

Once you have your items in an electronic form at, they will be available for future use and you will have the basis for item banking. If you are writing your items in a word processing program, it is helpful to print each item on an individual sheet of paper for review by your colleagues. Having each item on a separate sheet also facilitates reviewing and sorting the items into a test.

Advantages of Multiple-Choice Items

The multiple-choice format is the most versatile type of item format. Those who object to multiple-choice items usually object to all selected-response test formats in favor of constructed-response format questions. Although multiple-choice items do have limitations, they also have several advantages over constructed-response questions.

When written effectively, the multiple-choice format can be used to assess a wide range of learning outcomes across all cognitive levels. Multiple-choice exams are widely used for assessment in nursing education. They are adaptable to all types of subject matter, their scoring is accurate and efficient, and they provide students with practice for the types of items they will most likely encounter on licensure and certification exams.

The issue of content sampling on a test is addressed most efficiently by the multiple-choice format. When compared with constructed-response questions, multiple-choice items require much less time for recording answers. Therefore, multiple-choice exams can include many more items and afford a more representative sample of course content on a test than constructed-response items, particularly essay questions.

While the constructed-response format is susceptible to subjective scoring, multiple-choice items provide objective measurement of student achievement. The difficulty level of multiple-choice items, which contributes to test reliability, is easier to control than with essay questions. Multiple-choice exams are compatible with efficient and accurate computerized scoring and lend themselves to statistical item analysis, which enables the teacher to determine how well the items functioned with the group of students tested. In addition, item analysis data, which includes difficulty levels and discrimination indices of the items, provide valuable information for item revision. Last, but certainly not least, computer software can store multiple-choice items in an item bank for future use. Item banking, which is an invaluable tool for test development, is addressed in Chapter 14, "Instituting Item Banking and Test Development Software."

Limitations of Multiple-Choice Items

No item format is perfect. They all have flaws. Constructed-response items are easier to write than multiple-choice items, but they are time consuming to score and are susceptible to subjective scoring. On the other hand, multiple-choice items are time consuming to develop, particularly because it is challenging to compose plausible incorrect options.

Opponents of objective testing point out that the constructed-response format is a more accurate measure of a student's ability to apply knowledge because it requires students to construct their own response rather than to simply respond to a proposed answer. Another criticism of multiple-choice items is that they have a tendency to be written at the recall level. Even when multiple-choice items are written at higher cognitive levels, students might only need to recognize the correct answer; they do not need to organize and construct their own response. The format is also faulted because it is susceptible to guessing and tends to favor test-wise students who can spot the cues in poorly written items.

Well-developed multiple-choice items can refute all these criticisms. Effective multiple-choice items do not enable students to choose the correct answer by simple rote memory. Rather, they require the student to reason out the basis for selecting the correct response. Carefully designed multiple-choice items eliminate the cues that test-wise students depend on. They can be designed so that students have to use critical thinking skills to make the subtle distinctions necessary to reason out the correct answer.

The debate over the qualities of different item formats should not be the main focus of test developers. One format is not inherently superior to another. Remember the basic principle: Select the item format that is most suitable for measuring the desired learning outcome. For example, while it is important to take advantage of the flexibility and applicability of the multiple-choice format, it should not be used when the objective requires performance-based assessment (Miller, Linn, & Gronlund, 2009).

Multiple-choice items only fulfill their potential when they are constructed appropriately. The ability to write effective, high-level, multiple-choice items requires a skill that only develops with practice over time. The old adage, "Rome wasn't built in a day," certainly applies here. The guidelines in this chapter are designed to assist you to develop the skills you need to become a proficient multiple-choice test item writer.

Relevance of Multiple-Choice Items

The choice of item format must be directed by the specific learning outcome you are assessing. Whatever format you choose, the items should be designed to elicit knowledge related to the course outcomes at higher-order levels of thinking, as designated by the test blueprint. Multiple-choice items can be designed to address specific content and learning outcomes and are well suited for measuring achievement across cognitive levels (DiBattista & Kurzawa, 2011).

Documenting that a test is assessing, relevant content and objectives, not trivia, is an essential requirement for establishing content-related evidence of the validity of test results. Every test item should represent both course content and a course objective. When evaluating a test item, ask yourself, "How does this question relate to both the content and an objective on the test blueprint?" Only items that relate directly to the blueprint should be included on a test. Another important question to ask is, "Why is this information important for a nurse to know?" Questions that are dubious or inconsequential should be omitted. The multiple-choice format is easily adapted for measuring intended learning outcomes; it is your professional judgment that determines the relevance of individual items for the test.

Style Guide

Consistency of style is essential. Consistency improves test validity and reliability by decreasing ambiguity, increasing item quality, and increasing student respect for your tests. When all exams in a nursing program follow a style guide, a consistent and professional test appearance is created. Consistency of style also establishes the basis for developing an item bank. All items in a bank should follow a particular style so they create a professional impression when used together on a test.

A group consensus is necessary for adoption of a test and item-writing style guide. If you use a test development software program, the program dictates some of these decisions. However, it is helpful to start the process of developing a guide with some suggestions. Basic style suggestions are proposed in Appendix C, "Basic Style Guide." These basic style rules are the ones I found to be most conducive to the development of professional-looking tests. You will note that all the items presented in this book follow these style suggestions. Obviously, you should adapt your style to the needs of your individual group. The essential requirement is that all writers adhere closely to the agreed-upon style guide so the items look like they are professionally developed and that they belong together when used on a test.

This chapter contains more than 60 exhibit examples of items that illustrate the suggested item development guidelines. Box 5.3, "Exhibit Reference List" provides an organized reference list of all of these examples

Multiple-Choice Format

The multiple-choice format consists of two parts (see **Exhibit 5.1**):

Exhibit 5.1   Multiple-choice format

Question
All of these foods are on the lunch tray for a client who is following a low-residue diet. Which one should a nurse advise the client to remove?

A. Chicken noodle soup	Distractor
B. Mashed potatoes	Distractor
C. Broiled flounder	Distractor
D. Steamed broccoli	KEY

Incomplete Statement
All of these foods are on the lunch tray for a client who is following a low-residue diet. A nurse should advise the client to remove the

A. chicken noodle soup.	Distractor
B. mashed potatoes.	Distractor
C. broiled flounder.	Distractor
D. steamed broccoli.	KEY

---

1. The stem, which identifies the problem
2. The options, which present the response alternatives

The key is the option that is the correct answer, and the distractors are the options that appear plausible to the uninformed but are incorrect responses to the stem.

Although the multiple-choice format appears to be very straightforward, item writing is a demanding process. Many subtle intricacies are involved with developing multiple-choice items that provide trustworthy information on which to base decisions. Effective multiple-choice items reduce errors by minimizing the possibility of confusing the informed students—and at the same time minimizing the chance that the uninformed students will guess the correct answer. In this way, effective items increase item discrimination and the overall reliability of the test results.

Most faculty members have no difficulty in identifying what they want to test; however, many faculty members have difficulty crafting items. As with any skill, the more you write, the better you become. Following the guidelines presented here will set you in the right direction for developing new items, editing your old items, and improving items from textbook item banks. Chapter 11, "Interpreting Test Results," provides direction for improving your items based on item analysis data.

Stem Formats

The most important attribute of a stem is that it is stated clearly. The stem should present one problem that relates directly to a learning outcome. Referring to your learning outcomes every time you develop a stem ensures that each item is designed to assess the achievement of your course objectives. The stem should present the central idea with all the information needed to solve the problem. The students should not have to read the options to determine what problem the stem is presenting.

Multiple-choice stems can be framed as either a question or an incomplete statement (see Exhibit 5.1). While it is true that most experts prefer the question format, the completion format can be a viable approach for developing effective stems. Clarity is the most important quality of a stem. The students must clearly understand what the item is asking.

Question

Presenting the stem as a question is the preferred format for writing multiple-choice items. When the problem is formulated as a question, the item writer is compelled to state the problem clearly and completely in the stem. In real life, when we want a student to solve a problem, we ask a direct question. We do not propose an incomplete sentence and expect the student to finish our thought.

Asking a question is the most direct way to pose a problem. This method of presentation puts a minimum demand on reading skills and ensures that the problem is framed completely in the stem. It also decreases the possibility of introducing grammatical cues with the options. Although a question might require a longer response in the options, a stem that is written as a question is often more effective than framing the stem as an incomplete sentence. **Exhibit 5.2** is an example of a stem presented as a question.

Exhibit 5.2   Question stem format

Which of these instructions should a nurse give to a client who is taking digoxin?

Completion

In some situations, a stem can be presented more concisely as an incomplete sentence than as a question. The completion format increases the cognitive complexity of the item, however, because students have to rephrase it as a question before responding. This format may require some students to keep rereading the stem to identify which option completes the sentence correctly. Students lose time when they have to keep reading the stem. This situation poses a particular difficulty for students who are learning the English language (English language learners [ELLs]) and for students who have learning disabilities. Remember, the key objective of an achievement test is to identify what a student has achieved in a particular domain. A good item removes all obstacles that would interfere with a student's maximum performance.

Although there are arguments against the completion format, they are not sufficient to necessitate that this format never be used. The recommended approach is to attempt to write the stem as a question first; if you have difficulty keeping the problem clear and concise as a question, use the completion format. Make sure that each option completes the stem to form a grammatically correct complete sentence. In some cases, the completion format can do a better job of clarifying the problem than the question format. It is always a good idea to ask a colleague for advice when you find a particular item challenging to develop. The most important guideline is to use the format that works the best to make the item as clear as possible for the students. **Exhibit 5.3** shows a stem that uses the completion format.

Exhibit 5.3   Completion stem format

A nurse should monitor a client who is receiving intravenous potassium chloride for side effects, which include

---

Item Writing Guidelines

As Anderson (2003) describes it, item writing is a craft, a little bit art and a little bit science. The science provides the guidelines, while the art provides the flexibility to operate within the guidelines.

Guidelines and suggestions for developing multiple-choice items have been published by a host of experts in the field of classroom assessment (Anderson, 2003; Haladyna, 2004; Miller et al., 2009; Brookhart & Nitko, 2014; Popham, 2003; Reynolds, Livingston, & Wilson, 2008; Schoolcraft, 1989; Trice, 2000). While authorities in the field agree that there are no hard-and-fast rules for test development, there is also remarkable overlap and agreement in their suggestions for test and item development.

The guidelines presented here reflect both the suggestions of these authorities and my own experience with developing multiple-choice items that are dependable indicators of student achievement. These guidelines represent the aspects of item writing that are salient enough to be discussed and practiced. You must cultivate your own creative touch and combine it with these guidelines to develop your personal item writing style.

The level of detail presented in these guidelines might seem daunting at first. Actually, you will find that many of these suggestions reflect basic common sense and can be readily incorporated into your item-writing repertoire. Other suggestions are more easily understood once you actually start to implement them.

Incorporate these suggestions at your own pace. Begin slowly, but get started. Your tests will benefit from your effort.

These guidelines are not rules; rather, they are suggestions. Because testing specialists advocate these guidelines, however, you should seriously consider adopting them. The quality of your items will improve if you review these guidelines and gradually incorporate them into your own creative item-writing style. These guidelines are particularly helpful when reviewing the item analysis data. Chapter 14, "Instituting Item Banking and Test Development Software," discusses methods for using item analysis data in conjunction with these guidelines to further improve test items for future use.

General Guidelines

To yield reliable and valid results, achievement tests must be direct and meaningful measures of learning that provide students with the opportunity to display the knowledge they have acquired. The paramount requirement for test reliability is well-constructed test items; therefore, clarity is essential. Tests are not intended to assess a student's cleverness. We want students to spend test time figuring out the correct answer, not trying to figure out what the question is asking.

Anderson (2003) summarizes the rules for item writing: First, be clear; second, be reasonable; and third, do not give the answer away (p. 54). If students have attained a learning outcome, a test should afford them the opportunity to demonstrate that attainment. It is unfair if students answer incorrectly because of factors that are extraneous to the purpose of the test. These factors limit and modify student responses and prevent students from showing their true level of achievement. Unfair factors that might prevent students from performing at their best should be eliminated from a test.

A testing situation in itself is anxiety provoking—a factor that we obviously cannot completely eliminate. Although we cannot entirely remove the anxiety factor, we can take measures to modify it. Students will scrutinize each question for meaning (expressed and implied). Ambiguous items cause confusion and increase anxiety. Therefore, the precise meaning of every item should be communicated as efficiently as possible. This responsibility puts great demands on the vocabulary and writing skills of the item developer.

Concerns about clarity bring up the issue of reading comprehension. Achievement tests are not tests of reading comprehension. In fact, you should design your achievement tests to be below the reading ability of the students to avoid confounding the measurement of reading comprehension with the measurement of skill in the content domain. However, while it is important to avoid unfamiliar vocabulary, it is also important to include healthcare terminology. **Table 5.1** illustrates examples of vocabulary to include and to exclude from your test items.

In addition to minimizing complicated vocabulary, you should avoid bias in your test questions (Klisch, 1994). Be aware of vocabulary that can confuse students— ELL students are particularly susceptible to misinterpreting words or phrases they are not familiar with. **Table 5.2** provides several examples of words that could be easily misinterpreted by ELL students. Be especially careful when including foods

Table 5.1   Vocabulary for Item Writing

Examples of Vocabulary to Avoid	Examples of Vocabulary to Include
Circumvent	Circumoral
Ludicrous	Diaphoresis
Superfluous	Hematemesis
Domicile	Auscultate
Unequivocal	Opportunistic
Cryptic	Extravasation
Meander	Endotracheal
Embellish	Fibrillation

Table 5.2   Vocabulary That Can Be Confusing or Misinterpreted

Examples of Vocabulary to Avoid

Crackerjack	Nifty
Kibosh	Backbone
Stressed out	Value added
Cold turkey	A fifth of vodka
Green thumb	Blindsided
In concert with	Sponge cake

in a question because foods are often related to culture and may be unfamiliar to ELL students.

Another issue related to clarity is the use of homonyms, which are words that have more than one meaning. Students may misunderstand the meaning of the word or miss the meaning the teacher intended (**Exhibits 5.4** and **5.5**). Always double-check a thesaurus to identify if a word that has two meanings could confuse ELL students.

Exhibit 5.4   Confusing homonym

Which of these instructions should a nurse include when teaching a client who is scheduled to start taking furosemide?

A. "Take the medication before you retire."
B. "Limit the amount of fluid you drink each day."
C. "Be careful to arise slowly from a sitting position."*
D. "Don't drive while taking this medication."

The word retire *can confuse the students. Was the client going to bed or leaving his job? Also note: Only the generic name is included for medication, following the National Council of State Boards of Nursing (NCSBN) protocol for the National Council Licensure Examination (NCLEX) exam.*

Exhibit 5.5 Confusing homonym and colloquialism

A client says to a nurse, "I am really upset. The podiatrist just told me that I have to have an operation to remove a bunion. But I refused to have the procedure." Which of these responses should the nurse offer?

A. "There is no need to worry. That is a very minor procedure."
B. "I see you're tearing up. Let's talk about what's upsetting you."*
C. "I know the podiatrist has a very good track record for that procedure."
D. "The decision is up to you. You have to suit yourself."

There are two confusing homonyms in this item. Tearing *can refer to crying or to ripping something apart.* Suit, *in this case, means to "please." It is also used to describe a set of clothes. Both of these words could confuse ELL students. This item also uses a phrase that introduces bias.* Track record *is a colloquialism that may not be familiar to ELL students.*

Having a colleague critique your exams is a good way to minimize complicated vocabulary, decrease words that may introduce bias, and eliminate words that could be misconstrued by students. In fact, you should never administer a test that has not been reviewed by at least one of your colleagues. It is much better to identify flaws in the items before you administer the test than to have the students point out errors in the test. When asking colleagues to review an exam, be sure to remind them to review the incorrect options. Faculty members often have the habit of reading the stem and only the correct answer. The most effective approach is to give your colleague an unkeyed copy of the test to see whether you agree on the correct answer.

When developing items you must ensure that each item stands alone. Answering an item correctly should not depend on answering another item correctly. If students miss the first item in a group of connected items, they will miss all subsequent items in the group.

A student might well have been able to answer the second question if it were independent of the first item. When answering a question, students should not have to refer specifically to the answer that was given in a previous question, as **Exhibit 5.6** illustrates.

Exhibit 5.6 Connected items

1. A nurse should recognize that a client who has elevated intracranial pressure will most likely receive which of these medications?
   A. mannitol*
   B. digoxin
   C. indomethacin
   D. nadolol

2. The nurse should plan to monitor the client for side effects of this medication, which include

    A. hyponatremia.
    B. bradycardia.
    C. hematuria.
    D. agranulocytosis*

The answer to item 2 here depends on a correct answer to item 1. Therefore, item 1 has a higher scoring weight on the test. Students who miss item 2 because they answered item 1 incorrectly may have been able to answer item 2 correctly if it had been independent of item 1.

Most experts agree that the best approach to item writing is to compose the stem and the key first and then create the distractors that parallel the correct answer. Effective items are written so that the only difference between those who do well on the test and those who do not is the ability to use the knowledge that is being measured by the test items.

It is important to be especially careful about the grammatical structure of all options when you use the completion format. Because the correct answer is written with the stem, it usually completes the stem appropriately. It can be all too easy to overlook grammar when you are focused on writing believable distractors. Furthermore, if you change an item after you edit it, be sure to double-check the grammatical consistency of all options. If only one option is grammatically synchronized with the stem, the students will be inclined to choose it. This problem is not encountered with the question format, as illustrated in **Exhibit 5.7**.

Exhibit 5.7   Grammatical inconsistency, with revision

Grammatical Inconsistency
When assessing the health needs of a community, a nurse should consider that spirituality refers to an

A. participation in an organized religious group.
B. practices and rituals of a particular religion.
C. dimension that is outside the realm of health assessment.
D. individual's beliefs about the meaning of life and death.*

Grammatical Consistency
When assessing the health needs of a community a nurse should consider that spirituality refers to

A. participation in an organized religious group.
B. practices and rituals of a particular religion.
C. a dimension that is outside the realm of health assessment.
D. an individual's beliefs about the meaning of life and death.*

In the grammatically inconsistent example, the stem is consistent only with the correct answer. This provides the uninformed student with an obvious cue.

Exhibit 5.8 illustrates another type of grammatical error, the misplaced modifier. A misplaced modifier is a word or phrase that is placed too far from the noun it is describing. The result is a sentence that is confusing and often unintentionally funny. Because we want our test items to be clear and taken seriously, it is important to remove misplaced modifiers.

Exhibit 5.8   Misplaced modifiers

A nurse is caring for a client post gastric resection with a nasogastric tube.

Revised
A nurse is planning care for a client who had a gastric resection and has a nasogastric tube connected for continuous suction.

Be careful; misplaced modifiers can change the meaning of a sentence. Who has the nasogastric tube in the original, the client or the nurse? Make sure to structure your sentences so that the modifier is closest to the noun it is modifying.

A client was referred to a nutritionist with a serious weight problem.

Revised
A client, who has a serious weight problem, was referred to a nutritionist.

The author here intended to say that the client had a serious weight problem. However, the sentence says that the nutritionist has a serious weight problem. The revision clears up the confusion by placing the modifier close to the noun it is modifying, the client.

If you use the completion format, make sure you do not leave a blank at the beginning or middle of a stem. As **Exhibit 5.9** demonstrates, this action interrupts the students' reading continuity and makes the stem confusing and difficult to answer. It is much easier to understand a completion stem if the proposed answers are presented as conclusions to an incomplete statement.

Exhibit 5.9   Internal blank

Internal Blank
A nurse is caring for a client who has a normal-functioning, double-barrel, transverse colostomy. The nurse should document that the proximal stoma is producing _____ and the distal stoma is producing _____.

Revised
A nurse is caring for a client who has a normal-functioning, double-barrel, transverse colostomy. The nurse should expect the client to have which of these types of drainage from the distal stoma of the colostomy?

This question is really two questions. If a student answered the original item incorrectly, you would not be able to determine which part of the question the student did not understand.

Characteristics of Effective Stems

The stem is the core of a multiple-choice question. It introduces the student to the central problem being posed. Stems should be clear, succinct, and focused, and have a positive approach. If students cannot understand the stem, they will not be able to answer the question. The best stems depict a novel problem in a clinical setting that students must solve and do not paraphrase a textbook (which encourages rote learning). The stem should completely pose the problem to be solved; the student should not have to read the options to figure out what the question is asking.

Complete   Students should understand what the stem is asking before they read the options. After you write a stem, read it alone before you write the options. When reviewing a colleague's questions, cover the options and read the stem alone. Ask yourself, "What is the problem or potential problem that the stem is posing?" If you cannot determine what the stem is asking, it should be rewritten. **Exhibits 5.10** and **5.11** contrast incomplete stems with complete stems. The complete stem poses the complete problem for the student, while the incomplete stem requires the student to read all the options to determine what the question is asking.

Exhibit 5.10   Incomplete versus complete stems

Incomplete Stem
Steroids

A. pose a risk for immunosuppression.*
B. can cause renal shutdown.
C. increase metabolism.
D. alter pulmonary function.

Complete Stem
A nurse should advise a client who is taking an oral steroid preparation to report signs of adverse effects, which include

A. sore throat.*
B. urinary retention.
C. weight loss.
D. dyspnea

Exhibit 5.11   Incomplete versus complete stem

Incomplete Stem
Dehydration

A. leads to postural hypotension.*
B. results in hyponatremia.
C. causes Kussmaul breathing.
D. is associated with bradycardia.

(continues)

Exhibit 5.11   Incomplete versus complete stem (*Continued*)

Complete Stem

Which of these client manifestations should indicate to a nurse that the client is developing fluid volume deficit?

A. Bradycardia

B. Hyponatremia

C. Postural hypotension*

D. Kussmaul breathing

Succinct   While it is important to include all the information that is needed to solve the problem in the stem, you must keep your stems clear and to the point. One sentence is not necessarily the best choice if it is a complex sentence because complex sentences can confuse students. It is better to use two or more sentences if including all the information in one sentence makes the sentence too complex. The objective is to communicate the problem as efficiently and clearly as possible. Students should be able to read and answer each item in less than 1 minute.

The key to writing effective stems is to specify all the conditions necessary to have the intended response be the only correct answer to the problem while excluding any unnecessary information (see **Exhibits 5.12** and **5.13**). Extraneous information does not increase the cognitive level of an item; it increases ambiguity and lengthens the processing time that is required for students to understand what the question is asking.

Exhibit 5.12   Diffuse versus succinct stems

Diffuse Stem

A 58-year-old accountant has been experiencing substernal chest pressure on exertion for the past 6 months. He is now admitted to the cardiac care unit for diagnosis and management. Right jugular pulmonary artery and right radial lines are inserted. During the cardiac assessment, the nurse finds that the client has cold clammy skin, gray skin color, weak rapid pulse, and a blood pressure of 80/50 mm Hg. The nurse most likely interpreted the client's condition to be related to

Succinct Stem

A nurse is assessing a client who is experiencing severe substernal chest pain. The client is diaphoretic and has cold, clammy, gray-colored skin; a weak and rapid pulse; and a blood pressure of 80/50 mm Hg. Which of these actions should the nurse take?

The succinct stem decreases the reading time by almost half yet includes all pertinent information. Eliminating extraneous information focuses the student on the problem and makes the item more direct and easier to understand. The original item asks the nurse to recognize the cause of the problem. The revision requires the nurse not only to recognize but to do something about the problem.

Exhibit 5.13 Diffuse versus succinct stems

Ambiguous Stem

A client with hepatic cirrhosis has repeated massive paracentesis. Which concurrent nursing implementation will be most effective in reducing recurrence of ascitic fluid with fewest complications?

A. Administer salt-poor albumin intravenously*
B. Restrict dietary intake of protein foods
C. Administer thiazide diuretics by mouth
D. Encourage upright posture and mobility as tolerated

Succinct Stem

A client who has hepatic cirrhosis had several paracenteses with repeated recurrence of ascites. The client has all of these prescriptions. A nurse should recognize that which prescription will most effectively decrease the recurrence of ascites?

A. Administer intravenous salt-poor albumin to the client*
B. Restrict the client's dietary intake of protein
C. Administer the oral diuretic to the client
D. Maintain the client on bed rest

When you are revising an item, ask yourself, "What is the point of this question?" In this case, the item is testing an important concept; does the student understand the effect of option A? The succinct version specifies that the options are not nursing interventions but prescriptions, and it requires the student to identify which option is most effective for reducing ascites. Note that the term prescriptions *refers to any doctor's order on the NCLEX.*

Focused   Each item should serve one and only one purpose. Therefore, it is important to keep the stem focused on a single problem. While items should require students to progress through a problem-solving sequence, there should be only one problem to solve in a single question. If students incorrectly answer a question that includes more than one problem, the teacher will be unable to identify which problem the students missed.

Instructional information in the stem qualifies as extraneous information and can reduce the effectiveness of an item. Irrelevant material that does not contribute to the basis for answer selection only serves to complicate the reading comprehension of the item. Keep each item focused on the problem at hand, as the focused stem in **Exhibit 5.14** illustrates.

Exhibit 5.14 Unfocused versus focused stem

Unfocused Stem

Documentation is a critical component of the nursing process when caring for rape victims. Which of the following entries most accurately represents a woman who comes to the emergency room reporting that she has been raped by a former boyfriend?

Focused Stem

A woman who is admitted to an emergency department is sobbing. The woman has several bruises on her face and swollen, bloody lips. When a nurse asks the woman

(continues)

Exhibit 5.14 Unfocused versus focused stem (*Continued*)

---

what happened, the woman says, "My boyfriend says I had sex with his friend, so he beat me up and raped me. I would never cheat on him. I love him." Which of these documentations accurately reflects this interaction?

A. "The client has bruises on her face, as noted in the attached photo, and states that she was beaten and raped by her boyfriend."*

B. "The client will need encouragement to press charges for rape because she loves her boyfriend."

C. "A rape exam will be invalid because the client may have had sex with more than one partner."

D. "The client's boyfriend inflicted injuries to her face and raped her."

The purpose of an exam is to measure knowledge, not to provide instruction. The focused stem eliminates the instructional material and uses a client quote to provide a clearer description of what the client reported. The student must determine which option provides the most accurate documentation.

Positive Approach   Experts concur that negative stems should be avoided. At the very least, you should always attempt to reword a negative stem positively. The correct answer to a negative stem has to be a false statement.

It is very easy to misinterpret a negative question. Because students are usually focused on finding correct statements, a negative stem can easily confuse them. In addition, the anxiety generated in a testing situation can cause students to overlook a negative word in a stem. Even when students recognize a negative word, reading time is increased because these stems require a reversal of thought patterns. **Exhibit 5.15** demonstrates how a negative stem can be reworded as a positive stem and demonstrates the effectiveness of the positive approach for framing stems.

Exhibit 5.15 Negative versus positive stem

Negative Stem

A nurse is assessing a client who has pneumonia. Which of these assessment findings indicates that the client does NOT need to be suctioned?

A. Diminished breath sounds

B. Absence of adventitious breath sounds*

C. Inability to cough up sputum

D. Wheezing after bronchodilator therapy

Positive Stem

Which of these assessment findings, if identified in a client who has pneumonia, indicates that the client needs to be suctioned?

A. Absence of adventitious breath sounds

B. Respiratory rate of 18 breaths per minute

C. Inability to cough up sputum*

D. Wheezing before bronchodilator therapy

The negative stem in the first example is particularly confusing because the correct answer is also negative (absence). Although the positive stem tests the same concept, it is much clearer. It certainly is more important to know when a client needs to be suctioned.

Despite the evidence against negative stems, they are still used on national exams. Thus, it makes sense to accustom students to the use of negative stems such as the item presented in **Exhibit 5.16**. Remember that the point of a test is to determine what the student knows, not what the student can detect. Because we do not want a student to miss an answer because of carelessness or anxiety, it makes sense to alert the student that the correct answer is the incorrect option. I recommend that if you use this format you should highlight the negative word; bold, italicize, and capitalize so that negative words **REALLY** stand out, as the negative stem in Exhibit 5.16 illustrates.

Exhibit 5.16   Acceptable format for a negative stem

A nurse reviews self-care with a client who had a cataract extracted from the right eye this morning. Which of these statements, if made by the client, indicates that the client needs **FURTHER** instruction?

A. "I will avoid becoming constipated."
B. "I can take a short walk with my wife."
C. "I will stay on bed rest for three days."*
D. "I can watch the football game on television."

*When students take a test, their mind-set is to search for the correct option. When confronted with a negative stem. they can easily overlook the negative word and miss the question, even though they have mastered the material. One way to decrease this problem is to highlight the negative word, in this case, **FURTHER**.*

Only words that reverse the meaning of the stem should be highlighted. Once you start to highlight adjectives and adverbs, such as *first, last, most, least,* and *priority,* the impact of highlighting diminishes. Students are then more likely to overlook the emphasis put on the word. In addition, highlighting can become very subjective. Faculty members will not always agree on what to highlight, and the results will be inconsistent. Students will pick up on the inconsistency and might even argue that they missed a question because you forgot to highlight an adjective or adverb. Keep it simple. Highlight only those words that reverse the meaning of the stem so that the correct answer is the one incorrect option. As long as you explain in the test directions that students should read all options and select the best answer, students will not be placed at a disadvantage.

Present Tense   Keeping the problem in the present tense eliminates confusion—the problem in the stem should be happening now, not at some other point in time. It is particularly important to avoid the passive voice. Include events from the past or identify the client's history while asking the students to solve a problem that is happening now, as illustrated in **Exhibit 5.17**.

Exhibit 5.17   Passive voice versus present tense

Passive Voice

A 4-year-old child who had a tonsillectomy this morning has been assessed by a nurse. Which of these findings should be followed up by the nurse?

A. The child states, "My throat is very sore."
B. The child's swallowing has increased*
C. The child has not urinated
D. The child is drowsy

Present Tense

A nurse is assessing a 4-year-old child who had a tonsillectomy hour ago. Which of these findings, if identified in the child, is the priority for the nurse to follow up?

A. The child states, "My throat is very sore."
B. The child is swallowing repeatedly*
C. The child has not urinated
D. The child is drowsy

The initial item is poorly constructed and would be particularly confusing for ELL students. The revised item keeps the action in the present tense while identifying that the child had surgery in the past. The revised item also clarifies that all the findings should be monitored but that option B is the priority.

Qualities of Effective Options

The goal of a well-written test item is to have the stem and options be so clearly written that the informed students, although they are challenged, select the correct option and are not tricked into choosing an incorrect option. At the same time, all options should appeal equally to those who are uninformed (the low achievers on the test). When the low achievers choose the correct option and/or the high achievers choose the incorrect option, or if no one chooses a particular option, the test item is not functioning properly.

Keep the options succinct. Long options become a test of reading ability and tend to confuse the reader. If the options are longer than two lines, the question probably was not fully developed in the stem. As a general rule of thumb, keep the options shorter than one line and certainly shorter than the stem.

How many options should be offered in a multiple-choice question? If the distractors are effective, a higher number of distractors will yield a more discriminating item. Many standardized multiple-choice exams use four options. Good distractors are hard to write, however, and there is no magic in four options. Most important, you want to avoid distractors that trick or confuse high-achieving students or that fail to attract low-achieving students. You do not want students to get to the right answer by process of elimination due to the weakness of the distractors.

Four options reduce the chance of guessing, but it is better to use three options if you are unable to write a fourth option that is plausible. Having one correct answer and two plausible distractors is better than including a distractor that is implausible just to keep the number of options at four. In fact, if you use three options, you reduce the reading time per question and can include more items on the test. For example, if you administer a test that has 50 items with four options each, you could administer a 60-item test that had three options for each item in the same time frame. This approach allows you to sample a wider range of content from the course and increases the validity of the test results.

It is acceptable to include questions with both three and four options on a test. It is less confusing for students and more conducive to face validity to keep all items with a uniform number of distractors, however. The major difficulty with four options is posed with writing distractors. One of the goals of this chapter is to assist you with developing skill in the ability to write plausible distractors.

A key requirement for item plausibility is homogeneity—all options should look alike. Listing the options vertically allows the best visual comparison. They should all be approximately the same length or be listed in ascending length. If one of the options is of disproportionate length compared with the others, as shown in **Exhibit 5.18**, it causes a cuing error in the item. In some cases, it could attract students; in other situations, it could cause students not to select that option. In either situation, a student's choice of an option should not be related to cuing; it should be based solely on knowledge, or lack of knowledge, in the content area.

Exhibit 5.18   Disproportionate option length

A client says to a nurse, "I have a living will, but I haven't told my family because I don't want to worry them." Which of these replies would be appropriate for the nurse to make?

A. "You have a right to privacy about this matter."
B. "I won't tell your family, but I have to note it in your chart."
C. "I have to tell your doctor, but I won't tell anyone else."
D. "You should discuss this with your family and doctor so that if a health crisis did occur, they would have firsthand information of your wishes so that they could act as you would want them to."*

Option D is disproportionately long, providing a cue to its correctness.

Another requirement for item options is to place those associated with a value in numerical, chronological, or sequential order. Either ascending or descending order can be chosen. An answer that requires a numerical response causes confusion if the student has to hunt for the answer. It is much more effective to place such answers in sequential order. **Exhibit 5.19** illustrates the advantage of ordering options.

Exhibit 5.19   Option order

Disordered Options
A client is to receive quietane syrup 50 mg po bid. The bottle of quietane syrup contains 25 mg per 5 mL. How many milliliters of syrup should a nurse give the client for each dose?

A. 10*
B. 25
C. 5
D. 20

(continues)

Exhibit 5.19   Option order (*Continued*)

Ordered Options

A client is to receive quietane syrup 50 mg po bid. The bottle of quietane syrup contains 25 mg per 5 mL. How many milliliters of syrup should a nurse give the client for each dose?

A. 5

B. 10*

C. 20

D. 25

Notice how the disordered example causes the student to hunt for the correct answer. Keeping the options in order decreases confusion and reading time. Notice also that milliliters *is identified in the stem, so there is no need to repeat it in the options.*

Many test development software programs scramble options to create different versions of a test. If you want options to remain in a particular order, be sure to disable this feature for the item. If you are storing your items in hard copy, make a notation that the options should not be scrambled.

The more precisely you word your items, the more accurate they are. Therefore, it is important to provide appropriate labels for answers that relate to values such as vital signs or laboratory values. **Exhibit 5.20** illustrates how labeling values clarifies their meaning and limits student speculation.

Exhibit 5.20   Unlabeled versus labeled values

Unlabeled Values

Which of these laboratory results should a nurse recognize as suggestive that a client who is diagnosed with schizophrenia has developed an adverse effect of prescribed clozapine?

A. Blood urea nitrogen (BUN), 16

B. Platelets, 160,000

C. Creatinine phosphokinase (CPK), 55

D. White blood cells (WBCs), 3,200*

Labeled Values

Which of these laboratory results should a nurse recognize as suggestive that a client who is diagnosed with schizophrenia has developed an adverse effect of prescribed clozapine?

A. Blood urea nitrogen (BUN), 16 mg/dL

B. Platelets, 160,000/mm^3

C. Creatinine phosphokinase (CPK), 55 U/L

D. White blood cells (WBCs), 3,200 μ/L*

Positive Statements   As with stems, negativity should be avoided in the options (especially if a negative stem is used). Double negatives cause extreme confusion. Negative options are often used to increase item difficulty, but the problem is that they increase difficulty by tricking the students. Negative options are generally not acceptable distractors. **Exhibits 5.21** and **5.22** demonstrate the misleading quality of negative stems and negative options.

Exhibit 5.21   Negative options

Stem with Negative Options

When physically restraining a client, a nurse should consider all of these standards of care EXCEPT

A. obtaining the client's consent for the restraint.*
B. using the least restrictive device for the shortest time.
C. not keeping restraints on continuously.
D. applying restraints when nonrestrictive alternatives are not effective.

Negative options are particularly confusing when the stem is also negative. Options C and D both include negative terms, which make this question an exercise in logic rather than a true test of knowledge.

Revised

Which of these standards of care should a nurse include when caring for a client who is physically restrained?

A. Obtaining a signed consent from the client
B. Using the most restrictive device available
C. Removing restraints at regular intervals*
D. Alternating two different types of restraints

Exhibit 5.22   Negative stem with negative options

A nurse reviews self-care with a client who has chronic renal failure and an A-V fistula on the left arm. Which of these statements, if made by the client, should indicate to the nurse that the client needs ***FURTHER*** teaching?

A. "I will wear my watch on my left wrist."*
B. "I will not allow anyone to draw blood from my left arm."
C. "I will not have my blood pressure taken on my left arm."
D. "I will not carry heavy objects with my left arm."

Positive Stem

A nurse reviews self-care with a client who has chronic renal failure and an A-V fistula on the left arm. Which of these statements, if made by the client, should indicate to the nurse that the client understands the instruction correctly?

A. "I will wear my watch only on my left wrist."
B. "I will have blood drawn only from my left arm."
C. "I will have my blood pressure taken only on my right arm."*
D. "I will eat or write only with my right hand."

*The word **FURTHER** in the negative stem reverses the meaning of the stem so that the student must identify the incorrect option. The nots in the options reverse the meaning of the distractors. The correct answer is the only positive one. This is an extremely confusing item! The revision is positive and presents a straightforward approach in the item.*

Negative questions are seldom encountered in real practice; therefore, they lack practical relevance. Situations do arise in healthcare settings, however, where the wrong action can have dire consequences. Use a negative stem only when knowing what not to do is important.

Distinct Each option should be distinct. Retaining as much information as possible in the stem rather than in the responses reduces redundancy and reading time. Words or phrases that have to be repeated in the options should be in the stem, not in the options, as shown in **Exhibit 5.23**. The operating principle here is to keep reading time to a minimum.

Exhibit 5.23   Repetitive options

Repetitive
Which of these methods provides a quick estimation of the cardiac rate from the electrocardiogram of a client who has normal sinus rhythm?

A. Count the number of T waves in a 5-second strip and multiply by 6
B. Count the number of large squares in an R-R interval and divide by 10
C. Count the number of small squares between two P waves and multiply by 5
D. Count the number of QRS complexes in 6 seconds and multiply by 10*

Distinct
To obtain a quick estimation of the cardiac rate from the electrocardiogram of a client who has a normal sinus rhythm, a nurse should count the number of

A. T waves in a 5-second strip and multiply by 6
B. large squares in an R-R interval and divide by 10
C. small squares between two P waves and multiply by 5
D. QRS complexes in 6 seconds and multiply by 10*

The revised item eliminates redundancy and decreases the time needed for reading the question. This is an example of the completion format.

Another concern with maintaining the distinctness of the options is to avoid overlapping the options. Items should not be partially correct; that is, a correct response should not be part of a distractor. Structuring an item this way confuses students. Keep all the options mutually exclusive; when options overlap, more than one option may be correct. **Exhibits 5.24** and **5.25** present different applications for keeping options distinct.

Exhibit 5.24   Partially correct versus distinct options

Partially Correct Options
Which is the most effective approach for a nurse to take when approaching a suspicious client?

A. Cautiously extend the hand
B. Introduce oneself and state the reason for visit*

C. Extend a hand and state the reason for visit

D. Introduce yourself and extend hand

The actions in these options overlap. Including a correct component in a distractor confuses students. Each option should stand alone, with the correct option being the only completely correct answer.

Distinct Options

After introducing oneself, which of these approaches would be appropriate for a nurse to take when initially approaching a hospitalized client who is suspicious?

A. Offer to shake the client's hand

B. Explain the reason for the visit to the client*

C. Tell the client there is no need to be distrustful

D. Provide the client with a thorough orientation to the facility

Each option is distinct, the distractors contain only incorrect components, and there is only one clearly correct answer. Note that the action of introducing oneself is included in the stem.

Exhibit 5.25   Overlapping options

Overlapping Options

A nurse should explain to a client who is taking lithium that the dose must be individualized to maintain blood levels between:

A. 0.2 and 0.5 mEq/L.

B. 0.5 and 1.5 mEq/L.

C. 1.5 and 2.0 mEq/L.

D. 2.0 and 3.5 mEq/L.

Revised

A nurse should explain to a client who is taking lithium that the dose must be individualized to maintain blood levels at how many milliequivalents per liter?

A. 0.2–0.4

B. 0.5–1.5*

C. 1.6–2.5

D. 2.6–3.5

Each option stands alone. One option does not include another. Also note that you can remove mEq/L from the options by including milliequivalents per liter in the stem.

Homogeneous Appearance   For options to be equally attractive to the students, all options must be parallel in length, grammatical structure, content, and complexity. The more homogeneous the options appear, the more challenging the item. Homogeneity refers to appearance only; each option must be mutually exclusive and provide a clear and distinct choice. The correct option must be the only correct option, and the incorrect options must be undeniably wrong. **Exhibit 5.26** shows that the more the incorrect options look like the correct answer, the more difficult it is for the uninformed students to guess the correct answer.

Exhibit 5.26   Heterogeneous versus homogeneous options

Heterogeneous Options
Which of these nursing diagnoses would be the priority for this client?

A. Activity intolerance
B. Constipation
C. Hypertension
D. Fluid volume deficit*

Homogeneous Options
A client has all of these nursing diagnoses. Which one is the priority for this client?

A. Activity intolerance
B. Constipation
C. Anxiety
D. Fluid volume deficit*

Option C in the heterogeneous example is not a nursing diagnosis and is therefore inconsistent with the stem and the other options.

Opposite options pose a problem in multiple-choice items. If two options are opposites, the students will be drawn to decide between those two and ignore the other options. **Exhibit 5.27** shows how opposite distractors can provide a cue to test-wise students.

Exhibit 5.27   Opposite options

Opposite Options
A client has a Sengstaken-Blakemore tube connected to low wall suction. When the client develops respiratory distress, which of these actions should a nurse take?

A. Inflate the tube's esophageal balloon
B. Deflate the tube's esophageal balloon*
C. Decompress the tube's gastric balloon
D. Increase the amount of wall suction

Distinct Options
A client has a Sengstaken-Blakemore tube connected to low wall suction. When the client develops respiratory distress, which of these actions should a nurse take?

A. Lavage the tube with ice water
B. Deflate the tube's esophageal balloon*

C. Decompress the tube's gastric balloon

D. Increase the amount of wall suction

In the first example, options A and B are opposites, which attracts students to choose between only options A and B and ignore options C and D. By removing the incorrect opposite option, uninformed students are more likely to consider all four options as equally attractive. In addition, in the original question, option D is the only option that does not mention a balloon.

The Rule of Two Sets applies to opposite options. If similar structure or wording is included in two options, it must be used in all four options. If two options are opposites, you must use two sets of opposites. As the examples in **Exhibit 5.28** show, two similar options attract students and cause them to discount the two that are dissimilar, whereas two sets of opposite options decrease the guessing ability of the uninformed students.

Exhibit 5.28   Rule of Two Sets

One Set of Opposites

A nurse should monitor the client for side effects of the medication, which include

A. hypertension.

B. hypotension.*

C. insomnia.

D. palpitations.

Two Sets of Opposites

A nurse should monitor the client for side effects of the medication, which include

A. tachycardia.

B. bradycardia.

C. hypertension.

D. hypotension.*

In the first example, test-wise students are apt to ignore options C and D. The second example uses the Rule of Two Sets, in which two sets of opposites attract the uninformed student to all four options.

Homogeneous options use medical terminology and technical language consistently. If terminology is used in one option, it should be used in all options. **Exhibit 5.29** provides an example of how students are drawn to the answer that appears to be most technical.

Exhibit 5.29   Technical language

Technical Language

A nurse should carefully observe the client for which of these manifestations?

A. Pruritus*

B. Redness

(continues)

Exhibit 5.29   Technical language (*Continued*)

C. Bruises

D. Ringing in the ears

Revised

A nurse should carefully observe the client for which of these manifestations?

A. Pruritus*

B. Erythema

C. Ecchymosis

D. Tinnitus

Choice A, which is the correct answer, contains the only technical term in the first example. Students are most likely to choose the technical term even if they are not familiar with the material being tested. If either B, C, or D was the correct answer in the first example, the question would be a trick item. The revised example uses all technical terms, making the options homogeneous.

Avoid writing items that have very specific correct answers and very general distractors or very specific distractors with a very general correct answer, as **Exhibit 5.30** demonstrates. Students are attracted to select the option that is different. If one of the homogeneous options in these sets is the correct answer, the question is attempting to trick the students.

Exhibit 5.30   General versus specific options

General Options

Which of these measures is most important to include when caring for a client during the first hour after surgery?

A. Repositioning the client at regular intervals

B. Monitoring the client's cardiovascular status*

C. Orienting the client to the post anesthesia unit

D. Checking the client's ability to move the lower extremities

Specific Options

Which of these measures is most important to include when caring for a client during the first hour after surgery?

A. Repositioning the client at regular intervals

B. Monitoring the client's blood pressure*

C. Orienting the client to the postanesthesia unit

D. Checking the client's ability to move the lower extremities

Test-wise students will recognize that the correct answer is the global option, which is the heterogeneous one in the original question. The revised item contains four specific options, which decreases the opportunity of the test-wise student to answer the question correctly without having mastered the content.

Succinct   Succinctness of the options is just as important as succinctness of the stem, as **Exhibit 5.31** illustrates. Keeping key words in the stem eliminates repetition in the options. Repeating words in the options causes confusion and unnecessarily complicates the reading of the question. In addition, a distractor should not be partially correct.

Exhibit 5.31   Repetitive versus succinct options

Repetitive Options

Before administering digoxin to a client who has congestive heart failure, a nurse should check the client for

A. bradycardia, hypokalemia, and gastric upset.*
B. constipation, bradycardia, and hypokalemia.
C. hypokalemia, dry mouth, and bradycardia.
D. hypertension, bradycardia, and hypokalemia.

Succinct Options

Before administering a dose of digoxin to a client who has congestive heart failure, a nurse should monitor the client for bradycardia, hypokalemia, and

A. gastric upset.*
B. constipation.
C. dry mouth.
D. hypertension.

In the preceding question, checking for bradycardia and hypokalemia are in every option, so they belong in the stem.

Developing the Correct Answer

There should be one and only one correct answer for each question. Perhaps this statement seems too elementary to even mention, but frequently the key is a problem in classroom tests. Whether the correct answer is the only right answer or the best response, faculy should agree that the designated answer is the only correct one. Writing a referenced rationale for each of your items is the most effective way to ensure the veracity of the key. In addition, referenced items can be shared with your students for a very effective test review.

It is critical that the stem specifies all the necessary conditions that make the intended response the only correct answer. At the same time, avoid some of the factors that interfere with the effectiveness of your items.

First, it is important to randomize the key. The correct answer should be equally assigned to each option choice. If you consciously alternate the position of the correct answer when you write your items, it makes it easier to randomize the key when you assemble a test. It is counterproductive to alphabetize the options as some experts suggest. If you rewrite the options because of item analysis results, you will have to reorder the options, which will cause confusion when you try to associate data with the options in the future. Also, alphabetizing the options will be lost if you use a test development program that allows you to scramble options to create alternate forms of a test. You do not need another step to item writing. Just alternate between the available options when you write your items and randomization will not be a problem.

In addition to randomizing, you want to make sure that the key does not repeat the same letter more than three or four times. A string of six A's, for example, might make a student doubt that the seventh answer is also an A, even if it is. After you assemble your test, print out a key and check that the same letter is not repeated more than three times. If you identify a problem, move the questions around; do not change the order of the options. Changing the order of the options can cause great confusion with the key, especially if you have data associated with the items.

A helpful method for ensuring that your key does not become confusing is to put an asterisk at the end of the correct option. If you use a test development software program to compose your items, this step is unnecessary because the program maintains the key once you enter it. If you write your items in a word processing program, however, the key could become confusing if you rearrange the options for any reason. Having an asterisk at the end of the correct answer ensures that the key is correct no matter how often you cut and paste your options during test development. Note that the item examples in this text follow this suggestion.

Several cues can give away your correct answer to test-wise students. These cues include having a longer and more precise correct answer compared with the incorrect options, as in Exhibits 5.18 and 5.32, and phrasing the correct answer in textbook terminology, as in **Exhibit 5.32**.

Exhibit 5.32   Textbook language

A nurse should recognize that the manifestations of tuberculosis are related to

A. the production of lymphokine, which is stimulated by the immune response to the tubercle bacilli.*
B. a decrease in the white blood cells.
C. an inflammatory response.
D. the increased production of sputum.

Revised
Which of these manifestations would a nurse expect to identify when assessing a client who has active tuberculosis?

A. Anorexia and fatigue*
B. Pleuritic chest pain
C. Dyspnea on exertion
D. Prolonged expiratory phase

Textbook language cues students to select an option even if they do not understand the material. Also note that tubercle bacilli is mentioned only in the key, and the key is much longer than the distractors. The revision is clinically relevant. It asks the student to identify the manifestations.

Designing Effective Distractors

The art of writing effective multiple-choice items requires you to use your creativity and critical thinking skills. Crafting distractors presents the biggest challenge to most teachers. The goal of distractors is to discriminate between the students who are informed and those who are uninformed or have not mastered the course content and objectives. To discriminate effectively, all of the item's options must be equally attractive to those students who are uninformed or to students who have not achieved the desired outcome. If a distractor does not attract students, if the distractors attract the high-achieving students, or if more low achievers than high achievers choose the correct answer, the item is not functioning properly. It takes practice to develop expertise in crafting workable distractors; using the suggestions that follow will help you get started.

One method for increasing the difficulty of a multiple-choice item is to require the student to select the best answer. When you are asking for the one correct answer, the distractors should all be wrong. A question that asks for the best answer implies that all the options vary in degree of correctness, with only one option as the best answer. The difference between these two formats is illustrated in **Exhibit 5.33**.

Exhibit 5.33   Best answer versus correct answer

Best-Answer Format

A nurse should give priority to which of these short-term outcomes for a client who is experiencing a panic attack?

A. The client will have decreased symptoms of anxiety
B. The client will avoid frightening situations
C. The client will learn thought-stopping techniques
D. The client will remain safe during the episode*

Each option is a possible outcome, whereas option D is clearly the priority outcome at this time.

Correct Answer Format

Which of these questions would be appropriate for a nurse to ask when assessing a client for bulimia?

A. "How many times a day do you eat?"
B. "For how long have you been at your current weight?"
C. "Do you have particular food dislikes?"
D. "Do you ever eat in secret?"*

In this example, all the distractors are incorrect. Only option D is an appropriate answer. Because there is only one correct answer, the stem cannot ask for a best answer, such as "Which of these questions should a nurse ask first?"

Best-answer items tend to be more difficult and discriminating than questions that have distinctly incorrect distractors. Items that are written in the best-answer format are an effective strategy for developing critical thinking items. Chapter 6, "Writing Critical Thinking Multiple-Choice Items," elaborates on writing items using this format.

Plausibility   It is not enough for a distractor to be wrong; it must be plausible without being tricky (**Exhibit 5.34**). If high-achieving students choose distractors because they are tricky, the item loses its usefulness. At the same time, highly implausible or absurd distractors contribute nothing to the effectiveness of a test. Ideally, all incorrect options should appeal only to the uninformed student. The uninformed student should not be able to eliminate the incorrect options with certainty. Learning to write plausible distractors takes practice.

Exhibit 5.34   Implausible distractors

A nurse should recognize that which of these individuals is most likely to have a personality disorder?

A. An 18-year-old man who is beginning a new relationship and is unsure about whether he is ready for a long-term commitment

B. A 24-year-old woman who is unable to show emotion, has no friends, and is estranged from her family*

C. A dependable, loyal, 30-year-old man who expresses himself through art

D. A 43-year-old woman who describes herself as shy and reticent

Options A, C, and D are implausible, whereas option B is so obviously correct.

Common Misconceptions   You probably have lots of ideas for plausible distractors right at your fingertips. Keep a log of the common misconceptions that students express in clinical practice. Make a list of classroom questions that students frequently ask. Keep track of the incorrect responses that students supply on short-answer items. Common errors and beliefs of students translate into very believable distractors. **Exhibit 5.35** shows how common misconceptions can be translated into effective distractors.

Exhibit 5.35   Common misconceptions

When a client has a seizure, which of these actions should a nurse take?

A. Place an object in the client's mouth

B. Protect the client's head.

C. Restrain the client's extremities

D. Insert an airway into the client's mouth

This item recognizes that students who are not familiar with the content will be drawn to the common misconceptions identified in the distractors.

Sound Bites   A statement that relates to a situation that is close to the question but does not satisfy the requirements of the question will attract the uninformed students. Students who have not mastered the content will remember hearing or reading these facts but will be unable to apply the information correctly. The uninformed students will remember that you "said that in class," but they will not recognize that what you said does not apply to the question at hand. A sound bite that does not apply to the stem requires students to make a judgment related to the accuracy of the statement as well as its relevance, as **Exhibit 5.36** illustrates.

Exhibit 5.36   Sound bite

A client who has congestive heart failure says to a nurse, "I really don't understand what is wrong with my heart." Which of these explanations would be appropriate for the nurse to give to the client?

A. "There is a blockage in the arteries that supply your heart muscle."
B. "Your heart is having difficulty pumping enough blood for your body."*
C. "The impulses that direct the beating of your heart are acting randomly."
D. "There is a bulging in the major vessel that leaves your heart."

While options A, C, and D are responses that describe cardiac pathology, they do not apply to congestive heart failure. They look familiar to the uninformed student. Writing distractors that correctly explain another situation is much more effective than creating pathophysiology, such as "The blood is moving too rapidly through the left side of your heart."

Seeks Help Appropriately   Items that call for the nurse to seek assistance require the student to recognize when a situation requires the expertise of another healthcare professional. Because students hesitate to select the option, "call the primary care provider (PCP)," it makes a very poor distractor. When that option is the correct one, however, it works well because it requires the student to discriminate carefully among the alternatives to recognize when a situation requires the attention of the PCP. You might prefer to have the nurse take an action in the stem first, but calling the PCP is an acceptable format, as the question in **Exhibit 5.37** demonstrates.

Exhibit 5.37   Seeks help appropriately

A client who has esophageal varices develops hematemesis. Which of these actions should a nurse take immediately?

A. Obtain a specimen for blood gas analysis
B. Increase the client's oral fluid intake
C. Administer the client's prescribed lactulose
D. Notify the client's physician*

Quote the Nurse and/or the Client

Quote the nurse, quote the client. Use quotes liberally. Quotes represent real-life situations that a nurse would encounter in practice, and they also ensure that the material is not directly copied from a textbook. Do not sum up a situation for the students; quote the individuals depicted in the item. Let the students analyze the situation to determine what the problem is. The items in **Exhibits 5.38** demonstrates how effectively quotes work in a question.

Exhibit 5.38 Quotes

A client scheduled to receive chemotherapy for cancer asks the nurse about the most common side effect of chemotherapy. The nurse informs the client that the most common side effect of chemotherapy is

A. alopecia.
B. nausea and vomiting.
C. altered glucose metabolism.
D. increased appetite.

Revision
A client who is scheduled to receive chemotherapy for cancer treatment asks a nurse, "What side effects can I expect from this treatment?" Which of these responses should the nurse offer?

A. "Hair loss occurs with all chemotherapy."
B. "Nausea is common, but it can be treated."*
C. "Your blood sugar will fluctuate, so you will have to limit sweets."
D. "Most clients experience constipation that is manageable with laxatives."

Characteristics to Avoid

Cues are irrelevant and unintended clues to the correct answer that enable students to make the correct response without having the required ability. Cues have a negative impact on the reliability of a test.

An effective multiple-choice item eliminates these cues so that students are able to answer the question correctly only if they have mastered the concepts that the question requires. Grammatical inconsistency and homogeneity are two cues that were previously discussed. It is obvious that violating many of the guidelines presented in this chapter provides cues to the uninformed student. Several additional cues are identified in the subsections that follow. Your goal as an item developer is to avoid these cues to ensure that your items are providing the information you need to make decisions.

Verbal Associations Repeating key words from the stem only in the correct option provides a cue to test-wise students. Verbal associations connect the correct answer to the stem, as is seen in **Exhibit 5.39**.

Exhibit 5.39 Verbal association

Verbal Association
A nurse should recognize that the first step in resolving an ethical dilemma related to a client's advanced directives is to

A. recognize that an ethical dilemma exists.*
B. identify the moral point of view of the client.

C. assess the viewpoints of all involved parties.

D. determine the client's health status.

Revised

A nurse should recognize that the first step in resolving an ethical dilemma related to a client's advanced directives is to

A. recognize that a conflict exists.*

B. identify the moral point of view of the client.

C. assess the viewpoints of all involved parties.

D. determine the client's health status.

The word ethical *provides a cue because it is repeated only in the correct answer in the original question. The revised item changes the words* ethical dilemma *to* conflict, *which removes the cue.*

Qualifying Words   Qualifying words provide cues to students because they neutralize the option, making it a safe choice. Words such as *often, seldom, sometimes, usually,* and *generally* are most often found in the correct answer, as shown in **Exhibit 5.40**. These words qualify the key by indicating that the option does not have to be true all the time. Test-wise students recognize that if one option is not definitive, it is the safe choice. If you use qualifying words, keep the options homogeneous by including qualifiers in all options.

Exhibit 5.40   Qualifying words

When screening a group of senior citizens for hypertension, a nurse should understand that elderly clients who have hypertension

A. often have no symptoms.*

B. will refuse to accept treatment.

C. have an underlying cause for the problem.

D. respond more positively to medications than younger clients.

The qualifying word in the correct answer provides a clue because the option is more general. The key allows that some clients have symptoms, whereas the distractors are absolute.

Specific Determiners   Words such as *never, none, all,* and *always* are specific determiners. These words are the antitheses of qualifiers: They indicate that a situation is absolute. Because very few things in nursing are absolute, using specific determiners only in the incorrect answers provides a cue to test-wise students, as **Exhibit 5.41** shows.

Exhibit 5.41   Specific determiners

When planning care for an elderly client who is bedridden, a nurse should recognize that pressure ulcers

A. always result from the client's inability to ambulate.
B. develop when tissue is subjected to sustained pressure.*
C. can always be prevented by vigorous massage.
D. never develop if the client is well nourished.

Specific determiners rule out the possibility of an exception to the rule. The rule "Never say never" applies here. Pressure is also a cue in the stem.

Specific determiners are seldom used in the correct answer, and test-wise students are aware of this fact. These words are appropriate to use in the stem; however, they should be used sparingly in the options and then only when they can be used appropriately in the correct answer. Items should be written to test more than a student's ability to recognize that unequivocal statements are seldom true.

All of the Above   "All of the above" and "none of the above" are used most often when a teacher cannot think of a fourth option. "All of the above" is particularly helpful to test-wise students who are able to select the correct answer based on incomplete information (**Exhibit 5.42**). These students recognize that if they can identify two correct answers, then "all of the above" is correct; conversely, if they can identify that one answer is incorrect, then "all of the above" is incorrect. The use of "all of the above" should be avoided; it is much more effective to rephrase the question so that four plausible alternatives are provided.

Exhibit 5.42   All of the above

When assessing a client who reports having sleep deprivation, a nurse should assess the client for manifestations, which include

A. confusion.
B. slowed response time.
C. diminished reasoning skills.
D. all of the above.*

The test-wise student need only recognize that two of the options are correct to identify that the correct answer is "all of the above." Therefore a student who has incomplete understanding can guess the correct answer.

None of the Above   "None of the above" should be used sparingly, if at all. After all, if there is no correct answer to the question, why ask it in the first place? **Exhibit 5.43** clarifies how the use of "none of the above" as a distractor produces an ineffective item.

Exhibit 5.43   None of the above

Which of these components of the nursing process determines the extent to which the planned client outcomes have been achieved?

A. Assessment

B. Planning

C. Evaluation*

D. None of the above

Test-wise students know they should avoid the none-of-the-above option, which reduces the plausible options to three.

Some experts advocate the use of "none of the above" to decrease the chance of correctly guessing when the student must perform an operation to obtain the correct answer. Several authorities acknowledge the benefit of using this option when testing calculations in a multiple-choice format (Miller et al., 2009; Brookhart & Nitko, 2014; Popham, 2003).

The use of "none of the above" is recommended only when students are more likely to answer the question and then look at the options, such as with a math calculation, as shown in **Exhibit 5.44**. Students might be able to estimate the correct calculation answer on a multiple-choice exam. When you want to be confident that students can perform the calculations, use "none of the above" so that students cannot assume that the correct answer is included in the options. This alternative avoids giving clues to students when their incorrect solution is not among the options. When "none of the above" is an option, the students have to be certain that their solution is correct. If "none of the above" is not an answer choice, it is easier to guess without really knowing how to calculate. There is one caution to remember if you use "none of the above" as an option: The correct answer must be absolute. The answers for math calculation questions, for example, cannot be rounded up or down. Unless you specify in the stem that the answer is approximate, a rounded number is not absolutely correct and thus "none of the above" is the technically correct answer, even when you intend another option to be the correct answer. If you choose to use the none-of-the-above format for math calculation items, reserve it for answers that are absolute, such as the example in Exhibit 5.44.

Exhibit 5.44   None of the above for math

A nurse is preparing to administer 2 mg of a medication to a client. The medication is available in a vial that is labeled 1 mg/0.5 mL. How many milliliters should the nurse administer to the client?

A. 0.5

B. 1.5

C. 2.0

D. None of the above*

In this example, the student must be sure of the answer to recognize that "none of the above" is correct.

A problem with the none-of-the-above option is that students might not believe that this option is ever correct. If students do not believe that it is a viable choice, it will not work as an option. It is important to explain to students who are not used to the inclusion of the none-of-the-above option on a test that this choice is sometimes the correct option.

Multiple Multiples   The goal of item development is to make the question as clear as possible and to eliminate any extraneous factors that would confuse students. Multiple-multiple or complex multiple-choice items directly contradict this goal. The example in **Exhibit 5.45** shows just how confusing a multiple-multiple item can be. This item format is unnecessarily complex and is more a test of a student's logic ability than a direct and meaningful indicator of a student's achievement.

Exhibit 5.45   Multiple-multiple

A screening test for a disease is found to have a sensitivity of 90% and a specificity of 95%, which means that of the people who had the test

A. 5% of those who have the disease were identified as positive.
B. 95% of those who do not have the disease were identified as negative.
C. 10% of those who were identified as negative have the disease.
D. 90% of those who were identified as positive do not have the disease.

A. A and B are true, and C and D are false
B. C and D are true, and A and B are false
C. A and C are true, and B and D are false
D. B and C are true, and A and D are false*

This question is impossibly confusing. Even if the student can interpret the stem, an inordinate amount of time is needed to decipher what is being asked.

Revised
A screening test for a disease is found to have a sensitivity of 90% and a specificity of 95%. A nurse should interpret this as meaning that of the people who had the test

A. 5% of those who were identified as negative do not have the disease.
B. 10% of those who have the disease were identified as positive.
C. 90% of those who were positive do not have the disease.
D. 95% of those who do not have the disease were identified as negative.*

Trick Items   Trick items are designed by item writers who are under the false impression that any means of increasing item difficulty is acceptable (see **Exhibits 5.46** and **5.47**). The problem is that these items trick both low and high achievers, and therefore the item will not be an effective indicator of student achievement. These items lure students to second-guess themselves and to select an incorrect answer because of an extraneous cue. Students become understandably distrustful of faculty members who use tricks in their tests.

Exhibit 5.46   Trick item

A client who is receiving an intravenous infusion develops dyspnea and increased blood pressure. A nurse should recognize that which of these problems may be developing?

A. Infection
B. Air embolism
C. Fluid overload*
D. Hypovolemia

This question will confuse students. It is a trick item because an embolism is not associated with elevated blood pressure, but it is definitely associated with dyspnea. The inclusion of dyspnea in the stem will mislead students. The question would be more effective if it included several clear manifestations of fluid overload and/or if air embolism was left out of the distractors. Even the most experienced professional would not make a definitive diagnosis based on two manifestations. In addition, it is far more important to ask what a nurse should do when a client experiences an untoward reaction to an intravenous infusion.

Exhibit 5.47   Trick item

Which of these client manifestations would support a nursing diagnosis of fluid volume deficit?

A. Tachycardia*
B. Decreased respiratory rate with prolonged expiratory phase
C. Dysuria
D. Diaphoresis

Students may be drawn to select B because it is the longest answer. Exhibit 5.18 illustrates a disproportionately long correct answer that provides a cue to students. This example violates the same rule, but it is particularly unfair because it purposely tempts the student with a cue to the wrong answer.

Putting the Action in the Stem   Identifying what action a nurse should take in the stem and then asking the students to refine the action is an approach that results in a very easy item. It is difficult to break an action down into four believable options, and therefore the students only have to eliminate the obviously incorrect to identify the correct answer. A better approach is simply to ask the students to identify which action is appropriate in the stem and keep the options distinct from each other. **Exhibits 5.48** and **5.49** present examples that illustrate this type of question.

Exhibit 5.48   Action in the stem

Action in the Stem

In which of these positions should a nurse place a client who had a liver biopsy 1 hour ago?

A. Right side lying*
B. Left Sims
C. Prone
D. Supine

Actions in the Options

Which of these measures should a nurse include in the care plan for a client who had a liver biopsy 1 hour ago?

A. Monitor the neurovascular status of the client's affected extremity
B. Advise the client to maintain a right side–lying position*
C. Check the client's urine for occult blood
D. Instruct the client to move slowly when arising from a sitting position

The original question tells the student that the answer involves positioning. The student can then guess between plausible options. The revised question requires a higher level of discrimination from the student. The action is not indicated in the stem, so the student must choose from among a list of unrelated options.

Exhibit 5.49   Action in the stem

Action in the Stem

A nurse is assessing a client who had abdominal surgery today. What would the nurse expect to hear when auscultating bowel sounds?

A. Hyperactive bowel sounds
B. Hypoactive bowel sounds
C. Absent bowel sounds
D. Normal bowel sounds

Actions in the Options

A nurse is assessing a client who had abdominal surgery. Which of these findings should the nurse expect to identify?

A. Increased pulse rate
B. Decreased blood pressure
C. Absent bowel sounds
D. Subnormal urine output

No wonder every examinee answered this original question correctly. It is too easy. Once you remove the action from the stem, the item is more challenging.

Stating the action in the stem is such a common problem with teacher-developed items that I have included three additional examples to illustrate how dramatically these items can be improved if the actions are kept in the options. **Exhibits 5.50, 5.51, and 5.52** demonstrate the advantage of keeping the actions in the options, not in the stem. In addition, these exhibits introduce the concept of developing parallel items for use in future tests.

Exhibit 5.50   Action in the stem

Action in the Stem

When administering medication to a client via an intravenous heparin lock, a nurse should

A. flush the lock with 5 mL of bacteriostatic water.
B. flush the lock with 10 mL of 5% dextrose solution.
C. flush the lock with 2.5 mL of normal saline.*
D. flush the lock with 1 mL of atropine sulfate.

Actions in the Options

Which of these actions should a nurse take immediately before administering a medication to a client who has an intravenous heparin lock in the right arm?

A. Apply iodine to the lock insertion site
B. Aspirate the lock to check for blood return
C. Flush the lock with 2.5 mL of normal saline*
D. Elevate the client's right arm above the level of the heart

The original question tells the student that the answer involves flushing the lock. The uninformed student has to guess only the reasonable amount of solution to use. The revised question requires a higher level of discrimination from the student. The action is not indicated in the stem, so the student has to choose from among a list of unrelated options.

Exhibit 5.51   Action in the stem

Action in the Stem

A nurse should place a client who had a total right hip replacement 4 hours ago in which of these positions?

A. Supine, with the legs abducted*
B. Low-Fowler's, with the legs elevated
C. Left side lying, with the knees flexed
D. Right side lying, with the legs extended

Actions in the Options

A nurse is planning care for a client who had a hip replacement 4 hours ago. The nurse should include which of these measures in the client's care plan?

A. Checking the client's patellar reflexes
B. Observing the client's incision site for redness

(continues)

Exhibit 5.51   Action in the stem (*Continued*)

C. Positioning the client with the legs abducted*

D. Assisting the client to use a bedside commode

This example demonstrates the advantage of keeping the actions in the options. In the first example, the stem tells the student that the action is positioning. The student has only to remember which position. In the revised example, the student has to identify that positioning is the correct answer from a group of alternate activities. You could easily create a parallel item for use in a future test. Change the correct answer to an incorrect position and write a different correct answer.

Parallel Item

A nurse is planning care for a client who had a hip replacement 4 hours ago. The nurse should include which of these measures in the client's care plan?

A. Checking the client's patellar reflexes

B. Monitoring the drainage from the client's wound*

C. Positioning the client with the legs adducted

D. Assisting the client in using a bedside commode

Exhibit 5.52   Action in the stem

Action in the Stem

A client has been prescribed bed rest for a prolonged time. To promote the use of resistive isometric exercise for the client, the nurse should initiate

A. quadriceps setting.

B. gluteal muscle contraction.

C. moving the arms and legs in circle.

D. pushing against a footboard.*

Actions in the Options

Which of these instructions should a nurse give to a client who is scheduled to be in traction on bed rest for 6 weeks?

A. "You should flex your feet against the footboard at least ten times each hour."*

B. "Make sure you lie flat. You could develop a headache if you elevate the head of the bed."

C. "We will be checking your blood glucose level twice each day."

D. "It is very important that you restrict your fluid intake. Have only two liters per day."

In the original example, the student is told that the action is to implement resistive isometric exercises. The student does not even have to figure out why this is important. In addition, the only resistive exercise is the correct answer. In the revision, the student has to identify that deep vein thrombosis is a potential complication and that resistive isometric exercises are required. This item also offers an opportunity to write a parallel item.

Parallel Item

Which of these instructions should a nurse give to a client who is scheduled to be on bed rest with traction for 6 weeks for treatment of a back injury?

A. "You should pull up frequently on the overhead trapeze to maintain your upper body strength."

B. "Make sure you lie flat. You could develop a headache if you elevate the head of the bed."

C. "We will be checking your blood glucose level twice each day."

D. "It is very important that you have a fluid intake of at least two liters each day."*

Missing Information Item stems that do not provide adequate information to solve the problem present a serious issue in an exam. Obviously no one plans for an item to be incomplete, but sometimes the author can overlook important details. Although an incomplete item can be removed after the test is administered, the damage is done. When students encounter an item that they cannot answer, their first impulse is to assume that they have inadequate knowledge, which increases anxiety and can affect their performance on the rest of the test. **Exhibits 5.53** and **5.54** provide additional illustrations for why careful proofreading by a colleague is so important when you develop a test.

Exhibit 5.53   Missing information

Nursing interventions in the preoperative management of a child with Wilm's tumor include which of these interventions?

1. Restrict fluid intake.
2. Assess urine for blood.
3. Palpate the abdominal mass for changes.
4. Teach child and family about nephrectomy.

A. 1, 2, 3
B. 2, 3
C. 1, 2
D. 2, 4*

Revised
Nursing interventions in the preoperative management of a 4-year-old child who has Wilm's tumor and is scheduled for surgery in 2 days should include which of these actions? Select all that apply.

A. Restrict the child's fluid intake
B. Assess the child's urine for blood
C. Palpate the child's abdomen for changes
D. Teach child and family about nephrectomy
E. Monitor the child's intake and output
F. Maintain the child in low-Fowler's position

The original version of this item is missing essential information. What is the child's age and when is the surgery scheduled? Note that the original form of the item is written in the multiple-multiple format. The revision uses the multiple-response format, a format used in the NCLEX exams, which is also discussed in this chapter.

Exhibit 5.54 Extraneous and missing information

Your client has developed a deep vein thrombosis as a result of immobility from his spinal cord injury. He is receiving 950 units of heparin in 500 ml D5W. The client's lab data indicated that he needs more anticoagulation, and the doctor orders an increase of 3 units per kilogram per hour. You will set the pump at

A. 19.0 ml per hour.
B. 22.0 ml per hour.
C. 23.5 ml per hour.*
D. 24.5 ml per hour.

Revised

A client who weighs 165 pounds is receiving an intravenous infusion of 1000 units of a medication in 500 ml D5W via an infusion pump. The client's prescription is for 2 units of medication per kilogram per hour. The nurse should set the infusion pump to run at how many milliliters per hour?

A. 16.5
B. 33
C. 75*
D. 130

This item contains two characteristics to avoid. The original version has information that is not necessary for the problem solution and it omits information that is essential: The original neglects to tell us what the client weighs! The revision consolidates the information and provides the client's weight. Even if this question is removed from the test, the damage was done. Consider the anxiety of the students who attempted to answer the question before the error was noted. This example clearly demonstrates the necessity of proofreading.

Humor   Humor is an indispensable tool in the classroom; however, it is out of place on an exam. Although humor can decrease tension in the classroom, it can have the opposite effect in a testing situation, particularly with highly anxious test takers (Haladyna, 2004).

Students who do not get the joke on a test can become embarrassed and distracted by laughter during a test. ELL students in particular will have difficulty understanding the humorous intention of an item and can lose their focus when trying to interpret the meaning of such an item (Klisch, 1994). Consider how distracting it would be to have students around you laughing during an exam while you are struggling to decipher what a question is asking. In addition, using a humorous option decreases the number of plausible distractors and makes the test artificially easier. Haladyna (2004) points out that humorous questions might encourage students to be less serious about taking the test. The best approach is to save your humor for classroom instruction.

Alternate National Council Licensure Examination (NCLEX) Items

In April 2003, the National Council of State Boards of Nursing (NCSBN) introduced alternate item types in both the NCLEX-PN and the NCLEX-RN exams. NCSBN describes alternate items as questions that use technology to present items other than the standard four-option multiple-choice item. As with the standard multiple-choice items, alternate items are scored as either correct or incorrect; there is no partial credit on NCLEX (Wendt, 2003).

The current alternate item types include (National Council of State Boards of Nursing [NCSBN], 2016):

- Fill in the blank
- Point and click
- Multiple response
- Chart/exhibit
- Hot spot
- Ordered response
- Graphic options
- Audio format

The NCSBN maintains that these item formats do not affect the pass rate on the exams. The alternate items are additions to the current NCLEX test pools; they are not replacing the items that are in the current NCLEX exams. The difficulty level of these items is calibrated, just as the standard multiple-choice items are; they undergo the same rigorous quality control as do the standard four-option multiple-choice items; and they are all pretested and must meet the stringent criteria of the NCSBN before being used as a scored item on NCLEX (NCSBN, 2016).

Nursing faculty across the country are expressing concern about preparing their students for these item types so they are not penalized when taking the NCLEX. This concern reminds us of the ultimate goal of any educational program: to facilitate the students' ability to think. If the students can think, they can reason out any question that is proposed to them. However, it is important to acknowledge that an exam situation is stressful enough without being surprised by the type of items presented. Just as nursing students should be familiar with basic computer technology before they take the NCLEX, it is important that they be familiar with the alternate item types before they take the exam. Faculty do not need to be overly concerned if they do not have access to the technology needed to present these items to their students. The next section examines the different types of alternate items and discusses how you can adapt these formats, both to familiarize the students with them and to provide you with another tool for assessing student attainment of the objectives of your nursing program.

Another use for these alternate item formats is to use them in class to promote group discussion at the beginning or end of a lecture. This type of activity supplements your lecture and encourages active learning while introducing students to the alternative item formats.

These items are designed to test higher cognitive levels or critical thinking. Examples of each of the item types are presented here. Chapter 6, "Writing Critical Thinking Multiple-Choice Items," further examines alternate item types and discusses how these item formats can be used to assess critical thinking on classroom exams.

Fill-in-the-Blank

Fill-in-the-blank is a constructed-response item (discussed at length in Chapter 8, "Constructed Response Format: Developing Short-Answer and Essay Items"). The fill-in-the-blank items used on the NCLEX present a problem and require the student to type in the answer rather than selecting from among four answers. **Exhibit 5.55** provides an example of this type of item.

Exhibit 5.55   Fill in the blank

A nurse assesses a newborn at 1 minute after vaginal delivery. The nurse identifies that the infant has a lusty cry in response to stimulation, regular respirations, a pink body with bluish-colored extremities, a heart rate of 120/min, and good muscle tone with spontaneous flexion of the extremities. What Apgar score should the nurse assign to the infant? _____

The software that you currently use to scan your exams probably does not allow for scoring this type of item electronically. The simple solution is to include this type of question at the end of the test and hand-score the answers to add the results to the students' raw score. These items can also be used effectively as separate tests or quizzes, which are hand-scored. Although you may want students to show their work on the page, most experts advise against giving partial credit for a calculation problem because of the implications of calculating incorrectly in a healthcare situation.

Point and Click

This item type is also referred to as a hot-spot item. It involves presenting a problem with an illustration and asking the student to use the mouse to click on the area of the illustration that answers the problem. Refer to **Exhibit 5.56** for an example of a hot-spot item. You most likely cannot duplicate this technology with the current software available for test development; **Exhibit 5.57** illustrates how to adapt the format to fit the capabilities of today's popular software. A, B, C, and D represent different waves on the electrocardiogram. Although the student is able to select a response, this adaptation of the format introduces the student to the point-and-click format. This type of item represents another format that promotes classroom discussion and encourages critical thinking.

Exhibit 5.56   Point and click

A nurse is reviewing a client's electrocardiogram, as depicted below. Click on the area of the tracing that represents the T wave.

Exhibit 5.57   Point-and-click multiple-choice alternative

A nurse is reviewing a client's electrocardiogram, as depicted below. Which of these areas, as indicated by A, B, C, and D, represents the T wave on the client's electrocardiogram tracing?

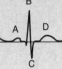

Multiple Response

Multiple-response items present a problem in the stem, as they do with a standard four-option multiple-choice question, and then direct the student to select all the options that apply. Instead of choosing the one correct answer, the student must identify all correct responses. There is no partial credit for these questions; the student must select all the correct options and none of the incorrect options to receive credit. Some software test development programs can score this type of item. If your program does not, hand-scoring is the best alternative.

An example of a multiple-response item appears in **Exhibit 5.58**. Refer again to Exhibit 5.45, which illustrates how this item format is preferred over multiple-multiple items.

Exhibit 5.58   Multiple-response item with rationale

Which of these manifestations, if identified in a client who is having an asthma attack, would indicate that the client is developing status asthmaticus? Select all that apply.

A. Inability to speak

B. Cyanosis

C. Bradycardia

D. Confusion

E. Retractions

F. Prolonged inspiration

Answer: A, B, D, E

Rationale: Status asthmaticus is characterized by chest tightness, tachycardia, breathlessness, cyanosis, confusion, retractions, prolonged expiratory phase, and rapidly progressing dyspnea. Therefore, options A, B, D, and E are correct.

Multiple-response items also provide excellent prompts for classroom discussion. Use one or two of this item format as a pre- or post-lecture quiz and have the students correct each other and discuss the results. This kind of exercise promotes critical thinking while familiarizing the students with an alternative item format. Additional examples of multiple-response items are illustrated in **Exhibits 5.59** and **5.60**.

Exhibit 5.59   Multiple-response item with rationale

A visiting nurse is assessing a client who has congestive heart failure. Which of these client findings should the nurse report to the primary care provider? Select all that apply.

A. Oxygen saturation 92%
B. Urine output of 25 mL/hr
C. Blood pressure of 116/72 mmHg
D. Recent weight gain
E. Confusion
F. Temperature of 99.0°F (37.2°C)

Answer: B, D, E

Rationale: Decreased urine output, weight gain, and confusion are indications of worsening heart failure. The circulation is decreased because the heart is failing, which leads to decreased perfusion of the kidneys, decreased urine output, and accumulation of fluid in the tissues (edema). Weight gain results from the edema, and confusion results from inadequate oxygenation of the brain. Options A, C, and F are not indications of worsening heart failure.

Exhibit 5.60   Multiple-response item with rationale

Which of these measures should a nurse include when preparing a client for a thoracentesis? Select all that apply.

A. Explain to the client that the procedure will require general anesthesia.
B. Check that the client has signed a consent form.
C. Advise the client not to cough during the procedure.
D. Tell the client to stay NPO for 12 hours before the procedure.
E. Obtain the client's baseline vital signs.

Answer: B, C, E

Rationale: Options A and D are incorrect. The client may receive a mild sedative before the procedure, but general anesthesia is not required. The client does not have to remain NPO before the procedure. Options B, C, and E are correct. The client will need to sign a consent form for this procedure, and baseline vital signs should be obtained. It is important to instruct the client not to cough during the procedure to avoid puncturing the lung.

Chart/Exhibit

This item type presents the student with a problem related to information in a chart. The student must analyze the information to answer the question. The NCLEX presents several tabs that each contain different pieces of information that mimic the current setup of a client's medical record. You can use this format model to determine whether your students can interpret information to solve a problem, as in **Exhibit 5.61**.

Exhibit 5.61 Chart interpretation with rationale

A nurse is preparing to administered digoxin to a client who has a serum digoxin level indicated in the chart below. Which of the actions listed below the chart should the nurse take?

Therapeutic Serum Digoxin Level	Client's Serum Digoxin Level
0.8 to 2 ng/ml	2.3 ng/ml

A. Document the finding and administer the digoxin
B. Hold the dose of digoxin and notify the physician *
C. Obtain the client's electrocardiogram before giving the digoxin
D. Administer the client's prn dose of Digibind

Rationale: Option B is correct; the client's digoxin level is above the therapeutic level so the client cannot safely receive the dose of digoxin. The nurse should hold the dose and notify the client's primary care provider. Options A, C, and D are not correct.

Graphic Interpretation

This format presents the student with a graphic instead of text. The students must interpret the graphic in the stem or select the correct graphic option to receive credit for the correct answer.

Exhibit 5.62 Graphic interpretation with rationale

A nurse is caring for a client who is admitted to an emergency department with crushing chest pain. Which of these actions should a nurse take first when the client's cardiac monitor has the reading below?

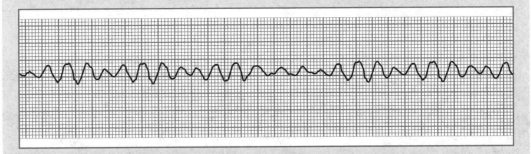

A. Administer prescribed epinephrine
B. Check the client's carotid pulse*
C. Start cardiopulmonary resuscitation
D. Prepare for immediate defibrillation

(continues)

Exhibit 5.62   Graphic interpretation with rationale (*Continued*)

Rationale: Option B is correct. The first action of the nurse when ventricular fibrillation (v fib) is noted on the cardiac monitor is to check the client's pulse to be sure the cardiac monitor is not malfunctioning. The nurse should then call for help while initiating CPR. The client must be defibrillated immediately once help arrives. If fibrillation continues for more than a few minutes, the client could suffer permanent brain damage. Defibrillation delivers a strong electrical current that depolarizes the myocardium and allows the heart's natural pacemaker to control the heart's rhythm. Epinephrine may be used for v fib that persists after defibrillation.

Ordered Response

Ordered response items require students to prioritize. The students must drag the options from one column to a second column in order of priority, as shown in **Exhibit 5.63**. As with the other alternate item formats, partial credit is not granted for ordered response items. The student must place the options in the correct order to receive credit for this item type. If your scanning program does not support scoring this type of item, you could set it up as a matching column. This format also lends itself to class discussion. Present an ordered response item at the end of a lecture and ask the students to discuss the order of the steps for a procedure, for example. A lively discussion is guaranteed and this exercise will familiarize the students with the ordered response format.

Exhibit 5.63   Ordered response

A nurse prepares to instill ointment into a client's eye. After explaining the procedure to the client and checking the five rights, the nurse takes all these actions. Drag the actions from the first column and place them in order from first to seventh in the second column. All the actions must be used.

A. Put on gloves	1.
B. Tilt the client's head back	2.
C. Wash the hands	3.
D. Ask the client to look up	4.
E. Apply a thin line of ointment on the inside edge of the lower lid	5.
F. Document the instillation	6.
G. Instruct the client to gently close the eyes and rub the lid lightly	7.

You must be very careful when you ask students to order actions in priority, particularly because there is no partial credit for items. The actions of explaining to the client and checking the five rights is included in the stem because there could be a difference of opinion about where these actions fit in the sequence.

While it is always important to ask a colleague to review your items, it is particularly important with the ordered response and multiple-response items. You should be sure that the answers are irrefutably correct before you include them on an exam.

Item Rationale

An effective method for increasing the validity of your multiple-choice items is to write a rationale for each question. A quality rationale includes a textbook reference and explains why the correct answer is correct and also why each of the distractors is incorrect.

This explanation should be kept with the item in an electronic file, either in an item banking program or in a word processing file. Writing rationales for your items not only increases the quality of the items and ensures the veracity of the key, it also provides a valuable resource for student test review. Rationales are particularly useful for alternative format items. These items are challenging, both for the teacher to compose and the student to answer. Writing a rationale helps to reduce ambiguity and ensure the correctness of the key. Exhibits 5.58 through 5.62 provide examples of items with rationales.

Question Difficulty

While it is important not to trick or confuse students, it is just as important to present them with questions that challenge them and that are trustworthy measures of their abilities. Chapter 3, "Developing Instructional Objectives," reviews the cognitive levels and notes that the levels of knowledge, comprehension, analysis, and application are particularly suited to the development of multiple-choice items. Item writers should strive to develop items at the higher levels of application and analysis. In fact, nursing exams should not include any items at the knowledge level; comprehension-level items should be the lowest cognitive level item included on a nursing exam. Appendix D, "Targeting Cognitive Levels for Multiple-Choice Item Writing," provides lists of verbs and examples of items at the different levels of cognitive ability.

An item writer can manipulate the difficulty of items. The important principle is that the difficulty of the item should relate directly to the content and instructional objectives being measured. Keeping distractors homogeneous increases the difficulty level of the question because students have to make fine distinctions. Using the best-answer approach also increases the difficulty of the item. Refer to Chapter 4, "Implementing Systematic Test Development," for a discussion related to planning test difficulty.

Framing Questions in Terms of the Nursing Process

Using the nursing process as a framework for item development poses several advantages for crafting quality multiple-choice items. In addition to increasing the face validity of the test, it increases the pertinence of the questions that you ask. If you have to put a nurse and/or a client in every stem, you have to think about the relevance of the question for nursing practice. This approach helps to eliminate trivia from your tests.

Another advantage of the nursing process approach is that it promotes the development of unique situations in which to frame nursing problems. While nursing process questions can be written at all cognitive levels, the format encourages item development at higher levels. Novel situations can be designed that require students

---

Box 5.1 Phases of the nursing process

Assessing: Obtaining, confirming, and communicating data about a client.

Analyzing: Selecting relevant data, and drawing inferences and conclusions to identify potential and/or actual problems that require nursing assistance. Includes identifying nursing diagnoses and communicating results of analysis.

Planning: Making plans with the client and family to set goals and establish outcomes to deal with the identified problems. Includes prioritizing and communicating the plan.

Implementing: Includes actions, such as communicating, teaching, performing, or assisting with activities of daily living, and informing client and/or family about health status to achieve the established outcomes.

Evaluating: Gauging the client's response to the planned actions and the movement toward or away from identified goals. Determining the extent to which client outcomes have been achieved.

---

to analyze and/or apply information in real-life clinical settings rather than simply to recall facts.

It is clear that the nursing process format is viewed as a valuable framework for item writing. The items on NCLEX exams are written in terms of the nursing process. The current plan (NCSBN, 2016) integrates items written in the framework of the nursing process across the categories of client needs.

Following the example of the NCSBN in developing your items makes perfect sense because their item development standards are held to the highest level. The nursing process format is viewed by the NCSBN, one of the most respected test developers in the country, as a valuable method for framing items that address nursing concerns. Following the lead of the experts when writing items to assess the content and objectives of your course is a logical approach to improving the quality of your multiple-choice exams. **Box 5.1** provides definitions of the phases of the nursing process that can be used to guide the development of multiple-choice items.

Item Shells

An item shell is a successful item with its content removed, leaving only the stem. Appendix E, "Sample Item Stems for Phases of the Nursing Process," provides suggested item stems that are framed in the context of the nursing process. Appendix F, "Sample Items Stems for Client Needs Using the Nursing Process Format," provides guidance for integrating the NCLEX client needs with the nursing process in your test items. These stems are successful items with their content removed, hence the term *item shell*. Substitute your content, and your stem is written. The challenge of writing the correct option and several plausible distractors still remains, but these stems set you in the right direction for writing items within the client need and nursing process context that assess higher-order thinking. These item shells can also help you to revise your original current items or those adapted from a textbook item bank. Using these shells helps you to focus on writing items that test material of importance rather than the recall of trivial facts.

Although stems are useful as prompts to get you started with developing your own items, do not mistake them for templates for all item writing. It is important to have variety in the structure of items on a test; we do not want all the questions to be too similar. Use the suggested stems as a starting point for developing your own item-writing strategy and remember, it is critical that every item on the test relate to your test blueprint.

Peer Review

Item review by your colleagues is critical for developing effective test questions. Chapter 4, "Implementing Systematic Test Development," addresses the need for blueprint review; item review is equally important. A relevant blueprint designates what the items on the test should address. It is the teacher, however, who must ensure that the items actually meet the requirements of the blueprint. The relationship of each item to the content domain must be verified to ensure that the test actually represents the content.

In addition to verifying that the items meet the blueprint, item review involves editing and determining whether the items meet the guidelines presented in this chapter. Circulating items among colleagues for opinions and suggestions is a helpful method for addressing blueprint issues and improving item quality. Omit the answer key from the items. If an expert in the content area is unable to answer the question, it most certainly needs to be revised. The objective is not to find fault or criticize but only to critique the items based on agreed-on criteria to increase the quality of the items. Remember to ask your colleagues to pay close attention to the wrong answers as well as the correct ones. Most problems that occur on a test are with the distractors. Make sure that the incorrect options are absolutely incorrect. The questions in **Box 5.2** summarize the guidelines presented in this chapter. Use these questions as a checklist for critiquing multiple-choice items.

Allowing an adequate time frame for blueprinting and item development increases the likelihood that the items address the test plan. It is unrealistic to expect members of a teaching team to devote adequate time to editing and carefully examining the relevancy of test items on short notice. In fact, you will not be able to do a careful job of analyzing items yourself if you do not allow enough time.

Refer to **Box 5.3** when you are looking for a specific item example.

Box 5.2   Criteria for item review

Item Review: Does the item reflect the principles of item development?

Overall:
Does the item specifically fit the blueprint?
Does the item reflect an objective established for the course?
Does the item deal with an important aspect of the course content?
Is the item testing information that is important for a nurse to know?

(continues)

Box 5.2   Criteria for item review (*Continued*)

Is the item worded succinctly?
Does the item stand on its own?
Does the item contain any cues?
Is the meaning of the item clear?
Does the item contain any spelling or grammatical errors?
Is the item original (not a direct textbook quote)?
Is the item written at an appropriate reading level?
Does the item address higher-level cognitive ability?
Does the item follow the style guide agreed on by the faculty?
If the guidelines are not followed, is the item effective?

The Stem:
Does the stem address an objective of the course?
Does the stem present a single, clearly formulated problem?
Is there a nurse and/or a client in the stem?
Is the problem clearly stated in the stem without having to read the options?
Does the stem provide all the necessary information to solve the problem?
Is the stem clear without extraneous information?
Does the stem use the nursing process format?
Is the stem stated so that there is one, and only one, correct answer?
Is the stem phrased to avoid repetitive words in the options?
If the stem contains a negative word, is it unavoidable and *HIGHLIGHTED*?
Is the stem longer than any of the options?

The Options:
Do the options overlap?
Are the options homogeneous? Are options placed in logical order?
Are distractors incorrect yet plausible?
Are there degrees of correctness for best-answer questions?
Are all distractors completely incorrect so that only one correct answer is provided?
Has the position of the correct answer been randomly placed?
Are all options grammatically correct and consistent with the stem?

Box 5.3   Exhibit reference list

Exhibit 5.1 Multiple-choice format
Exhibit 5.2 Question stem format
Exhibit 5.3 Completion stem format
Exhibit 5.4 Confusing homonym
Exhibit 5.5 Confusing homonym and colloquialism
Exhibit 5.6 Connected items
Exhibit 5.7 Grammatical inconsistency, with revision
Exhibit 5.8 Misplaced modifiers
Exhibit 5.9 Internal blank
Exhibit 5.10 Incomplete versus complete stem
Exhibit 5.11 Incomplete versus complete stem
Exhibit 5.12 Diffuse versus succinct stem
Exhibit 5.13 Diffuse versus succinct stem
Exhibit 5.14 Unfocused versus focused stem

Summary

Expertise in multiple-choice item writing is an ability that develops with practice over time. Because quality test items are essential for the validity and reliability of the results of your classroom exams, you need to develop this expertise. This chapter is designed to provide you with direction for becoming a proficient item writer. These guidelines are related only to the mechanical aspects of the item-writing process that can be discussed and practiced, however. While they provide important direction, your creativity and clinical expertise are just as important to successful item writing. To write multiple-choice exams that provide valid and reliable results, you need to cultivate your expertise in both aspects of the process. Chapter 6, "Writing Critical Thinking Multiple-Choice Items," specifically addresses how to call on your creative abilities when writing items that assess critical thinking. The chapters that follow provide additional guidance to assist you with objectively analyzing and improving your item-writing ability in both the selected-response and constructed-response item formats.

Learning Activities

1. Describe the advantages and disadvantages of the multiple-choice item format.
2. Write the following completion format stem in the question format using a chart for the client findings:

   A nurse is assessing a client who had repair of a fractured femur 12 hours ago. The nurse should recognize that the client may be developing a fat embolism when the client develops

   A. total cholesterol of 260 mg/dL.

   B. a pulse rate of 92/min.

   C. a respiratory rate of 28/min.*

   D. blood pressure of 100/68 mmHg.

3. Rewrite the item in Learning Activity 2, but this time have the nurse intervene to solve a problem.
4. Identify six qualities of an effective multiple-choice item. Write two multiple-choice items that incorporate those qualities.
5. Revise this stem and write an item that keeps the actions in the options: How should a nurse ambulate a client who is blind?
6. Revise this item with a positive stem: The nurse recognizes that all of the following can precipitate hypoglycemia in an individual who is taking insulin *except*:

   A. increased exercise.

   B. a stomach virus.

   C. skipping a meal.

   D. skipping an insulin dose.*

7. Develop five multiple-choice items, one for each of the formats below:
   - Multiple response
   - Chart/exhibit
   - Ordered response
   - Action in the options
   - Identify priority

8. Develop five multiple-choice items, one for each phase of the nursing process. Use the same client situation for each item and identify how each phase of the nursing process would apply to that client.

9. Develop eight multiple-choice items, one for each of the client needs. Relate each of the items to an objective in a course you are teaching or plan to teach.

Web Links

Bloom's Taxonomy

http://www.krummefamily.org/guides/bloom.html

https://en.wikipedia.org/w/index.php?title=Bloom%27s_taxonomy&utm_campaign=elearningindustry.com&utm_source=%2F

Revised Bloom's Taxonomy

http://www.utar.edu.my/fegt/file/Revised_Blooms_Info.pdf?utm_campaign=elearningindustry.com&utm_source=/how-to-write-multiple-choice-questions-based-on-revised-bloom-s-taxonomy&utm_medium=link

Educational Resources Information Center

http://www.eric.ed.gov

National Council of State Boards of Nursing

http://www.ncsbn.org

References

Anderson, L. W. (2003). *Classroom assessment: Enhancing the quality of teacher decision making*. Mahwah, NJ: Lawrence Erlbaum Associates.

Brookhart, S. M., & Nitko, A. J. (2014). *Educational assessment of students* (7th ed.). Upper Saddle River, NJ: Pearson Education.

DiBattista, D., & Kurzawa, L. (2011). Examination of the quality of multiple-choice items on classroom tests. *The Canadian Journal for the Scholarship of Teaching and Learning, 2*(2), 1–23.

Haladyna, T. M. (2004). *Developing and validating multiple-choice test items* (3rd ed.). Mahwah, NJ: Lawrence Erlbaum Associates.

Klisch, M. L. (1994). Guidelines for reducing bias in nursing examinations. *Nurse Educator, 19*, 35–39.

Miller, M. D., Linn, R. L., & Gronlund, N. E. (2009). *Measurement and assessment in teaching* (10th ed.). Upper Saddle River, NJ: Pearson Education.

National Council of State Boards of Nursing. (2016). *What the exam looks like*. Retrieved from https://www.ncsbn.org/9010.htm

Popham, W. J. (2003). T*est better, teach better: The instructional role of assessment*. Alexandria, VA: Association for Supervision and Curriculum Development.

Reynolds, C. R., Livingston, R. B., & Wilson, V. (2008). *Measurement and assessment in education* (2nd ed.). Boston, MA: Allyn & Bacon.

Schoolcraft, V. (1989). *A nuts-and-bolts approach to teaching nursing*. New York, NY: Springer.

Trice, A. D. (2000). *A handbook of classroom assessment*. New York, NY: Longman.

Wendt, A. (2003). The NCLEX-RN examination: Charting the course of nursing practice. *Nurse Educator, 28*, 276–280.

© Anteromite/Shutterstock

Writing Critical Thinking Multiple-Choice Items

6

"Man's mind stretched to a new idea never goes back to its original dimensions."

—OLIVER WENDELL HOLMES

Critical thinking is a complex process. Consequently, assessing critical thinking ability is a complex process that presents a unique challenge to nursing faculty. While the guidelines for multiple-choice item development presented in Chapter 5, "Selected-Response Format: Developing Multiple-Choice Items," form the essential basis for creating critical thinking multiple-choice items, that is only the beginning of the process. Writing critical thinking multiple-choice items requires that you think critically yourself—that you call on all of your own reasoning and creative skills to assist you in assessing the behaviors that represent the characteristics of critical thinking in your students.

Introducing Critical Thinking Items

Higher-level thinking can be applied to basic content. The premise that students should be gradually introduced to items that require higher cognition skills is flawed. What good is information if you cannot apply it? If students cannot solve problems involving fundamental concepts, how will they be able to solve problems involving complex client care? If they are in a basic course, they need to be thinking about the basic content. As they progress through a nursing program and the content becomes increasingly complex, they need to think about the complex course content. Students should be required to think critically all along the way as they progress from the basic to the more complex. How are they going to develop critical thinking skills if they are not required to think from the very first day of a nursing program? Multiple-choice exams in nursing education should contain only higher cognitive level items throughout the program.

This chapter includes 40 exhibits containing examples of items that illustrate the suggested critical thinking item development guidelines. Box 6.1 includes a reference list of the sample items included in this chapter.

Characteristics of Critical Thinking Items

Multiple-choice items can play an important role in a multifaceted approach to the assessment of critical thinking. To contribute effectively to that assessment, multiple-choice items must be focused on measuring higher-order thinking ability; recall and comprehension items cannot effectively assess the cognitive processes associated with critical thinking. Incorporating higher levels of cognition when developing items is the basic criterion for measuring critical thinking with multiple-choice items. This criterion applies to all formats of critical thinking measurement instruments. It is of particular concern in the development of multiple-choice items, however, because it is so convenient to write these items at the recall and comprehension levels.

Although the ability to address higher levels of cognition is a key attribute of effective critical thinking multiple-choice items, it is certainly not the only requirement. An appreciation of the characteristics of multiple-choice items that support their ability to assess critical thinking will assist you in developing these items successfully.

Critical Thinking and the Nursing Process

An effective approach for writing items to assess critical thinking in nursing is to develop them in the framework of the nursing process. Using the nursing process model increases the relevance of the question for nursing practice and also promotes the development of novel situations (see Chapter 5, "Selected-Response Format: Developing Multiple-Choice Items").

The stems in Appendix E, "Sample Item Stems for Phases of the Nursing Process", and in Appendix F, "Sample Item Stems for Client Needs Using the Nursing Process Format" provide a useful foundation for writing critical thinking multiple-choice items. Use these templates to assist in revising or developing new multiple-choice items. Writing items using the nursing process framework in a clinical setting will remove trivia from your exams.

Sequential Reasoning

Although the retention of information is required to determine the solution to a critical thinking problem, requiring the ability to use the information in a unique situation distinguishes a critical thinking multiple-choice question from an item requiring lower-level cognitive skills. Recall- or comprehension-level questions do not tap the abilities that comprise critical thinking skills. As the recall question in **Exhibit 6.1** illustrates, questions at the lower levels of cognition call for rote memorization. Students are called on to choose from the proposed options based on recollection; they are not required to solve a problem.

Exhibit 6.1   Recall question

The dose of intravenous heparin should be adjusted to maintain a client's activated partial thromboplastin time (APTT) at how many times the control?

A. Less than 1.5
B. Between 1.5 and 2.5*
C. Greater than 2.5 and less than 3.5
D. Between 3.5 and 4.5

This question simply requires the student to recall that the client's APTT should be between 1.5 and 2.5 times the control.

Sequential reasoning is the key to writing questions that require critical thinking. Sequential reasoning requires more than just simple recognition: It is a process of deliberation that requires at least two logical steps. Knowing is not enough; students have to remember and then analyze or apply their knowledge.

Critical thinking multiple-choice items are written at the cognitive levels of application and analysis. They require students to use sequential reasoning to solve the problem presented by the question. Appendix D, "Targeting Cognitive Levels for Multiple-Choice Item Writing," presents suggestions for applying cognitive levels to item writing. The guide in this appendix is designed to assist you in developing your multiple-choice items so they meet the basic criterion for critical thinking assessment: measuring the application and analysis levels of cognition. Be careful not to confuse the cognitive level of analysis with the nursing process phase of analysis. While questions related to the analysis phase of the nursing process are frequently written at the cognitive level of analysis, items can be written at the cognitive levels of analysis and application for all phases of the nursing process.

A critical thinking item requires students to draw on their nursing knowledge, to approach the problem from more than one viewpoint, and to apply concepts to select the alternative that proposes an appropriate (or the most appropriate) solution to the problem. Exhibit 6.1 is an example of a recall level item. **Exhibit 6.2** presents a revision of Exhibit 6.1 that demonstrates how to apply sequential reasoning to increase the cognitive level of an item.

Exhibit 6.2   Application question

A client who is receiving intravenous heparin has an APTT of 2.5 times the control. Which of these actions would be appropriate for a nurse to take?

A. Call the lab for a stat repeat of the test
B. Discontinue the client's heparin infusion immediately

(continues)

Exhibit 6.2   Application question (*Continued*)

C. Continue to monitor the client*

D. Alert the blood bank to have a unit of packed cells available

This question takes the recall question of Exhibit 6.1 one step further. In addition to asking the student to recognize that the APTT should be between 1.5 and 2.5 times the control for a client who is receiving heparin, it requires the student to apply that information. Notice that the question calls for the student to select an appropriate action from among the listed actions. This critical thinking item does not include the universe of all possible options. Although the client's APTT is within the range in this question, it is at the top of the range. The nurse could also check the client's vital signs or observe for adverse effects, such as hematuria. However, the question asks the student to discriminate among the options offered, and only one is appropriate

---

Writing Original Critical Thinking Items

Applying sequential reasoning is the key to writing original items that assess higher cognitive levels. Follow these three steps for developing multiple-choice items that assess critical thinking:

1. Use the blueprint to identify a competency that relates to both the course content and a course objective.
2. Confirm that the competency is essential for safe entry level nursing practice.
3. Use the nursing process framework and the objective's learning outcomes to develop an item that assesses critical thinking in the clinical setting.

Suppose you are planning to write an item to determine if the students can recognize the manifestations of dehydration, an important competency. One approach would be to ask the student to select decreased blood pressure, as the correct answer in the recall item in **Exhibit 6.3** shows. Instead increase the

---

Exhibit 6.3   Recall versus sequential reasoning

Recall

Which of these findings should a nurse expect to identify when a client is dehydrated?

A. Bradycardia

B. Hypotension*

C. Decreased hematocrit

D. Increased urine output

Critical thinking

A client says to a nurse, "I have been vomiting for the past 8 hours and I haven't been able to drink any fluids." Which of these client findings should the nurse expect to identify?

A. Decreased pulse rate

B. Elevated blood pressure

C. Decreased hematocrit

D. Increased urine specific gravity*

---

problem-solving steps by using a more remote manifestation, one that is not so obvious, one that involves analysis. The critical thinking example in Exhibit 6.3 is a good example of a question related to basic content that requires the student to think. First, the stem does not identify the diagnosis of dehydration. A client would not wear a sign around his neck that says "dehydration"—the nurse has to figure it out. Instead, the stem quotes the client describing events that would certainly result in dehydration. The student has to analyze the statement and determine that the client has a fluid volume deficit, which would lead to increased urine specific gravity.

Exhibit 6.4 presents another example of using sequential reasoning to write an analysis item. The competency—recognizing objective data—is a basic one but certainly an important one.

Exhibit 6.4   Recall versus sequential reasoning

Recall

Which of these assessment findings would be an example of objective data?

A. Anxiety
B. Tachycardia*
C. Orthopnea
D. Dizziness

Critical thinking

A nurse identifies all of these findings when assessing a client. Which one is an example of objective data?

A. The client states, "I feel very shaky and nervous."
B. The client has a pulse rate of 140/min*
C. The client states, "I have to use two pillows to sleep at night."
D. The client reports having frequent episodes of dizziness

The original item in Exhibit 6.4 is straightforward recall; the student only has to remember the definition. The critical thinking version of the item presents the client findings as a nurse would encounter them in a clinical setting. The nurse has to interpret observations and client statements to determine that a client is anxious, has tachycardia, has orthopnea, or is experiencing dizziness. In this question, the nurse's observations are identified, and the student must interpret them to determine which finding represents objective data.

A third example of using sequential reasoning to develop a critical thinking item is demonstrated in **Exhibit 6.5**. Again, the first example requires recall of a definition, while the critical thinking example presents factors identified in the recall question and requires the students to interpret what they represent. The students have to interpret what the factors are and then decide which one represents an internal factor that influences health.

Exhibit 6.5   Recall versus sequential reasoning

Recall
Which of the following is an internal factor that influences health?

A. Economic status

B. Living in an urban area

C. Emotional factors*

D. Occupation

Critical thinking
Which of these factors, if identified in a client's history, should a nurse recognize as an internal factor that influences health?

A. Losing one's job

B. Living in a poor neighborhood

C. Grieving the loss of a spouse*

D. Working as an asbestos remover

The critical thinking item illustrated in **Exhibit 6.6** requires the student to recognize the desired outcome of intravenous therapy for hypovolemia and then to identify which of the proposed responses indicate the therapeutic response. The stem correctly uses the word *should* because the student is asked to interpret the data that are presented. There is only one correct answer—there are no degrees of correctness among these alternatives! The distractors are all incorrect. Note that, although additional assessments could indicate a successful outcome, such as increased blood pressure, the nurse is interpreting the data at hand from among these alternatives.

Exhibit 6.6   Evaluate outcomes

A client who has hypovolemia is receiving an intravenous infusion. A nurse should identify that the infusion is having the desired effect if the client develops an increase in which of these assessments?

A. Thirst

B. Heart rate

C. Urine output*

D. Pulse pressure

This critical thinking item requires the student to recognize the desired outcome of intravenous therapy for hypovolemia and then to identify which of the proposed responses would indicate that therapeutic response. The most recognizable outcome of increased blood volume is elevated blood pressure. An item that requires critical thinking should require the student to think past the most obvious. This item does just that. The student has to think through the process based on an understanding of physiology. When blood volume is increased, the blood pressure rises and the kidneys receive increased perfusion, which results in an increase in urine output.

Revising Items to Assess Critical Thinking

While most faculty develop some of their own original items, many of the items that they include in their classroom exams are from textbook item banks or from exams that were previously used in the nursing program. These are valuable resources for item ideas, but there are often serious flaws that prevent these items from providing you with the information you need to make decisions about students (Clifton & Schriner, 2010; Masters et al., 2001). Once you determine that an item is not assessing trivial information, it can be revised to meet the criteria of sequential reasoning for a critical thinking item. Ask these three questions:

1. Is the item assessing a competency that is integral to the course domain and included in the blueprint?
2. Is the competency essential for safe entry-level practice?
3. Can the item be rewritten in the nursing process framework to challenge the students to use critical thinking in a clinical setting?

Refer to **Exhibit 6.7**. Although the competency is important for safe entry-level practice, the original item is simple recall. The student has to remember that laryngeal nerve damage is a potential complication of a thyroidectomy. Problem solving is not necessary; memorization is all that is required. The student does not even have to understand what laryngeal nerve damage is.

Exhibit 6.7   Recall revised to application

Recall

A nurse should monitor a client who has had a thyroidectomy for signs of

A. laryngeal nerve damage.*
B. increasing intracranial pressure.
C. carotid artery distension.
D. hypercalcemia.

Application

Which of these nursing measures should be carried out at regular intervals when caring for a client during the immediate postoperative period after a thyroidectomy?

A. Asking the client to speak*
B. Checking the client's pupillary response
C. Palpating the client's carotid arteries
D. Instructing the client to flex and extend the neck

Instead of asking for simple recall, this question asks the students to understand the potential complication and plan measures for early identification of the problem.

The revision in Exhibit 6.7 demonstrates how sequential reasoning increases the cognitive level to application. The student must know that laryngeal nerve damage is a potential problem and must understand what laryngeal nerve damage is in order to determine what to do about it. The revision requires the nurse to *act*, not just to *know*.

The original item in **Exhibit 6.8** asks for simple recall of a definition, while the revision asks the student to apply the understanding of what specificity is in an actual situation. The student has to remember the meaning of specificity and then interpret findings based on that understanding. Note that the revised item also presents two sets of opposites.

Exhibit 6.8   Recall revised to analysis

Recall

A nurse is aware that a screening test has high specificity. This means that the test

A. provides precise findings.
B. correctly identifies those who have a disease.*
C. accurately identifies those who do not have a disease.
D. has a high correlation with severity of disease.

Analysis

A nurse who is planning a health screening program identifies that a particular screening test has a specificity of 90 percent. The nurse should recognize that this indicates that the test accurately identifies

A. 10 percent of those who actually have the disease.
B. 10 percent of those who do not have the disease.
C. 90 percent of those who actually have the disease.*
D. 90 percent of those who do not have the disease.

Rather than asking for recall of a definition, this item asks the student to interpret findings based on an understanding of the definition of the term. Note that the revised item also presents two sets of opposites.

Exhibit 6.9 is an example of a recall item that includes *teaching in the stem*. Even though it is tempting to impart just one more pearl of wisdom, a test is not the time for teaching. Students are expected to know that "a priority for this client is to reduce *ICP*" because that is what a test is about! However, we cannot be sure if increasing ICP is the priority in the original because we do not know when the stroke occurred. Also, notice that the action (positioning) is in the stem. These flaws contribute to confusion for this item and the item being at the recall level.

Exhibit 6.9   Recall revised to application

Original

The nurse is caring for a client diagnosed with a stroke. A priority for this client is to reduce intracranial pressure (ICP). Which of these positions is indicated to assist in reducing ICP?

A. Turn the client's head to the right side
B. Elevate the head of the bed*
C. Turn the client's head to the left side
D. Extend the client's neck

Revision

A nurse is planning care for a client who had a stroke 18 hours ago. Which of these measures is the priority in the client's care plan?

A. Keeping the head of the client's bed at 90 degrees*
B. Monitoring the client's intake and output
C. Orienting the client to the surroundings
D. Providing the client with passive range-of-motion exercises

The revision identifies when the stroke occurred and asks the student to figure out that ICP is the priority in this client's care. Note that this is an example of a *best*-answer item, All of the measures can be included in the client's care, as all are correct, but elevating the head to decrease ICP is the priority, and thus the correct answer to this question.

The original item in **Exhibit 6.10** only requires the student to know. Knowing is not enough in a critical thinking item. Sequential reasoning requires at least two steps. In addition, *respiratory arrest,* the original option A, is problematic. Students could reasonably argue that this is a correct answer.

Exhibit 6.10   Recall versus sequential reasoning

Original

A client is recovering from peritonitis following a ruptured appendix. A nurse should continue to monitor the client for which of these complications?

A. Respiratory arrest
B. Umbilical hernia
C. Abscess formation*
D. Urinary tract infection

Revision A

A client is recovering from peritonitis following a ruptured appendix. Which of these measures should the nurse include in the client's care plan?

A. Checking the client for a positive Homan sign
B. Monitoring the client's temperature*
C. Assessing the client for hematuria
D. Providing the client with a high-fiber diet

Revision B

A client is recovering from peritonitis following a ruptured appendix. Which of these measures should the nurse include in the client's care plan?

A. Checking the client for a positive Homan sign
B. Monitoring the client's white blood cell count*
C. Assessing the client for hematuria
D. Maintaining the client in low Fowler's position

Revision A is a critical thinking item because it does not tell the student what the complication is. Rather, it requires the student to identify that the potential problem is infection and to examine the alternatives to determine which option relates to that problem.

Revision B in Exhibit 6.10 is an example of a parallel item. When you develop an effective item, it is always a good idea to write a variation of the revision. You only need to change the correct option to have a new item that can be used on a parallel form of a test or a future test.

Exhibit 6.11 demonstrates how three revised items can be developed from a recall item. The options in the original are not heterogeneous. The only action in the item is the correct answer. The distractors only require knowing—the correct answer requires the nurse to do something.

Exhibit 6.11   Recall revised to application

Original

Your client is receiving furosemide 40 mg BID. You

A. know that this drug is classified as an osmotic diuretic.
B. are surprised when the client experiences polyuria.
C. are especially concerned that the client will develop hypernatremia.
D. weigh the client QD.*

Revision A

Which of these measures should a nurse include in the care plan for a client who is taking furosemide?

A. Weighing the client daily*
B. Straining all of the client's urine
C. Monitoring the client for hematuria
D. Obtaining the client's apical-radial pulse

Revision B: Parallel Item

Which of these measures should a nurse include in the care plan for a client who is taking furosemide?

A. Instructing the client to take the medication at bedtime
B. Monitoring the client's blood pressure*
C. Withholding the medication if the client develops polyuria
D. Assessing the color of the client's urine

Revision C: Parallel Item

Which of these measures should a nurse include in the care plan for a client who is taking furosemide?

A. Advising the client to change position slowly*
B. Instructing the client to avoid sun exposure
C. Restricting the client's fluid intake
D. Monitoring the client for hematuria

The revisions require critical thinking. The student must identify the potential problems associated with furosemide and select the action that addresses one of those problems. This item lends itself to the development of parallel items, which will be very useful for alternate exams.

Another typical recall question is illustrated in **Exhibit 6.12**. As long as the students can remember the effects of hypoglycemia, they will answer this question correctly.

The revision requires the student to think and reason out what can cause hypoglycemia. Notice that the word *hypoglycemia* is not even mentioned in the stem. The student has to understand that too much insulin results in hypoglycemia and analyze the manifestations to determine which are related to hypoglycemia. The item requires sequential reasoning.

Exhibit 6.12   Recall revised to analysis

Original

Hypoglycemia, a condition of low blood sugar, can produce episodes of

A. palpitations, sweating, and tremors.*
B. polyuria, polydipsia, and weakness.
C. dehydration, thirst, and loss of skin turgor.
D. deep, rapid breathing, fruity odor on the breath, and nausea.

Revision

Which of these manifestations, if identified in a client who has insulin-dependent diabetes mellitus (Type I), should a nurse recognize as an indication that the client may have taken too much insulin?

A. Frequent urination and thirst
B. Nausea and anorexia
C. Shakiness and sweating*
D. Fruity breath odor and polyuria

Exhibit 6.13 is an example of a confusing item. Basic editing must come first in order to apply sequential reasoning to this item. First, we need a clear statement of the client's condition. How advanced is the client's heart failure? Also, the correct answer is the longest and it identifies four manifestations, while the distractors have three each.

The revision clarifies that the nurse is looking for signs of worsening heart failure. The student has to identify what occurs with heart failure and select the manifestations that indicate deterioration. The revised item includes only two manifestations for each option, which keeps the question succinct and less confusing. Note that the revision also removes the client's age, as this information is extraneous, it is not relevant for solving the problem. **Exhibit 6.14** is another example of revising a recall item to assess critical thinking. The original item requires only memorization. The question to ask when revising this item is, "How is this content clinically relevant?" The revision does demonstrate why applying this content in a clinical setting is basic for safe nursing practice. When you encounter a question such as this, ask yourself, "So what? Why does this matter in clinical practice?" Then develop a stem that presents a clinical situation that addresses the competency.

Exhibit 6.13 Confusing revised to analysis

Original

A 70-year-old male is being seen in the clinic for heart failure. Which of the following findings are you most likely to observe in this situation?

A. Shortness of breath, orthopnea, paroxysmal nocturnal dyspnea, ankle edema*
B. Rasping cough, thick mucoid sputum, wheezing
C. Productive cough, dyspnea, weight loss, anorexia
D. Fever, dry nonproductive cough, bronchial breath sounds

Revision

A nurse is assessing a client who has heart failure. Which of these findings would indicate that the client's condition is deteriorating?

A. Dyspnea and tachycardia*
B. Productive cough and weight loss
C. Wheezing and thick mucoid sputum
D. Fruity breath odor and lethargy

Exhibit 6.14 Recall revised to analysis

Original

The body organ from which the excretion of drugs and their metabolites primarily occurs is the

A. kidneys.*
B. intestines.
C. skin.
D. lungs.

Revision

Which of these clients is at highest risk for inadequate excretion of ingested medications and their metabolites?

A. A 24-year-old client who has kidney failure*
B. A 32-year-old client who has liver failure
C. A 54-year-old client who has intestinal obstruction
D. A 75-year-old who has benign prostatic hypertrophy

The original item in **Exhibit 6.15** is a good example of how a recall item measuring a basic competency can be revised to require critical thinking. The original item is extremely easy. Notice that the action is in the stem; the student only has to select true or false. The revision removes the action from the stem, removes the gender from the nurse, and uses distractors that are common misconceptions. It is not difficult, but remember we are asking students to think about very basic content. We are reinforcing their critical thinking skills.

Exhibit 6.15   Recall revised to application

Original

If at any time during hand washing the nurse suspects that he has contaminated his hands, he should begin again from the beginning of the procedure.

A. True*
B. False

Revision

A nurse suspects that the hands have been contaminated during hand washing. Which of these actions should the nurse take?

A. Rinse the hands for an extra 30 seconds
B. Put on gloves before providing client care
C. Start again from the beginning of the procedure*
D. Increase the temperature of the water

Another technique for revising recall items that are testing basic content is to create a unique situation, one that requires the students to consider if this situation might be an exception to the rule. The original item in **Exhibit 6.16** asks a straight-forward question, while the revision adds a few subtle circumstances that require the students to determine if the rule applies in this case. In the revision, the transporter is complaining loudly, and a second client is in jeopardy in the bathroom. Will these events alter the required action? The students have to think this through and decide.

Exhibit 6.16   Unique situation

Original

After preparing a preoperative injection for a client, a nurse says to a student, "Can you please give this for me." Which action should the nursing student take?

A. "I can give it if you watch me."
B. "Let me ask my instructor."
C. "You should ask another registered nurse to give the injection."
D. "I cannot give an injection that you prepared."*

Revision

A nurse enters a client's room to give a preoperative injection. The transporter is in the hall complaining loudly about waiting for the client. Suddenly a client calls from the bathroom, "Help, I feel like I'm going to have a seizure." The nurse hands the injection to a student who is in the room and says, "Give this for me. I have to help the client in the bathroom." Which of these responses should the student make?

A. "You give the injection. I'll help the client in the bathroom."*
B. "Okay, in this situation I can give the injection for you."
C. "I'll have to check with my instructor to see if I can prepare a new injection."
D. "Leave the injection on the nightstand. I'll help you with the client in the bathroom."

Application- and analysis-level items such as these are appropriate throughout a nursing program. Thinking is essential in nursing. The cognitive levels of the items should always be at a higher level throughout a nursing program. We must require students to think about concepts that become more complex as the students progress though the program.

Best-Answer and Priority Format

Chapter 5, "Selected-Response Format: Developing Multiple-Choice Items," introduced the best-answer format. The best-answer format is particularly suited to the development of critical thinking multiple-choice items because higher-level cognitive skills are required to determine which alternative is the best, the first, the priority, or the most important. Remember, it is necessary that all options vary in degree of correctness, with one being the best answer. If the distractors have no element of correctness, then do not use the best-answer format. With this format, shown in **Exhibit 6.17**, the student must first use sequential reasoning to solve the problem and then differentiate between the degrees of correctness of the proposed options to determine which option is the priority.

Exhibit 6.17   Best-answer critical thinking item

A nurse plans all these measures for a client who was rescued from a fire and has a deep burn injury of the chest and arms. To which of these measures should the nurse assign priority during the emergent phase of burn management?

A. Monitoring the client's respiration*
B. Assessing the client's peripheral circulation
C. Measuring the client's urine output
D. Preventing the client from developing infection

This question requires the student to identify the treatment plan for a client who has a burn injury. The student must identify the threat to the airway from this type of injury to discriminate between degrees of correctness among the options to select the best answer.

Exhibits **6.18** to **6.21** provide four more examples of items that require the students to determine the degree of correctness of a group of options to select the best answer.

Exhibit 6.18   Best-answer critical thinking item

Which of these nursing actions is the priority when a client who has a fever of unknown origin is to be started on intravenous antibiotic therapy?

A. Review the client's white blood cell count
B. Ensure that the client's blood culture is drawn*
C. Obtain the client's body temperature
D. Increase the client's oral fluid intake

All these interventions are important in the care of this client. The student must use sequential reasoning to determine that option B is the priority.

Exhibit 6.19   Best-answer critical thinking item

A client who is hospitalized for treatment of exacerbation of chronic obstructive pulmonary disease (COPD) has all of the these prescriptions. Which one should the nurse implement first?

A. ciproflaxin 500 mg po q 12 hours

B. methylprednisilone 100 mg IVPB q 4 hours

C. albuterol 5 mg via nebulizer q 4 hours*

D. quaifenesin 200 mg q 4 hours

The student must analyze the client's situation to determine which prescription should be implemented first. This item can be adapted to a variety of client situations where the student must determine which prescription to implement based on the client's situation.

Exhibit 6.20   Best-answer critical thinking, with rationale

Which of these assessments is the most effective way to determine the need for oxygen for a client who has emphysema?

A. Determine the client's level of fatigue

B. Check the client's hemoglobin level

C. Ask the client to rate respiratory distress on a scale of 1 to 10

D. Obtain the client's pulse oximetry reading*

Rationale: The pulse oximeter reading is the most effective way to determine the client's oxygen saturation level. The client who has emphysema should receive oxygen therapy based on this reading. Options A, B, and C are important assessments, but they are not effective measures for determining a client's need for oxygen.

Exhibit 6.21   Best-answer critical thinking, with rationale

A nurse finishes receiving a change-of-shift report for all of these clients at 7:15 a.m. Which client should the nurse assess first?

A. A 32-year-old client who is receiving humidified oxygen and is scheduled for a bronchoscopy at 9 a.m

B. A 46-year-old client who was diagnosed yesterday with laryngeal cancer and was awake and crying most of the night

C. A 55-year-old client who is scheduled to receive chemotherapy for treatment of lung cancer at 8 a.m. The client must receive premedication 30 minutes prior to receiving chemotherapy*

D. A 65-year-old client who has pneumonia and a temperature of 101.4°F (38.5°C) and is receiving intravenous antibiotics

Rationale: Option C is the priority. The client needs to receive the premedication so that the chemotherapy can start on time. Clients A and D are stable, and client B needs emotional support, which can be attended to once the physiological needs of the other clients are met.

Novel Problems

A critical thinking multiple-choice question must propose a novel problem for students to solve. If the students are familiar with the problem, the question is a recall item, even if an item appears to be at a high cognitive level. For this reason, only the teacher can determine the true cognitive level of an item.

If you use a situation as an example in class, you cannot convert it to a test item and use it on a test for the same group of students. If you translate a situation that occurred in the clinical setting with a group of students into a test item, you cannot use it on a test with that group of students. This is not to say that you should not use real-life experiences as models for test items; you certainly should. Just be careful that you bank those items for exams that will be given to a group of students who have not been exposed to the situation.

The more unique the situation in a question, the more its solution involves the use of critical thinking skills. A familiar or textbook situation requires only that the students use recall. Unique situations require that students analyze and synthesize information to determine a course of action, as **Exhibit 6.22** illustrates.

Exhibit 6.22   Unique situation

An elderly client is about to have a minor surgical procedure. The client says to a nurse, "I really don't know why it is so important for me to have this surgery." The nurse notes that the client has signed a consent form for the surgery. Which of these actions should the nurse take?

A. Discuss nonsurgical treatments with the client and document the discussion in the client's medical record

B. Reassure the client that this is minor surgery and that the surgeon has an impeccable reputation for performing only surgery that is beneficial for clients

C. Contact the client's adult children to determine whether they understand the need for the surgical procedure

D. Inform the surgeon that the client does not understand the need for surgery*

This situation introduces several factors that make it unique: the client is elderly, the procedure is minor, the consent is already signed, and the client is not yet medicated. The question requires the student to analyze the information to identify the important principle. Note that none of the information is extraneous. All the information in the stem works to establish a unique situation, and each of the options relates to the stem.

Identifies Situations That Require Modification

An important role of the nurse is to analyze a situation and intervene appropriately when necessary. **Exhibit 6.23** presents a situation that requires sequential reasoning to determine which finding requires intervention, and **Exhibit 6.24** requires the student to analyze the situation to determine which action to take immediately.

Exhibit 6.25 presents a supervision item that requires the student to identify which situation requires modification. In this case, the student has to identify which action the charge nurse should correct.

Exhibit 6.23   Situation requiring modification

A client is in the postanesthesia unit after having a transurethral prostatectomy with epidural anesthesia. The client has a Foley catheter attached to continuous bladder irrigation and is receiving an intravenous infusion of 5% normal human serum albumin solution. A nurse should initiate immediate action if the client

A. reports having low back pain.*
B. has a pulse oximetry reading of 94%.
C. is unable to move his lower extremities.
D. has clots draining in the bladder irrigation fluid.

This question requires the student to analyze the situation to identify which client response requires intervention and which are acceptable findings.

Exhibit 6.24   Situation requiring modification, with rationale

A client who has right-sided heart failure suddenly becomes agitated and restless. A nurse assesses the client as having bilateral crackles at the bases of the lungs and having tachycardia. Which of these actions should the nurse take immediately?

A. Prepare the client for intubation
B. Administer the client's prescribed morphine
C. Notify the client's primary care provider
D. Put the client in high Fowler's position*

Rationale: Early signs of pulmonary edema, which is a complication of congestive heart failure, include restlessness, anxiety, tachycardia, dyspnea, and crackles at the bases of the lungs. Initial treatment of pulmonary edema includes maintaining the client in high Fowler's position to aid in lung expansion, administering oxygen, and notifying the client's primary care physician (PCP). Intubation and mechanical ventilation may be indicated and morphine has a sedating effect that decreases the client's anxiety, but these are not the initial actions.

Exhibit 6.25   Supervision, with rationale

A charge nurse observes a staff nurse taking all of these actions when caring for clients who are receiving oxygen therapy. Which action should the charge nurse correct?

A. Using a Venturi mask to deliver a precise concentration of oxygen to a client who has COPD
B. Applying a nasal cannula to deliver oxygen to a client at 3 liters per minute without humidification
C. Deflating the reservoir bag of nonrebreather mask when checking the client's vital signs*
D. Using a simple mask with humidification to deliver oxygen concentration of 50% to a client

Rationale: A nonrebreather mask is used to deliver high concentrations of oxygen. It has a reservoir bag that is inflated with pure oxygen. The mask should not be deflated because the client will breathe in exhaled carbon dioxide. Options A, B, and D are all acceptable actions.

Delegating in a Situation

One of the important responsibilities of a professional nurse is to delegate client care responsibilities. While total client care is never assigned to assistive personnel, it is essential that students are aware of the parameters for appropriately delegating tasks to assistive staff. **Exhibit 6.26** presents a simple delegation question that is at the recall level. The revision of this item introduces a situation that requires the student to analyze the situation to determine if the delegation is appropriate. **Exhibit 6.27** is another example of delegating in a situation.

Exhibit 6.26   Delegating in a situation

Delegating

Which of these tasks can a nurse assign to an unlicensed nursing assistant?

A. Monitoring a client's pedal pulses
B. Assessing a client's abdominal girth
C. Recording a client's Foley catheter output*
D. Teaching a client to use an incentive spirometer

Revision: Delegating in a Situation

Which of these tasks can a nurse assign to an unlicensed nursing assistant?

A. Monitoring the pedal pulses of a 36-year-old client who had a femoral-popliteal by-pass graft
B. Assessing the abdominal girth of a 56-year-old client who has cirrhosis
C. Recording the Foley catheter output of a 68-year-old client who has pulmonary edema*
D. Teaching a 72-year-old client who has emphysema to use an incentive spirometer

---

Exhibit 6.27   Delegating in a situation

A nurse is planning staff assignments. Which of these tasks should a nurse assign to a nursing assistant?

A. Monitoring vital signs for a 24-year-old client who had an appendectomy 4 hours ago
B. Reviewing bleeding precautions with a 45-year-old client who is receiving intravenous heparin
C. Teaching a 65-year-old client who is receiving inhalation therapy for acute asthma how to use an incentive spirometer
D. Providing morning care for a 78-year-old client who had a hip fracture repair 3 days ago*

Both Exhibits 6.26 and 6.27 present questions that measure the ability to discriminate when delegating responsibility. Note that client ages are included in the options because this adds an additional piece of information that the students must evaluate. Also note that, while the clients' diagnoses are serious, the tasks delegated to the nursing assistants in the correct answers are appropriate. The more relevant information that you include in a stem, the more discriminating the students must be to distinguish the correct answer. Just be careful to exclude extraneous information.

Multiple-Response

The multiple-response format, as described by the National Council of State Boards of Nursing (NCSBN, 2016), is a straightforward approach for assessing critical thinking that replaces the old, confusing multiple-multiple format. The multiple-response format is a useful design for developing items for classroom exams. While students generally find this format to be very challenging, multiple-response items are actually a series of true–false items. What makes this format challenging is that students must select all the correct options and none of the incorrect ones in order to receive credit for a correct answer. It is important to introduce the students to the alternate item types so they will become comfortable with the format. In addition, it is a very useful format for assessing critical thinking in classroom exams.

Before you introduce this item type in an exam, however, try examples of them in a classroom at the end of a class discussion. Advise students to approach the item as a series of true–false questions. Examining the item as a group will prompt the students to interact and use critical thinking to solve the problem presented in the stem. **Exhibits 6.28** through **6.32** provide examples for using the multiple-response format to assess critical thinking in a classroom multiple-choice exam.

Exhibit 6.28   Multiple-response format

A nurse is caring for a client who is about to ambulate for the first time after having surgery 2 days ago. Which of these actions should the nurse take before getting the client out of bed? Select all that apply.

A. Obtain the client's recumbent and sitting blood pressure *

B. Check the client for Homan's sign.

C. Have the client sit on the side of the bed for several minutes.*

D. Obtain the client's apical-radial pulse.

E. Discontinue the client's intravenous infusion.

This is a good example of a question testing basic content that requires students to select all that apply.

Exhibit 6.29   Multiple-response format

A nurse is planning care for a client who had a right hip replacement 3 days ago. Which of these actions should the nurse include? Select all that apply.

A. Instructing the client not to cross the legs*

B. Keeping the client on strict bed rest

C. Advising the client to use a raised toilet seat*

D. Teaching the client to bend at the waist when picking up items from the floor

E. Explaining that the client will have to use an abduction pillow for life

This item uses the select-all-that-apply format to test basic knowledge about care for a client who had a hip replacement. Notice that the item has five options, which is the minimum for this item type. You can have as many as nine options, but don't get carried away or you will introduce confusion. Also, you do not have to tell students how many options should be selected. Remember, the item is wrong if students do not select all of the correct options or if an incorrect option is selected.

Exhibit 6.30   Multiple-response format

Original

A client in the intensive care unit after surgery has developed disseminated intravascular coagulopathy (DIC). Which of these assessment findings are related to the diagnosis of DIC? Check all that apply.

A. Petechiae and ecchymoses on the skin and mucous membranes*
B. Bounding peripheral pulses
C. Prolonged bleeding from venipuncture sites*
D. Prolonged prothrombin time (PT)*
E. Decreased platelet count, and elevated fibrin split products*

Revision

A nurse is assessing a client who is being treated for disseminated DIC. Which of these findings, if identified in the client, should the nurse recognize as a manifestation of DIC? Select all that apply.

A. Bounding peripheral pulses
B. Decreased PT
C. Oozing at intravenous sites*
D. Increased heart rate*
E. Petechiae over the chest*
F. Decreased platelet count*
G. Ecchymotic areas on the skin*

The original item in this exhibit is confusing. Some of the options contain more than one finding. Are they both correct or incorrect? Instead, the revision has options that contain only one finding each.

Exhibit 6.31   Multiple-response format

A client who was in a motor vehicle accident is brought to an emergency department. The client has a cervical collar in place and is bleeding from a laceration on the thigh. Which of these measures should a nurse include when planning care for the client? Select all that apply.

A. Apply a tourniquet to the client's leg
B. Assess patency of the client's airway*
C. Maintain the client in supine position*
D. Obtain the client's vital signs*
E. Restrict the client to a clear liquid diet
F. Obtain an order for an indwelling urinary catheter
G. Establish intravenous access*

Exhibit 6.32   Multiple-response format, with rationale

Which of these measures should a nurse include in the care plan for a client who has a chest tube water-seal drainage system connected to suction? Select all that apply.

A. Report bubbling in the suction control chamber to the doctor

B. Encourage the client to cough and deep breathe every two hours*

C. Maintain an occlusive dressing to the chest tubes at the insertion site*

D. Monitor the water seal chamber for fluctuations with respiration

E. Reporting drainage of more than 100mL to the doctor*

Rationale: Bubbling in the suction control chamber is expected. It indicates that the suctioning is working. The client should be encouraged to cough and deep breathe. An occlusive dressing is recommended at the chest wall insertion site. The water seal should fluctuate with respiration if there is no external suction, which is not the case in this situation. Drainage over 100 mL should be reported to the primary health care provider.

Chart/Exhibit

The NCSBN (2016) describes the chart/exhibit format as an item that requires the examinee to read a chart or exhibit to solve the problem presented in the stem. This format is a valuable design that can be adapted for assessing critical thinking in classroom multiple-choice exams.

Let's examine two basic examples. **Exhibit 6.33** presents a very straightforward recall question. The students have to remember a laboratory value to answer correctly. No action or thinking is required.

Exhibit 6.33   Fundamental chart interpretation

Original

What is the normal serum digoxin level for a client receiving digoxin therapy?

A. 0.5 to 2 ng/mL

B. 0.5 to 20 ng/mL

C. 5 to 2 ng/mL

D. 5 to 20 ng/mL

Revision

A nurse is preparing to administer digoxin to a client who has a serum digoxin level indicated in the chart below. Which of the actions listed below the chart should the nurse take?

Digoxin Serum Level

Therapeutic level   0.8 to 2 ng/mL

Client's level   1.9 ng/mL

A. Document the finding and administer the digoxin*

B. Hold the dose of digoxin and notify the physician

C. Obtain the client's electrocardiogram before administering the digoxin

D. Administer the client's prn dose of digoxin immune fab

The revised item introduces a chart, asks students to interpret the finding, and requires an action. This is not a difficult item. In fact, it is very basic, but it requires the students to think. If you introduce the students to items like this, they will get used to thinking and not merely remembering.

The chart in **Exhibit 6.34** would also be appropriate on a test for an introductory nursing course. The question requires the student to analyze the data and determine which laboratory finding requires follow-up, then select a nursing action that is appropriate for that finding. While it is basic content, it is a question that involves sequential reasoning.

Exhibit 6.34   Chart interpretation

A nurse assesses a client and identifies the client laboratory data illustrated in the chart below:

	Normal Range	**Client Value**
Na	135–145 mEq/L	147 mEq/L
K	3.5–5 mEq/L	4.0 mEq/L
Ca	8.4–10.2 mEq/L	9.8 mEq/L

Which of these actions should the nurse take?

A. Encourage the client to increase fluid intake*

B. Check the client's electrocardiogram tracing

C. Remind the client to go for a bone density test

D. Check the client's apical-radial pulse

This item requires sequential reasoning to solve a problem related to a very basic concept. The client's sodium level is elevated. The students first have to interpret the chart and identify that the sodium is elevated, and then select the appropriate intervention to deal with the problem. It is up to you to decide whether to include the normal lab values.

The chart in **Exhibit 6.35** demonstrates how the same basic approach that was used in Exhibits 6.33 and 6.34 can be used as content becomes more complex. Exhibit 6.35 involves sequential reasoning at a more complex level than the charts in Exhibits 6.33 and 6.34. Students have to know the action of levothyroxine, interpret the meaning of the chart, and then select the appropriate action. Chart interpretation is a valuable tool for designing items that require critical thinking. In fact, these item types are currently used on the National Council Licensure Examination (NCLEX) (NCSBN, 2016). **Exhibits 6.36** through **6.40** provide a variety of examples that can be used as templates for developing multiple-choice items that incorporate charts for assessing critical thinking.

Exhibit 6.35   Chart interpretation

When assessing a client who has been taking levothyroxine for 2 weeks, a nurse identifies the client data illustrated in the chart below

	4/10/10	4/25/10
Pulse	64/min	76/min
Weight	152 lbs	149 lbs
T_3	70 ng/dL	80 ng/dL
T_4	4 ug/dL	5 ug/dL

Which of these actions should the nurse take?

A. Administer the levothyroxine and document the assessment findings*
B. Postpone giving the levothyroxine and request a repeat of serum T_3 and T_4
C. Hold the levothyroxine and notify the physician of the assessment findings
D. Check the client's apical-radial pulse before giving the levothyroxine

Exhibit 6.36   Graphic interpretation, with rationale

A nurse reviews a client's electrocardiogram tracing, as indicated below.

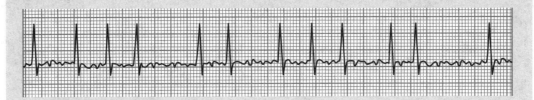

The nurse should document this tracing as indicating which of these arrhythmias?

A. Atrial fibrillation*
B. Ventricular fibrillation
C. Sinus arrhythmia
D. Premature ventricular contractions

Rationale: This tracing represents an arrhythmia/atrial fibrillation. An arrhythmia (also called dysrhythmia) is an abnormal rhythm of the heart, which can cause the heart to pump less effectively. Atrial fibrillation is a condition in which the electrical signals come from the atria at a very fast and erratic rate. The ventricles contract in an erratic manner because of the erratic signals coming from the atria.

Exhibit 6.37 Chart interpretation, with rationale

Prior to administering a calcium channel blocker to a client at 6 p.m., a nurse checks the client's blood pressure and reviews the client's previous blood pressures, as indicated in the table below.

6 a.m.	9 a.m.	12 p.m	3 p.m.	6 p.m.
120/88 mmHg	116/86 mmHg	118/84 mmHg	116/80 mmHg	94/66 mmHg

Which of these actions should the nurse take?

A. Hold the dose and notify the primary care provider (PCP)*

B. Administer the medication and document the blood pressure

C. Hold the dose and recheck the blood pressure in 30 minutes

D. Administer one half of the dose and reassess the client in 30 minutes

Rationale: Option A is correct. A client who is taking a calcium channel blocker requires careful monitoring of cardiac rates and blood pressure. In this case, the client's blood pressure has dropped significantly, and the PCP must be notified.

Exhibit 6.38 Chart interpretation, with rationale

A nurse assesses that a client has a respiratory rate of 12/min. The client's arterial blood gas results are documented in the table below. How should the nurse interpret these results?

	Client
pH	7.30
P_aCO_2	55 mmHg
HCO_3	26 mEq/L
P_aO_2	60 mmHg

A. Respiratory acidosis*

B. Metabolic acidosis

C. Respiratory alkalosis

D. Metabolic alkalosis

Rationale:

	Normal	Client
pH	7.35–7.45	7.30
P_aCO_2	35–45 mmHg	55 mmHg
HCO_3	22–26 mEq/L	26 mEq/L
P_aO_2	80–100 mmHg	60 mmHg

The pH is low, which indicates acidemia. The bicarbonate is normal and the P_aCO_2 is elevated. A high P_aCO_2 with a low pH indicates that the imbalance is respiratory acidosis. The client is hypoventilating and therefore retaining P_aCO_2.

Exhibit 6.39   Chart interpretation, with rationale

A client who has severe dyspnea is admitted to the hospital. The admitting nurse obtains the client's vital signs and history, completes a physical assessment, and reports the findings to the client's primary care provider (PCP).

Vital Signs	History	Physical Assessment
Pulse: 120/min	Completed a 12-hour airline	Hemoptysis
Respiration: 30/min	flight yesterday.	Pleuritic chest pain
B/P: 110/72 mmHg	Awakened from sleep this	Shallow breathing
Temperature: 99.4°F (37.4°C)	morning with sharp left-	Diaphoretic
	sided chest pain.	Anxious

The PCP writes prescriptions, which include all of these diagnostic tests for the client. Which one is the preliminary test that should be completed first?

A. Chest X-ray*

B. CT angiography

C. Electrocardiogram

D. Ultrasonography

Rationale: Information provided in the client's chart indicates the probability of a pulmonary embolism (PE). Initial evaluation for a pulmonary embolism includes the preliminary tests of chest X-ray and pulse oximetry. The chest X-ray may show focal infiltrates, atelectasis, or pleural effusion and will help exclude other diagnoses, but it is often nonspecific. ECG and arterial blood gases will help to rule out another diagnosis, such as a myocardial infarction More specific tests for diagnosing PE when preliminary tests are suspicious include:

- D-dimer testing
- CT angiography
- V/Q scanning
- Duplex ultrasonography

Exhibit 6.40   Chart interpretation, with rationale

A client who is in respiratory distress and complaining of chest pain is admitted to an emergency department. The admitting nurse obtains the client's vital signs and history, completes a physical assessment, and reports the findings to the client's primary care provider (PCP).

Vital Signs	History	Physical Assessment
Pulse: 120/min	Blunt force chest trauma	Diminished breath sounds
Respiration: 30/min	sustained in automobile	on right side
B/P: 96/72 mmHg	accident 1 hour ago.	Anxiety
Temperature: 99.4°F (37.4°C)		Dyspnea

(continues)

Exhibit 6.40 Chart interpretation, with rationale (*Continued*)

The PCP writes all of these prescriptions. Which one should the nurse question?

A. Arterial blood gases
B. Oxygen @4LPM via nasal cannula*
C. Portable chest X-ray
D. Prepare for thoracotomy

Rationale: It is important to read the question carefully. You are looking for the incorrect answer here. Option B is incorrect. It is recommended that a hospitalized client who is suspected of having a pneumothorax be treated with oxygen at high concentration. 100% oxygen should be administered immediately. Options A and C are correct. They are ordered to confirm the diagnosis as long as the client remains stable. Option D is also correct. Tension pneumothorax is a life-threatening event. A thoracotomy may be indicated to provide decompression if the client's condition deteriorates.

Summary

Developing critical thinking items is a challenge. The guidelines from Chapter 5, "Selected-Response Format: Developing Multiple-Choice Items," provide the framework, and the learning outcomes, established at the outset of the course, provide the natural basis for critical thinking multiple-choice item development. Your own creativity and critical thinking skills are needed to translate the specific behaviors that define these outcomes into items that assess higher-order thinking in the content domain, as specified in the test blueprint. This chapter builds on the basics and moves forward with direction and examples to help you improve your ability to create and evaluate critical thinking multiple-choice items. The key point is that multiple-choice items can play a valuable role in a systematic, multifaceted approach for the assessment of critical thinking learning outcomes.

In addition to providing you with direction for developing critical thinking multiple-choice items, the discussion in this chapter also reinforces the need for a comprehensive approach to the assessment of critical thinking. Although well-constructed multiple-choice exams can provide useful assessment information, there is certainly a need for a variety of approaches for assessing this complex construct. Students should be able to reason out their own solutions to complex questions, and it is important that faculty provide them with a variety of opportunities to do that. This chapter emphasizes that selecting the format that most effectively measures the outcomes you are assessing is fundamental to successful assessment of critical thinking. Chapter 7, "Selected-Response Format: Developing True–False and Matching Items," and Chapter 8, "Constructed-Response Format: Developing Short-Answer and Essay Items," propose suggestions for using these formats to assess critical thinking.

Refer to **Box 6.1** for a reference list of the sample items included in this chapter.

Box 6.1 Exhibit reference list

Exhibit 6.1 Recall question
Exhibit 6.2 Application question
Exhibit 6.3 Recall versus sequential reasoning
Exhibit 6.4 Recall versus sequential reasoning
Exhibit 6.5 Recall versus sequential reasoning
Exhibit 6.6 Evaluating outcomes
Exhibit 6.7 Recall revised to application
Exhibit 6.8 Recall revised to analysis
Exhibit 6.9 Recall revised to application
Exhibit 6.10 Recall versus sequential reasoning
Exhibit 6.11 Recall revised to application
Exhibit 6.12 Recall revised to analysis
Exhibit 6.13 Confusing revised to analysis
Exhibit 6.14 Recall revised to analysis
Exhibit 6.15 Recall revised to application
Exhibit 6.16 Unique situation
Exhibit 6.17 Best-answer critical thinking
Exhibit 6.18 Best-answer critical thinking
Exhibit 6.19 Best-answer critical thinking
Exhibit 6.20 Best-answer critical thinking, with rationale
Exhibit 6.21 Best-answer critical thinking, with rationale
Exhibit 6.22 Unique situation
Exhibit 6.23 Situation requiring modification
Exhibit 6.24 Situation requiring modification, with rationale
Exhibit 6.25 Supervision, with rationale
Exhibit 6.26 Delegating in a situation
Exhibit 6.27 Delegating in a situation
Exhibit 6.28 Multiple-response format
Exhibit 6.29 Multiple-response format
Exhibit 6.30 Multiple-response format
Exhibit 6.31 Multiple-response format
Exhibit 6.32 Multiple-response format, with rationale
Exhibit 6.33 Fundamental chart interpretation
Exhibit 6.34 Chart interpretation
Exhibit 6.35 Chart interpretation
Exhibit 6.36 Graphic interpretation with rationale
Exhibit 6.37 Chart interpretation, with rationale
Exhibit 6.38 Chart interpretation, with rationale
Exhibit 6.39 Chart interpretation, with rationale
Exhibit 6.40 Chart interpretation, with rationale

Learning Activities

1. Describe sequential reasoning. Identify the cognitive levels used to develop critical thinking multiple-choice items and explain how these levels require sequential reasoning.

2. Revise the following stems and develop four options to create an item that requires sequential reasoning:
   • Which of these findings should a nurse expect to identify when assessing a client who has hyponatremia?
   • A nurse is planning care for a client, who had surgery to create an ileostomy. Which of these measures should the nurse include during the immediate postoperative period?
   • Which of these measures is the priority in the management of care for a client who has severe renal colic?

3. Identify the questions you would ask when considering an item for revision. Answer those questions to revise the following three items.
   • Management of a client who has pneumonia includes all of the following EXCEPT:
   • A nurse should place a client who has asthma in which of these positions?
   • What is the most common complication of emphysema?

4. Revise the following item to require a chart interpretation:
   A nurse should observe a client who is in renal failure for
   A. metabolic acidosis.
   B. metabolic alkalosis.
   C. respiratory acidosis.
   D. respiratory alkalosis.

5. Develop one item in your area of expertise that requires students to prioritize.

6. Develop one item in your area of expertise that requires students to select all that apply.

7. Develop one item in your area of expertise that requires multiple response.

Web Links

Bloom's Taxonomy

http://www.krummefamily.org/guides/bloom.html

https://en.wikipedia.org/w/index.php?title=Bloom%27s_taxonomy&utm _campaign=elearningindustry.com&utm_source=%2F

Bloom's Taxonomy Revised

http://www.utar.edu.my/fegt/file/Revised_Blooms_Info.pdf?utm _campaign=elearningindustry.com&utm_source=/how-to-write-multiple-choice -questions-based-on-revised-bloom-s-taxonomy&utm_medium=linkEducational Resources Information Center

http://www.eric.ed.gov
National Council of State Boards of Nursing
http://www.ncsbn.org

References

Clifton, S. A., & Schriner, C. L. (2010). Assessing the quality of multiple-choice test items. *Nurse Educator, 35,* 12–16.

Masters, J., Hulsmeyer, S., Pike, M., Leichty, K., Miller, M., & Verst, A. (2001). Assessment of multiple-choice questions in selected test banks accompanying textbooks used in nursing education. *Journal of Nursing Education, 40*(1), 25–32.

National Council of State Boards of Nursing. (2016). *What the exam looks like.* Retrieved from https://www.ncsbn.org/9010.htm

Selected-Response Format: Developing True–False and Matching Items

"The greatest mistake you can make in life is to be continually fearing you will make one."

—ELBERT HUBBARD

In nursing education, as in many other disciplines, there is an unnecessary commitment to using the multiple-choice question format on classroom exams. This bias stems somewhat from the fact that so many professionally prepared standardized exams use only multiple-choice items. However, no item format is perfect for every situation. The cardinal principle applies to all testing situations: Avoid trivia and test only important concepts; then select the format that most effectively measures the outcomes you are assessing.

This chapter reviews true–false and matching exercises, two selected-response item formats whose value is often overlooked for efficiently assessing a number of important learning outcomes.

The True–False Item Format

A true–false (binary choice, alternate response) question presents a statement that requires the student to judge whether the statement is true or false, correct or incorrect, or right or wrong. The true–false format is often criticized for several reasons, but as Ebel and Frisbie (1991) maintain, the criticisms often relate to poorly constructed items, not to an inherent inferiority of the format. As with all item formats, developing quality true–false items requires practice; the most important skill one needs to develop is the ability to write clearly and succinctly.

163

Advantages of the True–False Item Format

The true–false item format has many advantages; most important, it can be used to measure higher cognitive levels when the items are constructed properly. True–false items provide an objective measurement that can sample a wide range of content simply and directly; in fact, they can sample a greater amount of material in a given time period than any other format. When compared with four-option multiple-choice items, a student can answer 50% more true–false items in the same amount of time. For example, a 75-item true–false test could be administered in the same time frame as a 50-item, four-option, multiple-choice test. Thus, the true–false format allows a broader sampling of course content than the multiple-choice format. In addition, true–false items are adaptable to all types of subject matter, can be developed to assess higher cognitive levels, are compatible with computerized scoring, produce reliable results, and can be analyzed and stored in an item bank for future use using test-development software.

Disadvantages of the True–False Item Format

The advantages and disadvantages of every format must be considered when selecting which one to use on a test. The results of true–false tests are not as reliable as multiple-choice tests. True–false items do not discriminate as well as multiple-choice items. They can lead to trivia testing, can be irrelevant, and can stress recall when poorly constructed. It is important to consider these limitations but also to recognize that the limitations can be counteracted.

The most consistent criticism of true–false items is that they are easy because they are conducive to guessing. Many experts discount the use of the format because students have a 50% chance of guessing the correct answer. However, as Brookhart and Nitko (2014) maintain, a distinction needs to be made between informed and blind guessing. Informed students realize that thinking is a better basis for determining the correct answer than blind guessing. In fact, the chance of obtaining a score of 80 on a 20-item exam using blind guessing alone is actually 2 in 1,000 (p. 160).

The true–false format is also criticized for being ambiguous and focusing on simple recall, which encourages memorization and rote learning. However, these criticisms relate only to poorly constructed true–false items, just as they would apply to poorly constructed items in any format. This chapter presents strategies to help you craft higher cognitive-level, discriminating true–false items.

While there are a variety of opinions about the value of the true–false item format, experts agree that it should be used only when there is a clear-cut true or false answer to the question. The statement must be indisputably correct or incorrect; adding qualifiers to a statement that is not clearly true or false results in a confusing item. The difficulty with writing these statements is seen as a disadvantage of this format.

However, these disadvantages are not only associated with the true–false format. Crafting items in any format requires practice. The first principle to remember is that the first draft of an item is often not acceptable. After you write an item, put it aside for a while and then review it again. Write a rationale for the correct and incorrect choices to be sure that you can defend the intended correct answer. Ask a colleague, preferably one who has test-writing experience, to critique it for you. Even then, be ready to edit it again after you actually administer the test.

Many of the guidelines discussed in Chapter 5, "Selected-Response Format: Developing Multiple-Choice Items," and Chapter 6, "Writing Critical Thinking Multiple-Choice Items," also apply to developing items in the true–false format. This chapter adapts some useful guidelines and offers additional ones that apply specifically to the true–false format. These suggestions will improve your ability to craft effective true–false items.

Guidelines for Developing True–False Exams

The importance of testing important concepts and avoiding trivia has been emphasized repeatedly in previous chapters. This principle cannot be overstated. To help determine the relevance of the material you plan to test, ask yourself, "Is mastery of this concept required to meet a course objective?"

Once you decide what to test, the next challenge is to develop exams with items that provide reliable information so that you can make decisions about student achievement in the domain you are testing. The suggestions that follow will help you develop skill in developing true–false test items that provide trustworthy information.

A number of expert educators (Ebel & Frisbie, 1991; Miller, Linn, & Gronlund, 2009; Brookhart & Nitko, 2014; Popham, 2003; Reynolds, Livingston, & Wilson, 2008) provide suggestions for developing true–false exams, and these suggestions overlap. The guidelines that follow reflect both the suggestions of experts and my own experience with developing true–false exams:

- Every question should test both content or concept and a course objective. This procedure eliminates trivia from your tests.
- The items should test only one idea. If you have more than one problem in the question and a student answers incorrectly, you will not know which problem the student could not solve.
- Make sure that the statements are indisputably correct or incorrect without qualifications. Compose a rationale in defense of the correct answers.
- Remove unnecessary words. Express the statements clearly and precisely. The goal is to determine if the students have attained the course objectives, not to see if they can decipher the questions.
- Have an approximately equal number of true and false as correct answers on the test. False items are more discriminating than true items because students tend to accept rather than reject a statement. Therefore, some experts suggest using more false items than true ones on an exam. Just be careful to avoid a pattern that prompts students to select the false response when they are in doubt about a question.
- Keep the length of all true–false statements approximately the same. Teachers often have the tendency to write longer true statements, which serves as a cue for test-wise students.
- Avoid patterns. Students look for patterns, so check the key before you print the test. Patterns such as T-T-F-F-T-T-F-F or T-F-T-F-T-F-T-F, for example, provide an obvious cue for test-wise students.
- Avoid repeating the same answer more than four times in a row. A long string of true answers (T-T-T-T-T), for example, could cause students to doubt their selection because the long string does not look right.

Characteristics of Effective True–False Items

Once you have determined the format for the overall exam, it is time to begin developing the individual items. The examples in **Exhibits 7.1** to **7.8** reflect the suggestions of several experts for writing true–false items (Ebel & Frisbie, 1991; Miller et al., 2009; Brookhart & Nitko, 2014; Popham, 2003; Reynolds et al., 2008).

Pairs   Effective items can be written in pairs. Writing true–false items in pairs, one true and one false, will help identify any ambiguity in the statements. Unless you can write a parallel but opposite statement, the statement does not make a good true–false item.

Exhibit 7.1   Pairs of items

T   F   A nurse should instruct a client who has chronic venous stasis to elevate the legs when sitting.

T   F   A nurse should instruct a client who has chronic venous stasis to sit with both feet on the floor, spread shoulder-width apart.

T   F   A nurse should advise a client who is taking furosemide to increase dietary potassium intake.

T   F   A nurse should advise a client who is taking furosemide to decrease dietary potassium intake.

These parallel items ensure that there is no ambiguity in either of the pairs. If you can write only the false version of the statement by using the word not, the statement is not a good candidate for a true–false item. Of course, only one of the pairs can be used on a test. Save the alternative for future use.

Ambiguity and Precision   Ambiguity causes confusion. The goal is to provide enough information while using simple, clear language that communicates precisely what you expect the student to know.

Exhibit 7.2   Ambiguous versus unambiguous statements

Ambiguous

T   F   A nurse should instruct a client who has elevated blood pressure to seek immediate medical attention.

Unambiguous

T   F   A nurse should instruct a client who has a blood pressure of 190/120 mmHg to seek immediate medical attention.

The first form of the question is not precise; it cannot be answered. How elevated is the client's blood pressure? It is important to be as specific as possible to avoid ambiguity. By specifying the client's actual blood pressure, the unambiguous version clearly indicates that the client needs immediate attention.

Exhibit 7.3   Ambiguous versus unambiguous statements

Ambiguous

T   F   Acceptance of one's own death represents the Maturity Stage of development.

Unambiguous

T   F   According to Erikson, acceptance of one's own death represents the Maturity Stage of development.

The first item cannot be answered. Referencing Erikson as the source of the stages of development adds the clarifying information necessary to remove ambiguity from the item.

One Idea   Keep the items focused on one problem to solve. One of the purposes of a test is to identify what a student does or does not know. If a student incorrectly answers a question that contains more than one idea, you cannot determine which idea the student did not understand.

Exhibit 7.4   Multiple ideas versus single concept

Multiple Ideas

T   F   Dyspnea is a common manifestation of left-sided heart failure, while weight gain is a common manifestation of right-sided heart failure.

Single Concept

T   F   Dyspnea is a common manifestation of left-sided heart failure.

T   F   Weight gain is a common manifestation of right-sided heart failure.

If a student answers the multiple-idea question incorrectly, we cannot determine which concept the student does not understand, or if the student does not understand both concepts. The single-concept format provides clearer information.

Important Concepts Writing   Items that assess trivial knowledge is easy, yet trivia provides you with irrelevant information. Challenging items that focus on important information are more difficult to write, but they help you determine whether students are attaining the objectives.

Exhibit 7.5   Trivial versus important concepts

Trivial

T   F   The incidence of encephalitis is 1 in 200,000 people.

Important Concepts

T   F   A nurse should position a client who has encephalitis with the head of the bed elevated 30 to 45 degrees.

One would have to ask, "Who cares?" in response to the first question. What relevance for nursing care does this memorized fact have? The revised question is clinically significant when one considers that encephalitis can cause elevated intracranial pressure.

Plausible Incorrect   As is the case with multiple-choice questions, an implausible incorrect answer contributes nothing to a test. The wrong answer, or false statements, should look acceptable to students who have only superficial knowledge, without confusing the high achievers.

Exhibit 7.6   Implausible versus plausible statements

Implausible

T   F   A living will documents that a client is requesting a lethal injection to end his suffering.

Plausible

T   F   A living will is a document that verifies that a client who has a terminal illness wants his health care proxy to make decisions when he is no longer able to.

When an item is implausible, students do not need to have mastery of the material to answer correctly. Both statements are false, but the students only need to use common sense to answer the first question correctly.

Common Misconceptions   Use common misconceptions that appear plausible to students with only cursory understanding, but do not confuse those who have achieved the outcomes. These statements identify those who have not mastered the material. A good source for common misconceptions is the incorrect answers that students fill in on short-answer or fill-in-the-blank questions. These formats are reviewed in Chapter 8, "Constructed-Response Format: Developing Short-Answer and Essay Items."

Exhibit 7.7   Common misconception

T   F   The primary responsibility of a nurse caring for a client who is having a seizure is to prevent the client from biting the tongue.

A common misconception of the general public is that something should be put in the mouth of a client who is having a seizure to prevent the client from biting or swallowing the tongue.

Exhibit 7.8   Common misconception

T   F   A mother calls an emergency department and says to a nurse, "My son just swallowed drain cleaner." The nurse should instruct the mother to give syrup of ipecac to make the child vomit.

Although this child should not be made to vomit, laypeople often believe this is the universal solution to poisoning.

Flaws to Avoid With True–False Items

Exhibits 7.9 to **7.16** illustrate common flaws associated with developing true–false items.

Negative Statements   Most of us have been tripped up at some time by a negatively worded question on a test. Negative statements can be so confusing that students who have achieved the outcome may miss the correct answer because they misread the statement. When this happens, the validity of the test results is marred. It is especially important to avoid negative stems with true–false items because of the double negative that results with the false option.

Exhibit 7.9   Negative statement for a true response versus positive statement for a false response

Negative Statement for a True Response
T   F   A client who is taking warfarin sodium should NOT eat green leafy vegetables.

Positive Statement for a False Response
T   F   A nurse should instruct a client who is taking warfarin to include broccoli and spinach in the diet.

The answer to the first question is "Yes, he shouldn't." This is a confusing response. It is clearer to state the question positively and require a false answer. Keeping the statements positive decreases confusion and improves the validity of your test results.

Exhibit 7.10   Negative statement for a false response versus positive statement for a false response

Negative Statement for a False Response
T   F   Bradycardia is NOT a side effect of digoxin.

Positive Statement for a False Response
T   F   A nurse should instruct a client who is taking digoxin to monitor the pulse for tachycardia.

A negative statement for a question that has a false response as the correct answer presents a student with a double negative that is confusing to answer. Keep the statements positive, especially if false is the correct response.

Specific Determiners   As with multiple-choice items, words like *always, never, none,* or *all* indicate that a statement is absolute. Very few phenomena always happen. Test-wise students know these words are associated with false statements. Ebel and Frisbie (1991) recommend using specific determiners in a true statement, referred to as using specific determiners in reverse, to attract the uninformed students. Just be sure that the true statement is *always* correct.

Exhibit 7.11 Specific determiners/false correct versus specific determiners/true correct

Specific Determiners/False Correct

T F Clients who have meningitis always have a petechial skin rash.

A test-wise student knows that unequivocal statements are seldom true and can recognize this as a false statement without having mastered the knowledge.

Specific Determiners/True Correct

T F A nurse should always assess a client who is being assessed for meningitis for a petechial skin rash.

The word always *in this statement is correct. A test-wise student who has superficial knowledge could not depend on cues alone to answer this question correctly.*

Qualifying Words Test-wise students expect qualifying words to be used in true statements. These words make the true option a safe choice. Again, Ebel and Frisbie (1991) suggest using these words in reverse to distinguish knowledgeable students. Words such as *usually, sometimes, seldom,* or *often* can be used in incorrect statements to assess more closely what students have learned.

Exhibit 7.12 Qualifying words/true correct versus qualifying words/false correct

Qualifying Words/True Correct

T F Clients who have cancer and are treated with chemotherapy usually develop side effects.

A test-wise student will recognize that the word usually *indicates that this statement is true, without having mastered the knowledge.*

Qualifying Words/False Correct

T F When assessing a 78-year-old client who is being treated for cancer, a nurse should recognize that older clients seldom develop side effects from chemotherapy.

The word seldom *in this statement makes the item incorrect. A test-wise student could not depend on cues alone to answer this question correctly.*

Partial Truth Avoid items that fall between true and false or are partially true. When items are not clear cut, the information they yield is ambiguous because you cannot determine exactly what the student did or did not know.

Exhibit 7.13 Partial truth

T F Because a client's blood pressure is the most important indicator of an impending stroke, it should be checked as part of a physical assessment.

T F A nurse should recognize that a client who has a blood pressure of 190/88 mmHg is having a stroke.

A client's blood pressure should be checked as part of a physical assessment; however, the reason is not because it is the most important indicator of an impending stroke. The first item muddies the waters because it is partially correct, whereas the second version is clearly false.

Textbook Statements   Copying textbook statements encourages rote memorization. Recall items do not identify achievement. Questions should be written at least at the comprehension level to determine whether or not a student understands the material.

Exhibit 7.14   Textbook statements

Textbook Statement

T F The electrocardiogram is a graphic reproduction of the electrical activity of the myocardium as the cardiac impulse is transmitted through the conductive tissue of the muscle.

This type of textbook statement promotes rote memorization. To test for comprehension, the statement should be paraphrased.

Paraphrased Textbook Statement

T F A nurse should explain to a client that an electrocardiogram provides a reading that represents the electrical activity of the heart.

This statement paraphrases the first statement to provide a better indication of student understanding of the concept.

Exhibit 7.15   Trick question

Trick Question

T F Before administering a 5 mg oral maintenance dose of digoxin to a client, the nurse should check the client's pulse.

This question is misleading. The dose of digoxin is too high. Is the purpose of the item to determine whether the student knows the importance of checking the pulse? If so, the dose should be appropriate or not included.

Revised Statement

T F Before administering the oral maintenance dose of digoxin to a client, a nurse should check the client's serum potassium level.

This statement is clearly true because it is not complicated by an incorrect statement.

Avoid Teaching   Many teachers cannot stop themselves from using one more opportunity to teach! However, teaching is not appropriate in a test. Those last words of wisdom only add verbiage to the statement, making it longer to read.

Exhibit 7.16   Teaching in a question

Teaching in a Question

T F Cyanosis is a bluish discoloration of the skin and mucous membranes. A nurse should monitor the hemoglobin level of a client who has cyanosis.

Teaching is unnecessary in a test; in fact, it can provide cues for the correct answer.

(continues)

Exhibit 7.16   Teaching in a question (*Continued*)

Revised Statement
 T   F   A nurse should monitor the hemoglobin level of a client who has cyanosis.

This statement requires the student to know what cyanosis is before deciding if it is necessary to monitor the client's hemoglobin.

Forms for True–False Item Writing

Ebel (1972) suggests 12 forms for writing true–false items. Although Ebel does not include these forms in subsequent editions of his text, they provide very useful guidelines for developing true–false items to match learning outcomes. Ebel's item models (pp. 183–185) are applied to items that assess nursing outcomes in **Box 7.1**. While the factual form is at the recall level, the other 11 provide useful models for writing true–false items at higher cognitive levels.

Box 7.1   Ebel's item models applied to nursing

Factual items present a fact in a declarative sentence.

• Surgical incisions heal by primary intention. (T)
• Urinary incontinence promotes maceration of the skin. (T)

Generalization items ask students to determine whether a statement is true or false for a group or part of a group.

• All clients who have a diastolic blood pressure greater than 120 mmHg should be referred for immediate follow-up. (T)
• Elderly clients always have poor nutritional status. (F)
• Many clients have difficulty following a weight-loss diet. (T)
• Most people who lose their job experience a prolonged period of depression. (F)
• The majority of clients who have abdominal surgery develop atelectasis. (F)

Comparative items examine how facts, treatments, events, principles, or concepts compare with each other.

• When compared with a newborn, the apical pulse for a 10-year-old child is slower. (T)
• Diet is more important than exercise when treating a client who is obese. (F)
• There should be no difference between a client's apical and radial pulse rates. (T)
• Both chemotherapy and radiation therapy can cause leucopenia. (T)
• Clients who are receiving chemotherapy are at higher risk for developing tissue fibrosis than clients who are receiving radiation therapy. (F)

Conditional items question the limitations and conditions under which an action can be taken, an event occurs, or a decision can be made.

• Unlicensed assistive personnel (UAP) can obtain a client's vital signs, but only a nurse can interpret the measurements. (T)
• If a client who has diabetes mellitus participates in strenuous exercise, the client will need to take additional insulin. (F)
• If a client's popliteal pulses cannot be palpated, a nurse should use a Doppler ultrasound probe to assess the pulses. (T)
• When the pumping action of the heart is weak, the blood pressure increases. (F)
• If a blood pressure cuff is too narrow, the client's blood pressure reading will be falsely low. (F)

Relational items assess how concepts, facts, treatments, events, and principles relate to each other.

- The higher a client's blood pressure, the more likely the client is to develop heart disease. (T)
- Decreased peripheral circulation increases the risk for infection of a foot ulcer. (T)
- Increasing the temperature of the water increases the effectiveness of hand-washing. (F)
- The more a client perspires, the more likely the client is to develop hypernatremia. (T)
- The higher a client's intelligence, the more receptive the client will be to teaching. (F)
- The fewer medications a client takes, the longer the client will live. (F)

Explanatory items ask for reasons why phenomena occur or actions are appropriate.

- The main reason for lubricating the nostrils of a client who is receiving oxygen is to provide humidification. (F)
- Because pain is subjective, a nurse's observations of the client are the most reliable indicator of the client's pain. (F)
- When a client is taking digoxin (Lanoxin) and furosemide (Lasix), the client should be encouraged to increase the intake of potassium. (T)
- The main purpose for wearing sterile gloves when changing a surgical dressing is to prevent contamination of the wound. (T)
- One factor that contributes to a client's increased risk for developing colon cancer is genetic. (T)
- Even though a client who has cancer has a thorough understanding of the prescribed treatment, the client may refuse to comply. (T)

Exemplary items require the students to determine if the item presents a legitimate example of the phenomena or situation.

- An example of parallel play is when two 6-year-old boys play a board game. (F)
- A paradoxical effect occurs when a client falls asleep after taking a sedative. (F)
- A client states, "I feel dizzy whenever I rise quickly from a sitting position." This statement indicates that the client has orthostatic hypotension. (T)
- An increase in systolic blood pressure is a sign that a client who sustained a head injury is developing increased intracranial pressure. (T)

Evidential items call for evidence about the truthfulness of a statement.

- Evidence-based practice is based on documented evidence for the success or failure of an intervention. (T)
- Findings from (a particular) study demonstrate that blood pressure is always decreased immediately after a back massage. (F)
- A nurse should identify that a client who has an arterial blood gas result of pH, 7.30; $PaCO_2$, 55 mmHg; HCO_3, 24 mEq/L, is exhibiting respiratory acidosis. (T)
- A nurse should recognize that decorticate posturing in an unconscious client is associated with lesions of the corticospinal tracts. (T)

Predictive items question what can be expected to occur in the future.

- A person who smokes two packs of cigarettes per day has double the risk for developing lung cancer as the person who smokes one pack of cigarettes per day. (F)
- Getting a client out of bed on the first postoperative day decreases the risk of the client developing phlebitis. (T)

(continues)

Box 7.1 **Ebel's item models applied to nursing** *(Continued)*

- Clients who have Alzheimer's disease usually die from suicide. (F)
- A client who has a spinal cord injury at the level of C6 should be able to self-transfer to a wheelchair. (T)

Procedural items ask the student to identify the steps in a procedure.

- A nurse should use a large cuff when obtaining the blood pressure of a client who is very thin. (F)
- The first step that nurses should take before initiating every procedure is to wash their hands thoroughly. (T)
- It is essential that a nurse never recap a needle after giving an injection to a client. (T)
- After injecting a medication into an intravenous solution bag, the nurse should gently rotate the bag. (T)

Computational items require the students to determine the accuracy of a calculation.

- A client whose intravenous infusion is regulated to deliver 360 mL of intravenous fluid in 3 hours will receive 240 mL in 2 hours. (T)
- A nurse prepares to administer 75 mg of a medication to a client. The medication is supplied as 100 mg in 50 mL of solution. The nurse should give the client 37.5 mL of solution. (T)

Evaluative items determine whether or not an intervention is the priority, is appropriate, or is successful.
- Observing a client self-inject insulin is the best way to determine whether the client is following the correct procedure. (T)
- The first action that a nurse should take when a client is found to be unresponsive is to check the client's pulse. (F)
- Assigning a client to a private room is the most important measure for preventing infection in a client who has a serious burn injury. (F)
- Measuring hourly urine output is a priority in the care of a client who has acute renal failure. (T)

Types of True–False Items

In addition to the straightforward approach exemplified in the previous examples, true–false items can be written in a variety of formats. The objective is to use the format that suits the content and objectives you are measuring. One important principle is to make sure that the instructions clearly communicate exactly how the students should respond to the question. Two examples of alternative true–false formats that are applicable to nursing exams are multiple true–false and correction items.

Multiple True–False or Cluster This format requires that students answer a group of items that all relate to an initial statement. When writing in this format, make sure the clusters are clearly separated from each other and that all items relate to the initial statement. This format is essentially the same as the multiple-response format described in Chapter 6, "Writing Critical Thinking Multiple-Choice Items." **Exhibit 7.17** provides an example of a multiple true–false item.

Exhibit 7.17   Multiple true–false statements

Mark each of the actions following the statement as follows: A for include, or B for do not include. Which of these instructions should a nurse include when preparing a client to have a colonoscopy?

A   B   "You will have several X-rays taken before the procedure."

A   B   "You must fast after midnight the night before the test."

A   B   "You should have someone pick you up after the procedure."

A   B   "You will have to eat a soft diet for 24 hours after the test."

A   B   "You need to take a strong laxative the day before the test."

Correction   The correction true–false item requires students to determine whether the statement is true or false and then to correct the false statements to make them true. The words that must be replaced are underlined in the statement. Make sure you decide how the items will be scored and explain the scoring to the students before you administer the test. Refer to **Exhibit 7.18** for examples of correction true–false items.

Exhibit 7.18   Correction items

Decide whether each statement below is correct or incorrect. If it is incorrect, change the underlined words to make the statement correct.

T   F   A nurse should instruct a client who is taking furosemide to increase the dietary intake of sodium.

T   F   A nurse should instruct a client who has diabetes mellitus (type 1) to have a snack before exercising.

T   F   When a client who has a newly applied cast on the right leg complains of unrelenting pain in the right leg, a nurse should elevate the client's right leg.

Despite the popularity of the multiple-choice format, the case is being made for using additional formats for paper-and-pencil or computer-administered classroom tests. The important issue is to identify unique ways to assess learning outcomes. Can our students think? How can we assess students' ability to think?

The discussion so far demonstrates that the true–false format is a useful tool for assessing understanding and higher-order thinking in a direct and efficient manner. True–false items provide a versatile and often overlooked format for assessing outcomes in nursing education. Refer to **Box 7.2** for a checklist when reviewing your true–false exams.

The main objective of a test is to determine student ability in a particular area. Teachers are not in the business of training students to be adept at a certain type of test format. Therefore, faculty should focus on the advantages and disadvantages of a variety of item formats when developing an exam. The selection of a particular format should depend solely on its ability to assess the objectives and content of the course. The discussion in the next section examines the selected-response item format, referred to as the matching exercise.

Box 7.2   Checklist for true–false exams

- Is true–false the appropriate format for testing these concepts and objectives?
- Does every item test an important concept?
- Does each item test only one concept?
- Is the correct answer clear, without partial truths?
- Have you written a rationale to justify that the answer is indisputably correct?
- Is every statement written succinctly, with all unnecessary words removed?
- Is there approximately the same number of true and false correct answers?
- Are the statements all of similar length?
- Have you avoided patterns and repeating the same answer more than four times consecutively?
- Have you avoided textbook statements?
- Are the incorrect answers plausible?
- Have you avoided negative statements?
- Have you avoided specific determiners and qualifying words?
- Have you avoided teaching in the statements?
- Have you included common misconceptions as incorrect options?

Matching Exercise

A matching exercise consists of two parallel columns: One column contains the premises (the problems to be answered) and the opposite column contains the responses (the answers to the problems). The students are required to make an association between the premise and a response, and match that association between the two columns based on a set of specific directions. Each premise is scored as a separate item.

Advantages of the Matching Exercise

The matching exercise is an objective format that assesses learning outcomes; in fact, it has the unique ability to identify associations between two sets of concepts. The matching format identifies relationships among concepts, principles, and facts. It is a useful format to follow in place of having several multiple-choice items with the same alternatives. Matching exercises are efficient because the same set of responses is used for a cluster of premises.

Disadvantages of the Matching Exercise

When matching items are constructed carelessly, they encourage rote memorization by the students, which is the problem with all the selected-response formats we have examined. The key issue with all formats is to construct the items so they are not merely measuring rote memorization. One of the strengths of the matching format can also be a disadvantage: It can be difficult to write a group of premises that are homogeneous enough to fit with the same set of responses.

Guidelines for Developing Matching Exercises

Most guidelines for developing multiple-choice and true–false items apply to matching exercises. Particularly important is the requirement for avoiding trivia and testing only the important concepts from the course, but a few additional suggestions will improve the quality of your matching exercises. The guidelines discussed here reflect the suggestions of experts (Brookhart & Nitko, 2014; Ebel, 1972; Miller et al., 2009; Popham, 2003; Reynolds et al., 2008) and my own experience with developing matching exercises.

- Write clear and explicit directions for matching the elements in the premise and response columns.
- Always include instructions about whether a response can be used once, more than once, or not at all.
- Keep the content in the matching exercise homogeneous. The material has to be related in order for the responses to be plausible for all the premises.
- List the premises in the left column and list the responses in the right column.
- Make sure there is only one correct or best response for each premise.
- Always present novel examples of the premises to identify higher-level student abilities. Examples that the students are familiar with are really only testing recall.
- Be mindful of grammatical accuracy. Ensure that all premises are grammatically consistent with all responses.
- Avoid negative premises. As is true with all other item formats, negative statements cause confusion and provide inconsistent statistical results.
- Keep the premises longer than the responses. The premise should present a statement or phrase that requires a match from the response column.
- Make sure all responses are equal in length.
- Write options that are plausible and equally attractive to the uninformed student.
- Arrange the responses in a systematic fashion, such as alphabetically. If there is a logical, quantitative order, such as dates or numbers, arrange them in ascending or descending order.
- Avoid providing cues to the students; be sure to have homogenous premises and responses so that each response is a plausible answer for every option.
- Assign numbers to the premises and letters to the responses. Each premise is a scored question, so they should be numbered in sequence.
- Include one or two more responses than premises. If the number of premises and responses are exact, a student could identify a correct answer through the process of elimination.
- Develop a manageable list of premises and responses. The list of premises should not exceed 10. Even with 10 premises and 11 responses, the student has to consider 110 combinations.
  - You may need to limit the number of responses to four or five if you are electronically scoring the exam. Check the ability of your scoring program.
  - Keep the entire matching exercise on one page. Turning back and forth between pages to find answers increases confusion.
  - Ask a colleague to review your matching exercise, without the key.

See **Exhibits 7.19** and **7.20** for examples of matching exercises. Refer to the checklist in **Box 7.3** to review the final form of your matching exercise.

Exhibit 7.19   Example of a matching exercise

Directions: For each nurse's statement in column A, select the therapeutic communication technique that the statement represents in column B. Each technique can be used only once.

Column A

Nurse's Statement

1. "I'm not sure I understand that."
2. "Can you tell me how this experience has been for you?"
3. "You may feel dizzy after this procedure."
4. "Tomorrow we'll review what we discussed today about breastfeeding."

Column B

Communication Technique

A. Giving information
B. Acknowledging
C. Providing general leads
D. Summarizing
E. Seeking clarification

Exhibit 7.20   Example of a matching exercise

Directions: For each medication in column A, identify an adverse effect from column B. Each adverse effect can be used only once.

Column A

Medication

1. digoxin
2. furosemide
3. theophylline
4. warfarin sodium

Column B

Side Effect

A. Bradycardia
B. Dehydration
C. Hematuria
D. Tachypnea
E. Thrombophlebitis

Box 7.3   Checklist for matching exercises

- Is a matching exercise the most appropriate format for testing these concepts and objectives?
- Is the entire matching exercise contained on one page?
- Is the content in the matching exercise homogeneous?
- Are the premises listed in the left column and the responses in the right column?
- Are numbers assigned to the premises and letters to the responses?
- Have you included explicit directions for matching the premise and response columns?
- Have you indicated how many times a response can be used?
- Are all responses grammatically consistent with all the premises?
- Have you avoided negative premises and responses?
- Have you listed the responses in logical order or alphabetically?
- Are the premises longer than the responses?
- Are the responses all brief and equal in length?
- Is every response a plausible answer to every premise?
- Are there one or two more responses than premises?
- Is the list of premises limited to 10 options?

Summary

Teachers can select from an assortment of format options when developing classroom exams. This chapter reviews the advantages and disadvantages of the true–false and matching exercise formats. While these item types are criticized for being prone to testing rote memorization, they can be written to assess higher cognitive levels. The key issues are to select the item format that is best suited for assessing the important concepts and principles of a course and to maximize the advantages and minimize the shortcomings of the format when developing your questions.

When the selected-response item format seems to be missing the mark for your assessment needs, you may consider using a constructed-response type item for developing a test. These items require the student to construct a response to a statement or question. Chapter 8, "Constructed-Response Format: Developing Short-Answer and Essay Items," discusses the development of two types of constructed-response items; completion or short-answer questions and essay questions.

Learning Activities

1. Explain the advantages and disadvantages of the true–false item format. Will you use this format when developing classroom exams? Explain why or why not.
2. Write a 10-item true–false exam. Use the checklist in Box 7.2 to review the exam.
3. Explain the advantages and disadvantages of the matching column format. Will you use this format when developing classroom exams? Explain why or why not.
4. Develop a matching exercise with 10 premises and 11 responses. Use the checklist in Box 7.3 to review the question.

Web Links

Colorado State University: Composing true–false questions
http://teaching.colostate.edu/tips/tip.cfm?tipid=155
Educational Resources Information Center
http://www.eric.ed.gov
National Council of State Boards of Nursing
http://www.ncsbn.org
Park University: Quality True–False Items
http://www.park.edu/cetl/quicktips/truefalse.html

References

Brookhart, S. M., & Nitko, A. J. (2014). *Educational assessment of students* (7th ed.). Upper Saddle River, NJ: Pearson Education.

Ebel, R. L. (1972). *Essentials of educational measurement* (2nd ed.). Englewood Cliffs, NJ: Prentice Hall.

Ebel, R. L., & Frisbie, D. A. (1991). *Essentials of educational measurement* (5th ed.). Englewood Cliffs, NJ: Prentice Hall.

Miller, M. D., Linn, R. L., & Gronlund, N. E. (2009). *Measurement and assessment in teaching* (10th ed.). Upper Saddle River, NJ: Pearson Education.

Popham, W. J. (2003). *Test better, teach better: The instructional role of assessment.* Alexandria, VA: Association for Supervision and Curriculum Development.

Reynolds, C. R., Livingston, R. B., & Wilson, V. (2008). *Measurement and assessment in education* (2nd ed.). Boston, MA: Allyn & Bacon.

Constructed-Response Format: Developing Short-Answer and Essay Items

© Anteromite/Shutterstock

"Writing is thinking on paper."

—WILLIAM ZINSSER

It is clear that, when you are selecting an item format for a test, it is most important to select the format that measures the course objectives most effectively and directly. Ebel and Frisbie (1991) suggest that you consider the verb in the instructional objective when deciding which item format to use for assessment. Objectives that have verbs such as *design, graph, develop,* or *explain* are probably assessed most accurately with constructed-response items that require the student to create the answer (p. 122).

The greatest criticism of the selected-response format is that it affords the student an opportunity to guess the correct answer. Constructed-response items, on the other hand, decrease the chance of guessing because students must supply the answer and use their writing skills to demonstrate understanding of the topic in question. This chapter offers suggestions for capitalizing on the advantages and minimizing the disadvantages of the two traditional types of the constructed-response format: short-answer and essay items.

Short-Answer or Completion Item Format

A short-answer item requires the student to provide an answer to either a direct question or an incomplete sentence. The student must supply a word, a phrase, or a sentence to complete the statement or answer the question. Short-answer items include completion items, where the student has to complete an incomplete sentence, and fill-in-the-blank items, where the student must supply a word that is missing from a sentence.

Advantages of the Short-Answer Item Format

The major advantage of short-answer items is that they require students to produce an answer, not just recognize the correct answer from a list of potential answers. Having partial knowledge can help students respond correctly to a selected-response item, while partial knowledge is less likely to be helpful when students have to construct a response to the answer.

Short-answer items are fairly easy to construct, they are efficient to correct, and a large number of items can be asked in a limited amount of time. Although they are used most frequently to assess basic recall and understanding of material, they can be used to assess higher-level student ability, such as interpreting data, applying rules, solving problems, balancing equations, or completing calculations (Brookhart & Nitko, 2014).

Disadvantages of the Short-Answer Item Format

Critics of short-answer items point out that, although they diminish the ability of the students to guess the correct answer, they tend to assess factual knowledge, which encourages students to memorize. Critics also note that the questions must be worded very carefully to avoid ambiguity, which could result in more than one correct answer and complicated scoring.

Spelling ability can also be a disadvantage of the short-answer format. If credit is taken off for misspelling, the students' scores will reflect spelling ability as well as achievement of the content. Even if spelling is not considered in the scoring, the teacher must decide if a misspelled word actually represents the correct answer (Miller, Linn, & Gronlund, 2009).

Additional weaknesses are inherent in this format: Only a limited content range can be assessed; scoring requires more time than with selected-response items; there is always a risk that the scoring can be subjectively influenced; and short-answer items do not lend themselves to statistical analysis, as do selected-response items.

Guidelines for Developing Short-Answer Items

It is important, once again, to emphasize the need to test significant concepts and to avoid trivia, a guideline repeated by many experts. In addition to focusing on what is important in a course, these experts offer a variety of suggestions for maximizing the strengths and minimizing the weaknesses of the short-answer format. This section summarizes and expands on the recommendations of educational experts (Brookhart & Nitko, 2014; Ebel & Frisbie, 1991; Miller et al., 2009; Reynolds, Livingston, & Wilson, 2008) to help you develop skill in writing items in the short-answer format.

- Provide the students with clear and concise directions.
- Word the questions carefully so there is only one answer. More than one correct answer is possible if the question is ambiguous, so ask yourself if the question can be interpreted more than one way.
- Word the question so that the answer will be as short as possible.
- Think of the answer first, and then write the question.
- The direct-question format is preferred over the completion format. Writing in the question format forces the author to be clear and unambiguous.

- If an incomplete sentence provides a clearer approach, word the sentence so there is only one blank at the end of the sentence.
- Avoid copying statements from a textbook. Verbatim textbook statements encourage rote memorization.
- Have only one blank in the sentence; multiple blanks cause confusion.
- The answer should be a key word or concept, not an irrelevant word in the sentence.
- Keep all the blanks the same length. Varying the lengths of the blanks provides a cue about the length of the answers to test-wise students.
- Make sure the blanks are long enough to accommodate the students' answers.
- Provide a space for recording answers on the right margin of the page. This allows for convenience when scoring.
- Use appropriate grammar and sentence structure. Grammatical cues can help test-wise students to narrow down a response.
- For computational items, specify the degree of precision required and the units in which the answer should be expressed.
- Have a colleague review and answer your items before you use them in a test.
- Develop a list of all possible correct answers and use a scoring key to give partial credit when more than one answer is required.
- Give credit when students provide an answer that is correct but is not on your scoring list.
- Clearly communicate your scoring criteria to students.

Characteristics of Effective Short-Answer Items

Specifically Worded   If the items are worded ambiguously, more than one answer could be correct. In fact, students who know the answer may answer incorrectly if they misinterpret the question. **Exhibit 8.1** demonstrates the importance of stating the question clearly and precisely so that a specific word or a brief phrase can be the only correct answer.

Exhibit 8.1   Precisely worded question

Ambiguous

Which diagnostic study should all women over age 50 years have?

Several diagnostic studies are recommended for women 50 years and older. There is a variety of correct answers, including some that may not apply to your course objectives.

Precisely Worded

Identify two gynecologic diagnostic tests that all women over age 50 years should have annually.

1.
2.

This version of the question specifically asks the student to identify two gynecologic diagnostic tests that all women should have.

Question Format   The question format is generally preferred over the completion format because it is the most straightforward and least confusing approach. The completion format can be confusing and time consuming to answer because the student has to translate the item into a question. Framing the item as a question requires a high degree of specificity so that the item that results is clear and unambiguous. **Exhibit 8.2** illustrates how the question format improves the quality of an item.

Exhibit 8.2   Question versus completion format

Completion Format

1. A 78-year-old woman says to a nurse, "When I was young, I was two inches taller." The nurse should recognize that the woman's height loss is most likely due to

    _____.

The completion format requires the student to rephrase the statement as a question. When an item can be written as a question, the question format is preferred as the more direct format. As written, this question could have more than one correct answer. For example, aging or heredity could arguably be correct.

Question Format

A 78-year-old woman says to a nurse, "When I was young, I was two inches taller." The nurse should recognize that the woman's height loss is most likely due to which musculoskeletal disorder?

1.

The question format, which is the more direct format, improves the quality of this question by clarifying that the teacher wants the student to identify the musculoskeletal disorder that is related to the woman's problem.

Completion Format   While the question format is often the preferable choice, the completion format is sometimes a better option. Brookhart and Nitko (2014) explain that, when a question suggests the need for a longer answer than the teacher requires, the incomplete sentence is a better choice. In **Exhibit 8.3,** the completion format is preferred.

Exhibit 8.3   Completion versus question format

Question Format

1. What activity is a nurse involved in during the evaluation phase of the nursing process?

This question implies that the teacher is asking for a detailed answer. Short-answer questions should be just that—short!

Completion Format

1. During the evaluation phase of the nursing process, the nurse compares data with

    _____.

The completion format can communicate the teacher's intent more clearly here and keep the answer brief!

Important Words   The words that are omitted in a completion item should be key words. You should ask the student only to supply an important fact, as illustrated in **Exhibit 8.4**. A good suggestion is to think of the answer first and then write the question.

Exhibit 8.4   Important words

Irrelevant Words

A nurse should expect a client who has dementia to have a (history) of being inattentive.

The words that are omitted should be key words or important concepts. You want students to focus on what is important. This item also has additional plausible answers (fear, denial, risk), so the item may not assess what the teacher intended.

Important Words

A nurse should expect a client who has dementia to have a history of

_____.

Although there are several possible answers to this question, they are all manifestations of dementia. Therefore, the intended objective is being assessed. The teacher will need to create a list of acceptable answers, or the teacher could convert this to a list question.

Adequate Information   Make sure that a completion question is detailed enough so that knowledgeable students have enough information to answer the question. Too many blanks, as shown in **Exhibit 8.5**, can leave the students trying to figure out what the question is asking instead of trying to answer the question.

Exhibit 8.5   Inadequate versus adequate information

Inadequate Information

1. Using a(n) _____ that is _____ will result in a blood pressure reading that is falsely _____.

How can you answer a question when you cannot figure out what the question is asking? There are too many blanks in this item. This item also presents a potential scoring dilemma because of the possibility that students will be partially correct.

Adequate Information

1. Using a blood pressure cuff that is too small will result in a blood pressure reading that is falsely _____.

Now the students can understand the question, and there is only one clear-cut answer.

Lists   A list question requires a student to respond with a set of answers to a question. The teacher may require a complete list or a partial list. The test directions must clearly explain the scoring method. In nursing, the list question is a valuable format, particularly for questioning students about manifestations of health alterations. A list question is useful for testing comprehension, as in **Exhibit 8.6**. Lists can also be crafted to assess higher-order thinking, as **Exhibit 8.7** demonstrates.

Exhibit 8.6 Short-answer lists

Example I

Identify four manifestations that a nurse should expect to identify when assessing a client who has untreated diabetes mellitus.

1.
2.
3.
4.

Because there are more than four manifestations of diabetes mellitus, the teacher would have to prepare a list of acceptable answers. Each answer counts as one point.

Example II

Identify four manifestations that a nurse should expect to identify when assessing a client who has untreated diabetes mellitus.

A.
B.
C.
D.

This question is the same as the first example; the difference is in the scoring. The answers in Example I are worth one point each. In Example II, the student must identify four manifestations to earn one point. The test directions must clearly explain the scoring method.

Exhibit 8.7 Short-answer lists to assess higher-order thinking

---

Example I

Identify three measures that a nurse should include in the care plan for a client who has the following arterial blood gas analysis results: pH, 7.47; $PaCO_2$, 44 mm Hg; HCO_3, 40 mEq/L.

This question requires more than memorization. The student must interpret the blood gas results and then decide what to do for the client. Each answer counts as one point.

1.

2.

3.

Example II

Identify three measures that a nurse should include in the care plan for a client who has the following arterial blood gas analysis results: pH, 7.47; $PaCO_2$, 44 mm Hg; HCO_3, 40 mEq/L.

This question is the same as the first example; the difference is in the scoring. The answers in Example I are worth one point each. In Example II, the student must identify three measures to earn one point. This exhibit is another example of why the test directions must explain the scoring method clearly.

Computation   Asking students to record an answer for a calculation problem eliminates the possibility of guessing that the multiple-choice or true–false item format offers. The degree of precision and the units of expression required must be identified. **Exhibit 8.8** presents two sample computation items.

Exhibit 8.8   Computation

Show all of your work for this question:

A client has an order to receive 400 mL of an intravenous (IV) solution every 8 hours. A nurse uses an IV setup that has a drop factor of 60 gtts/min to run the infusion. The nurse should regulate the IV to run at how many drops per minute?

1. _____

This item provides the student with all the necessary information and specifies the desired unit for the answer.

* * * * * *

Show all of your work for this question:

The recommended pediatric dose of digoxin (Lanoxin) is 0.03 to 0.04 mg/kg/day. What is the maximum dose in milligrams that an infant who weighs 24 pounds could receive in 1 day?

1. _____

This item provides the student with all the necessary information and specifies the desired unit for the answer. Also, because the answers are numbered and the questions are not, it is important to separate the questions clearly. This example uses a line of asterisks (*****) to separate the items.

Box 8.1 provides a checklist for making sure that your short-answer questions are worded correctly.

Box 8.1   Checklist for short-answer items

- Is the short answer the most appropriate format for these concepts and objectives?
- Does every item address an important course concept?
- Does each item test only one concept?
- Are the questions succinct, with all unnecessary words removed?
- Have you avoided textbook questions?
- Are the questions worded so that the answer will be as short as possible?
- Have you avoided negative questions?
- Have you avoided teaching in the questions?
- Is there only one blank in every question?
- Are the response lines long enough for the answers?
- Have you identified all possible responses to every question?
- Have you checked the questions for grammatical cues?
- For computational items, have you specified the degree of precision and the units to use for the answer?
- Have you clearly communicated the scoring criteria to the students?
- If the completion format is used, is it the most appropriate format?
- Has a colleague reviewed and answered the test items before you actually put them in a test?

Essay Question Format

An essay question requires students to construct an original composition to respond to the issues presented in a question. While essay questions can be designed to assess comprehension-level learning, they are also very well suited for assessing more complex abilities because they require the students to construct their own responses.

As we have examined with previously discussed item formats, every item format has assets and liabilities. The decision about which type to use should depend on how well the format matches the learning goals.

Forms of Essay Questions

Freedom of response is the defining characteristic of the essay question, which allows teachers to assess complex reasoning and thinking skills. Freedom must be somewhat limited, however, in order to direct the students to respond to the expectations of the teacher who is assessing the students' complex reasoning and thinking skills.

Restricted Response   Restricted-response essay items are designed to limit the content of the students' answers. The question directs the student to analyze and present a solution to a unique problem that allows the teacher to make decisions about students' ability in a certain aspect of very complex learning (Brookhart & Nitko, 2014).

A restricted-response item poses a specific problem and requires students to present directed and specific responses to solve the problem. These questions should direct students to solve unique problems so that higher-order thinking abilities can be assessed.

Exhibit 8.9 presents several examples of restricted-response essay items. These items direct students' responses to address specific areas of course content.

Exhibit 8.9   Restricted-response essay questions

- Describe the five phases of the nursing process and provide an example of a nursing activity that represents each phase.
- Compare right-sided and left-sided heart failure. Include the pathophysiology, causes, and manifestations of each.
- Identify three types of reactions that a client could develop when receiving a blood transfusion. Describe four manifestations of each type of reaction and identify four nursing measures to prevent complications of a transfusion reaction.
- Explain the pathophysiology of insulin-dependent diabetes mellitus. Identify three manifestations and explain how they are related to the pathophysiology.
- Discuss the difference between respiratory acidosis and respiratory alkalosis. Include in your answer (a) a description of the pathophysiology of both abnormalities, (b) three manifestations of each abnormality, and (c) three nursing interventions to prevent the complications of each abnormality.

Extended Response   Extended-response essay items offer students the opportunity to organize and express their own ideas. When the purpose of the exercise is to assess students' subject knowledge, the question must describe the general purpose of the plan that the student is expected to develop (Brookhart & Nitko, 2014).

As is discussed later in this chapter, it is important for the teacher to share the expectations for proficiency in an essay question with students. The proposed scoring criteria should be shared with students before the exam.

Exhibit 8.10 presents several examples of extended-response essay items. These items direct the student to respond freely while limiting the response to addressing the key issues for demonstrating proficiency in the content area. Many of these questions would be best suited for an out-of-class assignment, to allow students adequate time to formulate and organize their thinking.

Exhibit 8.10   Extended-response essay questions

- Discuss whether or not you agree that complementary and alternative medicine (CAM) therapies demonstrate a holistic healing approach to improve client care. Include four examples of CAM therapies and identify their relevance to nursing practice.
- Discuss the importance of the nursing process in delivering nursing care. In your discussion, use specific examples to compare the theoretical approaches of systems theory, problem solving, and the scientific method with the nursing process model.
- Devise a plan for implementing computer-based charting on a busy critical care unit where the staff members range widely in computer ability and resistance to change. Create your own hypothetical situation, describe the actions you would take, and explain the principles behind your actions.
- Explain the impact that a nurse can have on the self-concept of a client who is undergoing body image changes. Include a discussion of the significance of the nurse's self-concept. Create a hypothetical nurse–client interaction and explain the principles behind the nurse's actions.
- Compare Erikson's stages of development, Maslow's hierarchy of needs, and Piaget's stages of cognitive development with each other. How are they similar and how are they different? Select aspects of each to formulate a developmental model on which you would base your nursing care.

These extended-response essay items require the students to use a combination of skills. They require students to express their own ideas, develop logical arguments, explain their thoughts coherently, and solve problems. This type of assignment would be best addressed as an out-of-class assignment.

Advantages of the Essay Question

In the real world, you must construct your own solutions to problems; you are not given a variety of options from which to choose. The essay is the ideal format for asking students to respond to authentic real-world situations to evaluate their ability to translate understanding to clinical practice.

As with the short-answer format, the essay question requires the students to develop their own responses to a question rather than to select from a group of possible options. Because no options are given, guessing is eliminated. Although they are both considered to be constructed responses, the essay question differs from the short answer in its length and complexity. While the short-answer format is criticized for encouraging memorization, one characteristic of the essay format is that it discourages memorization. The essay question is used most effectively to assess higher-order thinking, including the analysis, application, synthesis, and evaluation levels of cognition. The ability of essay items to assess critical thinking is discussed later in this chapter.

The essay question is relatively easy to construct. It can examine students' ability to organize, express, and defend their ideas; it can be developed directly from the learning outcomes for the course; and it can be used for measuring critical thinking ability.

Disadvantages of the Essay Question

The essay has similar weaknesses as the short-answer format. First, only a limited content range can be assessed. While the multiple-choice test can require students to answer 50 items in an hour, the same time frame would allow only 4 or 5 short or 1 or 2 long essay items. Therefore, the essay format should be used to assess depth of knowledge rather than breadth of content knowledge.

The most serious limitation of the essay format is the unreliability of the scoring. Essay tests have a lower reliability than constructed-response exams, and they do not lend themselves to statistical analysis, as do selected-response items. Numerous studies indicate that poor reliability is often related to the subjectivity that can influence the scoring of an essay. Not only can interrater reliability be poor, teachers are subject to scoring the same responses differently at different times (Miller et al., 2009). Ebel and Frisbie (1991) identify three conditions that lead to the low reliability of essay exams:

1. Limited content sampling
2. Indefiniteness of the tasks required
3. Subjectivity of the scorers

Essay questions require less time to develop than constructed-response items. Unless the questions are precisely constructed, however, they can be misinterpreted by the students and thus will not measure what the teacher intended. Scoring an essay exam also requires more time than do selected-response items. In fact, essay tests can be very time consuming to score; this is a particular concern when class size is large.

Although students cannot guess on an essay exam, those who are good writers can bluff in an attempt to obtain partial credit. When students have not achieved the outcomes, they often attempt to inflate their grades with tactics such as writing in general terms that could apply to any situation, restating the question, or stating the importance of the topic (Miller et al., 2009). In contrast, those students who have poor composition ability, or have difficulty writing under stress, may lose points even when they have mastered the material.

The essay format has serious limitations. In fact, Miller and colleagues (2009) suggest that the essay question be used only for measuring learning outcomes that cannot be measured satisfactorily by objective items. The next sections of this chapter provide suggestions for developing and scoring essay exams that maximize the advantages and minimize the disadvantages of the essay format.

Guidelines for Developing Essay Items

Experts offer a variety of suggestions for improving test-writing and scoring ability to maximize the strengths and minimize the weaknesses of the essay format. As with all question formats, the importance of testing significant concepts is the foundation for high-quality essay items. This section summarizes and expands on the recommendations of educational experts (Brookhart & Nitko, 2014; Ebel & Frisbie, 1991; Miller et al., 2009; Reynolds et al., 2008) to help you develop skill in writing and scoring essay items.

- Restrict the use of essay items to objectives that cannot be measured by supplied response-type items.
- Develop the questions using the course learning outcomes as a framework. Each question should be designed to require achievement of a course objective.
- Use conditions and situations that are realistic.
- Be as precise and specific as possible when explaining the criteria required to demonstrate achievement. Provide enough information so there is no doubt about what you are asking student to do.
- Make sure students can interpret the questions. Students should not have to guess what your expectations are.
- Instruct students not to rephrase the question in their answers to minimize bluffing.
- Write a sample response to the question and develop a scoring key or rubric.
- Ask a colleague to read the question and write a response.
- Allow students more time than you believe they need to answer the questions.
- To increase the content sampling, include several questions that require short answers rather than one or two that require a long answer.
- Keep choices to a minimum or you will have different subtests that are not comparable. Many experts discourage offering options altogether, arguing that when students select different questions, they are taking different tests. If you choose to allow optional questions, allow the students to answer four of five questions, not two of six.
- Indicate a point value for each question on the test so students are aware of the value for each question.
- Tell the students how much time they should spend on each item so that they can pace their response time and not be caught without time to answer the last question on the test.
- Alert students to the time remaining during the test.

Refer to **Box 8.2** for a checklist for developing essay items.

Box 8.2 Checklist for developing essay items

- Is an essay item the most appropriate format for testing the concept?
- Does the item address a course objective?
- Are the questions worded so students understand exactly what is expected of them?
- Are the questions realistic?
- Have you avoided negative questions?
- Have you allowed more time than you feel is necessary to answer the question?
- Have you told students how much time they should spend on each item?
- Have you developed a sample response for the question?
- Have you developed a scoring rubric for the question?
- Have you clearly communicated the scoring criteria to students?
- Has a colleague reviewed and answered the questions before you actually put them in a test?

Suggestions for Scoring Essay Items

- Keep the students anonymous. Increase the reliability of the results of your essay items by using a number identification instead of names on the test. This will avoid introducing subjective bias of the students' ability.

- Use a predetermined scoring key or rubric to make sure you evaluate for content, not writing style.

- Share the scoring rubric with students before the test.

- Read a random sample of papers to estimate the overall quality of the student responses.

- Select a set of papers that demonstrate performance at each of the levels on the rubric. Refer to these anchor papers while scoring to ensure consistency of grade assignment.

- Read the questions in order. For example, read and score the first question for every student before rearranging the order of the papers and reading the second question.

- Note each student's score on a separate piece of paper. Read every question twice, rescore, and check to see whether your score agrees with your first impression.

- Ask a colleague to score a sample of the questions and compare the results with your decisions. This is a time-consuming but excellent way to improve the reliability of the scoring.

- Avoid taking off points for grammatical mistakes or handwriting. The purpose of the test is to evaluate student mastery of course material, not to judge writing ability. If you decide to consider grammar in the scoring, make sure no one fails because of writing ability.

Developing Essay Items to Assess Critical Thinking

The first step for assessing critical thinking is to decide which format is best suited for assessing the behaviors that represent your definition of critical thinking. While a variety of formats are appropriate for assessing critical thinking, the essay format is certainly well suited for this purpose.

A well-developed essay item requires students to engage in higher-order thinking. The abilities to compare, contrast, analyze, infer, draw conclusions, and evaluate information are some of the characteristics that can be assessed by essay items.

When developing an essay question to assess critical thinking, it is important to consider the level of cognition that the desired student response requires. Although comprehension questions are often appropriate and can have a high difficulty level, they are not appropriate for assessing critical thinking. **Exhibit 8.11** provides a sample of comprehension essay stems.

Exhibit 8.11   Comprehension essay stems

Comprehension

- Describe the pathophysiology of. . . .
- List four side effects of. . . .
- Summarize the two main ideas of the. . . theory of. . . .
- Identify the two main predisposing factors for. . . .

Although these items are appropriate for assessing student understanding of concepts, they are clearly comprehension and do not assess critical thinking.

Items that require ability at the cognitive levels of application, analysis, synthesis, and evaluation are best suited for assessing critical thinking in nursing. **Exhibit 8.12** provides examples of stems that incorporate the abilities associated with higher-order thinking that can be used to craft test items that assess critical thinking.

Exhibit 8.12   Critical thinking essay stems

Application

- Identify three nursing measures to include in the care plan for a client who. . . .
- Describe a client situation that illustrates the theory of. . . .
- (Present a client scenario) Identify three educational needs and how you would meet them.
- (Present a client scenario) Discuss two potential complications. Identify three nursing interventions to prevent each complication.

Analysis

- (Present a client scenario) Based on the assessment data, write three nursing diagnoses. Specify the defining characteristics for each diagnosis.
- (Present a client scenario) Explain why the client developed each of these manifestations.
- (Present a client scenario) Identify three factors in the client's history and explain how they precipitated. . . .

(continues)

Exhibit 8.12 Critical thinking essay stems (*Continued*)

Synthesis

- Develop a care plan for a client who. . . .
- Create a scenario that illustrates. . . leadership style.
- Create a teaching plan for a client who has. . . .
- (Present a scenario) Develop a plan to deal with the conflict in this situation.
- Create a scenario that illustrates an ethical dilemma and present two different approaches for dealing with it.

Evaluation

- (Present a client scenario) Describe how a nurse would determine whether the treatment plan for this client is successful.
- (Present a scenario) Critique each of the nurse's decisions in this situation. What alternate approaches would you take to be equally or more effective?
- (Present a scenario) Identify the ethical dilemma in this situation and discuss if the nurse handled it appropriately. What alternate approach would you take?
- Identify five measures to include in the care plan for a client who has . . . . What evidence would you look for to determine the effectiveness of the interventions?
- (Present a client scenario) Identify three client manifestations that indicate that the treatment plan is not having the desired effect. What alternate approaches would you suggest?

Scoring Rubrics

A rubric is a guide for scoring constructed-response items. Scoring rubrics identify the criteria that the scorer must consider when determining the quality of a student's response. All rubrics combine the evaluation criteria used to judge the students' performance with a rating scale to indicate the level of performance (Brookhart & Nitko, 2014; Miller et al., 2009; Reynolds et al., 2008). Scoring rubrics are useful tools to guide the evaluation of students' responses to essay questions.

When developing a rubric, it is important to define clearly both the rating scale and the criteria. Categories such as "excellent," "good," or "fair" provide little direction for the teacher and minimal guidance for students. Statements describing the characteristics of each score category must be included so it is clear, to both student and teacher, to which category the response belongs (Miller et al., 2009).

A rubric requires the instructor to clarify the important components of an assignment. Using a scoring rubric keeps the influence of extraneous factors, such as writing ability or mechanics and rater subjectivity, to a minimum, thus enhancing grading consistency across instructors. Sharing the rubric with students before administering the test helps them understand clearly what is expected of them, which enhances the validity of the test.

The two types of rubrics most commonly used for scoring essay responses are the holistic and the analytic. Both methods increase the objectivity of the scoring by ensuring that the same standards are applied when scoring every test.

Holistic Scoring Rubrics

Holistic scoring rubrics require the scorer to determine the degree to which a student's overall essay satisfies a set of predetermined evaluative criteria; all the elements in the essay are considered in a combined manner. These rubrics associate quality ratings with descriptions of the characteristics of the response that deserves the rating. The student's response receives a score based on how closely it matches the score's description (Brookhart & Nitko, 2014; Ebel & Frisbie, 1991; Miller et al., 2009; Reynolds et al., 2008).

Holistic rubrics can be constructed and used to score a set of essays more rapidly than analytic rubrics. They are preferred when there is an overlap between the elements of the response or when students are required to create a response to which there is no definitive answer (Brookhart & Nitko, 2014). However, they do not provide students with the specific feedback on their strengths and weaknesses that an analytic rubric offers.

Analytic Scoring Rubric

An analytic scoring rubric focuses on the individual elements of the ideal response to an essay question and assigns scores for each of the elements separately. The final score is a total of the points assigned to each element. Those scores are then totaled to provide an overall score (Brookhart & Nitko, 2014; Ebel & Frisbie, 1991; Miller et al., 2009; Reynolds et al., 2008).

The clear advantage of the analytic method is that it provides information about students' strengths and weaknesses. This is helpful feedback for students, and it also provides the teacher with information for improving teaching strategies. The drawback with analytic rubrics is that they can be time consuming to create.

Developing Scoring Rubrics

Both holistic and analytic rubrics are valuable tools for assessment. The first step for creating a scoring rubric is to clearly identify the criteria that must be displayed to demonstrate proficiency in the assignment. These criteria should be descriptions of the work, not judgments about the work. Start by writing a description that represents the top level of performance. Once the top level is identified, you can then decide whether the scoring of the assignment is best facilitated by a holistic or analytic rubric (Moskal, 2000).

In both cases, you need to define the levels of performance that represent the various score levels. Once you have defined the criteria that represent the highest level of performance, the next step is to define the criteria that represent the lowest level of performance. The contrast between the highest and lowest levels should then suggest a middle level (Moskal, 2000). For five levels, you would identify criteria between the highest and the middle and the lowest and the middle. In the end, you should be able to identify meaningful distinctions between criteria that indicate different score levels.

Moskal (2003) recommends that scoring rubrics be designed so that the connection between the rubric and the grade you assign to the essay is immediately apparent to students. If you use a holistic rubric, provide students with a summary explanation. If you use an analytic rubric, make sure the scores associated with each level are identified clearly on the rubric worksheet. It makes sense to include a copy of the student's individual rubric report with the grades assigned when you return the graded essay.

Table 8.1 provides an example of a holistic scoring rubric worksheet, and **Table 8.2** provides an example of an analytic rubric scoring worksheet. Both rubrics are developed for scoring the extended response essay in Exhibit 8.10, and both are based on a 100-point possible total score.

Table 8.1   Holistic Scoring Rubric Worksheet

Compare Erikson's stages of development, Maslow's hierarchy of needs, and Piaget's stages of cognitive development with each other. How are they similar and how are they different? Select aspects of each to create a developmental model on which you would base your nursing care.

Score Level	Criteria	Student's Score
90–100 points	Describes theories precisely and accurately. Presents explicit comparisons of strengths and weaknesses, with specific examples from all three theorists. Personal model is well organized, cohesive, and logical and incorporates aspects from each theorist.	
80–89 points	Descriptions of theories general but consistently accurate. Makes general comparisons of strengths and weaknesses of theories and uses some specific examples. Personal model reflects all theorists but lacks organization and cohesiveness.	
70–79 points	Description of theories not consistently accurate, with a few inaccuracies. Comparisons of strengths and weaknesses of theories limited, with few specific examples. Personal model undeveloped. References all theorists.	
60–69 points	Descriptions of theories have numerous inaccuracies. Comparisons of strengths and weaknesses of theories limited, with no specific examples. Personal model incomplete, with references to only one or two theorists.	
Below 60 points	Descriptions of theories awkward and inaccurate overall. Does not compare similarities and differences. Personal model incomplete and lacks reference to theorists.	

Total points = 100

Table 8.2   Analytic Scoring Rubric Worksheet

Compare Erikson's stages of development, Maslow's hierarchy of needs, and Piaget's stages of cognitive development with each other. How are they similar and how are they different? Select aspects of each to create a developmental model on which you would base your nursing care.

Possible Score	21–25	16–20	11–15	6–10	0–5	Score
Description of developmental stages	Precise descriptions of theories	Descriptions general but consistently accurate	Descriptions need improvement, contain few inaccuracies	Descriptions have numerous inaccuracies	Descriptions awkward and inaccurate overall	
Identification of similarities	Makes explicit comparisons between the three theorists, uses specific examples	Comparison of theorists general, uses some specific examples	Comparisons limited, with few specific examples	Comparisons limited, with no specific examples	Does not compare similarities	
Identification of differences	Makes explicit comparisons between the three theorists, uses specific examples	Compares the theorists, uses some specific examples	Comparisons limited, with few specific examples	Comparisons limited, with no specific examples	Does not compare differences	
Personal developmental model	Well-thought-out and logical model, incorporates aspects of each theorist	Model lacks organization, reflects all theorists	Model undeveloped, references all theorists	Model incomplete, references only one or two theorists	Model incomplete, lacks reference to theorists	

Total points = 100

Summary

A variety of format options is available for developing classroom exams. This chapter reviews the advantages and disadvantages of the short-answer and essay formats, and discusses strategies for maximizing the effectiveness of the constructed-response format.

Although essay items are valuable for requiring students to think on paper and discouraging memorization, they are limited by their ability to test only a limited amount of material. This chapter demonstrates how the fundamental principle of test development applies to the constructed-response item format: The best approach to ensure fair assessment of students is to select the item format that is best suited for assessing the behaviors that you are examining. This chapter also reinforces the importance of including a variety of formats in the overall assessment plan in order to accurately assess the diverse abilities required in a nursing course.

Learning Activities

1. Consider a course you are teaching or plan to teach. Develop two objectives with learning outcomes that can be measured with short-answer questions. Write 10 short-answer items to measure the objectives.

2. Compare the completion to the question format for short-answer items. Write one question in the completion format and one in the question format for the same topic.

3. Develop an extended-response essay question. Use Tables 8.1 and 8.2 as templates to develop a holistic and an analytic scoring rubric for the question.

4. Write three restricted-response essay questions for a topic of your choice.

Web Links

iRubric: Rubric Development Tool

http://www.rcampus.com/rubricshellc.cfm?mode=gallery&sms=home&srcg oogle&gclid=CI-914-G15ICFQKhlgodQBSUAg

Park University Faculty Resources: Developing Essay Items

http://www.park.edu/cetl/quicktips/essay.html

Park University Faculty Resources: Grading Rubrics

http://www.park.edu/cetl/quicktips/rubrics.html

References

Brookhart, S. M., & Nitko, A. J. (2014). *Educational assessment of students* (7th ed.). Upper Saddle River, NJ: Pearson Education.

Ebel, R. L., & Frisbie, D. A. (1991). *Essentials of educational measurement* (5th ed.). Englewood Cliffs, NJ: Prentice Hall.

Miller, M. D., Linn, R. L., & Gronlund, N. E. (2009). *Measurement and assessment in teaching* (10th ed.). Upper Saddle River, NJ: Pearson Education.

Moskal, B. M. (2000). Scoring rubrics: What, when, how? *Practical Assessment, Research & Evaluation, 7*(3). Retrieved from http://PAREonline.net/getvn.asp?v=7&n=3

Moskal, B. M. (2003). Recommendations for developing classroom assessments and scoring rubrics. *Practical Assessment, Research & Evaluation, 8*(14). Retrieved from http://PAREonline.net/getvn.asp?v=8&n=14

Reynolds, C. R., Livingston, R. B., & Wilson, V. (2008). *Measurement and assessment in education* (2nd ed.). Boston, MA: Allyn & Bacon.

© Anteromite/Shutterstock

Assembling, Administering, and Scoring a Test

CHAPTER 9

"Be prepared, be sharp, be careful, and use the King's English well."

—Robert N. C. Nix

If you are following the guidelines proposed in this book, you have devoted valuable time and effort to crafting your exam. You have carefully developed a blueprint based on your objectives and course content, and you have painstakingly written, edited, and reviewed items. You have made this effort to create a trustworthy instrument that will provide you with valid and reliable evidence of student learning. However, you are not finished yet! The final steps are just as important as the initial procedures for establishing the validity and reliability of your test results.

The goal of every test is to provide students with an opportunity to demonstrate their best performance. The processes of assembling, administering, and scoring a test can influence student performance and introduce measurement error that will negatively affect the validity and reliability of your test results. A systematic approach to these processes enhances the likelihood that the results of the test will be valid, reliable, and useful (Miller, Linn, & Gronlund, 2009).

Assembling a Test

Once your items are written, edited, and reviewed for relevancy to the test blueprint, you are ready to assemble the test. Teachers often have the misconception that putting a test together is a simple clerical task. In fact, if careful attention is not devoted to the process of assembling a test, much more time will be spent correcting mistakes after the test is duplicated or, even worse, administered.

The final appearance of your test is important for establishing the reliability and validity of the interpretations you make based on the test results. While a professional appearance lends face validity to your exams; tests that are illegible, carelessly typed, or collated incorrectly are subject to increased measurement error. Poorly designed tests confuse and annoy students, increase their test anxiety, and give the impression that you have carelessly prepared the exam. Teachers expect students to exercise care when completing written work. In fact, some teachers deduct credit from students who have grammatical or spelling errors in their written work. Teachers should hold themselves to an even higher standard than the one to which they hold their students. Remember, nothing you write will ever be more carefully scrutinized than your exam questions.

Arranging Items

Test development software streamlines the test development process. The programs track all items with their data and also provide a printout of whatever information you request. The software can sort and arrange the items by whatever criteria you require. One of the important features of test development software is that the item and its accompanying data are never separated. Chapter 14, "Instituting Item Banking and Test Development Software," discusses the advantages of test development software to manage this process electronically.

If you are not yet using test development software, you can write the items in a word processing program and organize them in folders according to the course content. Dedicate a separate page to each item. Include the item, rationale, instructional objective, learning outcome, and content measured by the item on the page. When you are ready to assemble the test, you can print the items, one item to a page, to expedite the sorting and arranging of items. This approach also facilitates item retrieval for editing, revising, and entering item analysis data after the test.

When sorting items for a test, group items together that have the same format. This is not an issue if the test consists entirely of one item format type, such as multiple choice. However, if you include more than one format type on the same test, such as an essay or short answers with multiple choice, keep all items of the same type together with a specific set of directions preceding each item group of the same format.

Some experts recommend grouping items that measure the same content topics in a test. For example, items related to endocrine health alterations would be kept together in an exam that contains items related to the nursing care of clients who have a variety of health alterations. However, arranging a test so that items related to the same topic are grouped together fosters recall. Instead, scramble the items. Requiring the students to use information to solve problems that vary from one question to the next is a more realistic approach. After all, they will be required to solve a continuously changing array of problems when they practice nursing. In fact, it makes sense to include items that require the students to select priorities for clients who have several health alterations, as long as each of the health alterations was included in the course content.

Consider the key when arranging items. You do not want the correct answer to be the same letter for more than three or four questions in a row, nor do you want a letter to be omitted as the key for several consecutive items. Students pay attention to the key; they may refer to it for cues to the correct answer or second-guess themselves if a letter is repeated. Because you do not want students to be misled by the pattern of a key, print out the key to check that the correct answer is evenly distributed among all the possible letter options. If you see a pattern that could mislead the students, scramble the order of the items until the key looks neutral.

The easiest way to ensure that all the answer options are equally represented in your item bank is to keep track of where you put the correct answer as you write the questions. Some test developers suggest that you alphabetize the options. This approach could become very complicated for several reasons. First, if you use test development software to produce several versions of the test, some students will receive the options in alphabetical order, and others will receive a scrambled option order. Suppose you decide to edit the options based on the item analysis data: Will you have to alphabetize the revised options or start your new options with the same letter as the one you are replacing? What happens to the data associated with the original options? It will be lost if you rearrange the options. Keep it simple; alternate the correct answer letter as you write the questions. Check the bank occasionally to determine whether the letter options are represented equally and rectify the situation as you add items to the bank.

It is not advisable to move the location of a correct answer in an item to solve the problem of randomizing a key. The distractors should be left in the position assigned to them by the item writer. As you remember from Chapter 5, "Selected-Response Format: Developing Multiple-Choice Items," strategies are associated with ordering options. In addition, manually reordering options increases the potential for introducing error into the key and causes confusion when storing the data associated with the options. Instead of reordering the options, consider the letter representing the correct answer as one criterion when organizing the items on a test.

Some test development software programs attempt to decrease cheating by scrambling the order of the options to create different test versions. If you want different test versions but do not want the order of your options scrambled, select a software program that enables you to scramble the order of the items while maintaining the order of the options. In any event, avoid manually reordering the options of an item. Most programs allow you to turn off the scrambling option for an individual item. This is helpful when you want the item to be presented to all students in the same order, as with an item whose options are arranged from smallest to largest value.

Experts generally agree that items on a test should proceed from easier to more difficult (Brookhart & Nitko, 2014; Miller et al., 2009; Robinson Kurpius & Stafford, 2006). For example, the National Council Licensure Exam (NCLEX) presents the students with a relatively easy item for the first question on the test (National Council of State Boards of Nursing, 2006). This arrangement helps to decrease anxiety and frustration and has a motivating effect on students. Even well-prepared students can become anxious when confronted with difficult items at the beginning of a test.

It is not possible to arrange every item on a classroom test in ascending order of difficulty; however, you should at least start the test with several of the easier items. Students who encounter very difficult items at the beginning of a test can become discouraged. In fact, they may even spend excessive time laboring over these difficult items and run out of time before they reach items at the end of the test that they would have been able to answer. If you are creating multiple forms of a test by scrambling item order, be sure to keep the first few items the same for every form so that every student encounters the same easier items at the beginning of the exam.

When including items on a test, it is important to have a range of difficulty level for each content area and objective on the test. For example, a test that includes all of the difficult items in one content area and all of the easy ones in another content area would not provide valid results. Because all the blueprint categories are important, even if they are weighted differently, the difficulty levels should be distributed across the questions that are included in each category.

If you use test development software, manipulating the test items is as simple as clicking your mouse. If your items are in a word processing program, you must cut and paste them to create the test. Remember to keep track of the data included on the page with the item in the word processing program when you cut and paste. Using test development software or the cut-and-paste option means that there is no longer any need for a test to be typed. Once your items are developed, they can be copied easily from the test development software or word processing program where they are stored. **Exhibit 9.1** summarizes the key points for arranging the items on a test if you are not using test development software.

Exhibit 9.1 Arranging items on a test

- Print each item on separate sheet.
- Group items of the same format together.
- Scramble the items. Avoid grouping items by content area.
- Randomize the key among the letter options.
- Avoid repeating the same letter in the key more than three or four times.
- Start the exam with several easier items.

Editing and Proofreading

Professional test developers not only have expert panels to review their blueprints, items, and assembled exams, they also employ professional editors and experienced word processors to ensure that their tests are polished before they are published. Although classroom teachers seldom have these resources, it is important that your tests have a professional appearance to ensure face validity. Poorly edited tests reflect poorly on you. They tell the students that you do not care or that you lack the competence to write clearly and correctly.

There is nothing more distracting or anxiety provoking than the need to make several corrections on the blackboard at the beginning of a test or to explain typographical errors or omissions to the students. Chapter 5, "Selected-Response Format: Developing Multiple-Choice Items," reviews the principles for ensuring that your items are grammatically correct and consistent. It is also important to review the entire test once it is assembled. Exams that have a professional appearance convey the message to students that quality is important in both teaching and testing. Therefore, it is imperative that every teacher who produces a test carefully proofreads the test once it is assembled.

Before finalizing a test, take the test yourself. This enables you to key the test and check for errors. Call on the expertise of your colleagues. After you have taken and reviewed the test, provide your colleagues with an unkeyed test copy to edit and proofread and ask them to answer the questions as a final check of the clarity of the items. Make sure you remind your colleagues to read all options to verify that the correct answer is the only correct answer. Ask them to note whether there is any shred of truth in any of the distractors. Educators often tend to focus on the correct answer when reviewing a colleague's exam and may overlook problems in the incorrect options that the students will surely identify. The final version of the test should also be proofread for spelling, punctuation, and grammatical errors. Make sure that all items on the test appear to belong together, that the style and formatting are consistent, and that all questions are written in the present tense. Discrepancies can creep in, especially if different people write the items or if you have adapted the items from a textbook test bank.

It is also important to check the test for cueing. Cueing within items was discussed in Chapter 5, "Selected-Response Format: Developing Multiple-Choice Items"; cueing occurs when one question gives away the answer to another. In addition to giving away the correct answer, cueing can also lead students to choose the incorrect answer by misleading them. To eliminate cueing, look for the same or similar options in two items that are near each other. Check to see whether an option is the correct answer for one item and is repeated as the incorrect answer for another nearby item. Inspect the items to determine whether one provides the answer for another. Examine the questions to make sure that two of them are not asking the same thing. Tests developed by more than one person, for example, in an integrated nursing exam where adult and pediatric questions are on the same test, are especially prone to cueing. When items cue each other, one item may have to be removed from the test, or the two items may have to be separated in the test. **Exhibit 9.2** summarizes the key points for editing and proofreading a test.

Exhibit 9.2   Editing and proofreading a test

- Allow adequate time.
- Inspect for spelling, punctuation, and grammatical errors.
- Examine for consistency of style and formatting.
- Check that all questions are written in the same tense.
- Analyze for cueing. Take the test yourself.
- Ask a colleague to review the test.
- Remind your colleague to read both correct and incorrect options carefully.
- Complete the key by reading the answers out loud to a colleague.

Formatting Tests

Several technical issues are related to formatting items on a test. The best approach is to develop a single format for all the nursing courses in a program and then take the time to check that each test follows this format. This not only gives a uniform and professional appearance to all exams but also facilitates the transfer of items from one course to another when content adjustments are made between courses.

As mentioned previously, items of different types should be grouped together, preceded by clear instructions for the particular type of item. A matching column should be completely contained on one page (or one screen for a computerized exam). Completion-type items must have adequate space for the student to respond. True–false items should be numbered on the page next to the response line. Follow the examples provided in the exhibits in previous chapters when formatting these item types.

There are several widely accepted suggestions for formatting a multiple-choice test. First, you should allow adequate room for each item on the page, with a double space between items; for computerized exams, each item should be placed on a separate screen. Number the items sequentially throughout the test and list their answer options in a vertical column under the stem, with each option preceded by a letter; numerous examples of formatted items that follow this template are provided in Chapter 5, "Selected-Response Format: Developing Multiple-Choice Items":

1. Question or incomplete statement
   A. First option
   B. Second option
   C. Third option
   D. Fourth option

Make sure that the stem and options are kept together on the same page and that margins are available for students to mark items they want to revisit. A computerized test should have a mechanism that allows students to return to a question they want to revisit. Remember, this is not the NCLEX where students are not allowed to return to previous items. Classroom exams present the same items to all the students. The students are graded based on their responses to a defined set of items. Therefore, they should be allowed to return to an item they want to reconsider because their score depends on their answers to all of the questions

Do not print a paper-and-pencil test on both sides of a page. This practice can cause confusion and distraction for the students, particularly if the stem is on one side of a page and the options are on the other. If your institution requires that tests be copied on both sides of a page, be extra careful to keep all the stems on the same page with their associated options, and staple the test in two places down the left-hand side of the test, so it opens like a book. This prevents the students from having to flip the pages back and forth and decreases confusion.

It is very important that you check and recheck your exams for proper formatting and make any editorial and proofreading changes before submitting them for copying or entry for computerized administration. Taking the time to review the test carefully before it is administered facilitates a seamless process on exam day and ultimately improves the reliability of your exams. Refer to **Exhibit 9.3** for a summary of the key points for test formatting.

Exhibit 9.3   Formatting a test

- Develop a uniform format.
- Double-space between items.
- Use a separate screen for each item on a computerized exam.
- Number items sequentially throughout the test.
- Keep an entire matching column on one page or one screen.
- Number true–false items next to the response line.
- Allow enough space for completion and short-answer items.
- List multiple-choice options vertically under the item's stem.
- Precede each multiple-choice option with a letter.
- Keep each multiple-choice stem with all options together on the same page or computer screen.
- Provide margins on each side of the page.
- Print the exam on *one* side only of a page if possible.
- Staple the test down the left side, as in a book, if you must print it on two sides.
- Double-check the formatting and proofreading before copying.

Providing Directions

Not only is a good test a well-planned collection of items but it also includes a set of rules that must be clear to students. Clear test instructions are essential for students to be able to demonstrate their maximum ability. If directions are not understandable, the test will not accomplish its purpose.

Students should be told about any special directions before the day of the test. They should know what materials are allowed, such as calculators or scrap paper; what materials are not allowed, such as cell phones or electronic pagers; and what they are required to bring to the test, such as pencils or student identification.

Print the directions for the test on a cover sheet so that the students can refer to them during the test. A cover sheet prevents students from reading the questions while you are distributing the tests, and it helps them to focus when you read the directions out loud. Also provide space on the cover sheet for the students to print and sign their names. A signed cover sheet facilitates the tracking of tests for added security, ensures that the students are aware of the directions, and enables you to locate an individual's test should any questions arise after the exam. The cover sheet can be the first screen of a computerized exam or it can be distributed in printed form. Directions for classroom exams should not be elaborate but should include at least these points:

1. Basis for scoring: Identify how many items are on the test and how much credit is given for each correct response. Explain if any items are included for extra credit. If your test includes more than one item format, advise the students of this at the beginning of the test and group the individual formats together in separate sections. Print specific directions and the basis for scoring immediately before each individual test section.

2. Time limit for the test: Explain the time constraints for the test in the written directions. In addition, after reading the test directions out loud, announce the exact times that the test begins and ends. Assure your students that ample time

is available for completing the test. It is usually helpful to announce to students when half of the allotted time has elapsed. To avoid creating stress by surprising students, however, it is important to tell students at the beginning of the test that you will be making a time-remaining announcement. It may also be beneficial to periodically write the time remaining on the classroom backboard. Time is a major concern for students. To reduce their anxiety, be sure that students understand exactly how you will communicate the time remaining to them. In addition, it is most helpful to have a large wall clock in the test room.

3. How to select answers: Advise students to read carefully to determine whether they are to select the best answer or the correct answer. Remind them to read all the options. It is also crucial to ensure that students clearly understand how their answers should be recorded on the scannable form. Pay special attention to direct students to keep track of their responses. If they skip a question, there should be a system to ensure that they do not fill in an answer in the wrong spot on the answer sheet or fail to return to the screen of the omitted item in a computerized test.

Always advise students to use caution when changing answers. Although educators have been warning students for years about the detrimental effects of changing answers, this advice appears to be a myth. Several studies indicate that students are actually more likely to change their answers from incorrect to correct than from correct to incorrect (Nieswiadomy, Arnold, & Garza, 2001). While some students have the tendency to second-guess themselves, which can result in changing a correct answer to an incorrect one, it is wise to advise the students that they should change an answer if they believe their initial selection was incorrect. It is critical for students to be aware of the results of their own pattern. If they consistently lose points when changing an answer, they should avoid the practice. Most important, the students need to be aware of their own test-taking flaws and take action to correct them.

In an effort to mimic the NCLEX format, some nursing faculty prohibit students from returning to a previously answered question to change an answer. This practice should be discouraged. The NCLEX is a computer adaptive test, as Chapter 15, "Preparing Students for the Licensure Exam: The Importance of NCLEX," discusses. The students receive an individualized exam based on the difficulty level of the questions they answer correctly. Some students pass the exam on as few as 75 questions, while others answer as many as 265 questions. Passing is not based on a percentage-correct score. On a linear classroom exam, all the students take the same test. Passing is based on a predetermined percentage-correct score of a limited number of questions administered in a limited amount of time. Therefore, students should be encouraged to "go with what they know": move steadily through the test, avoid spending too much time on difficult items, and return to items about which they are unsure.

4. Consequences for guessing: Explain to students whether they lose credit for incorrect answers. Correction for guessing is sometimes used on standardized tests. However, it is not usually recommended for classroom tests because these tests are already subject to much more measurement error than standardized tests. If you choose to use a scoring program that allows you to correct a student's score for guessing, make sure that the students understand exactly what the implications are for guessing.

The test cover sheet in **Exhibit 9.4** includes all the criteria for a complete cover sheet with test directions for a paper-and-pencil test. Use it as a model for developing a cover sheet for your exams.

Exhibit 9.4   Sample cover sheet with directions

Exam Number
School of Nursing
Fundamentals of Nursing Care
Examination I
Spring 2017

Keep this test booklet closed until the proctor tells you to start the test.

This is a closed-book test that consists of 50 questions. Each question is worth 2 points. You have 60 minutes to complete the test. Calculators must be checked by the proctor. No other electronic devices are allowed in the testing room.

Select the one option that best answers each question. There is one correct answer for each question. There is no penalty for guessing. Do not waste time on a question that you find difficult. Skip it and return to it when you have reached the end of the test. Avoid wild guessing. Use the knowledge you have to answer every question, even when you are not perfectly sure of your answer. Stay calm and confident, and you will be successful. Good luck!

Follow these directions carefully:

- Check that your test has 14 pages in the correct sequence.
- Use only a number 2 pencil.
- Remove the scannable answer sheet that is inserted in this booklet, and fill in the identifying information in the top left-hand corner.
- Check to be certain that the exam number on your answer sheet matches the number on your test booklet.
- Circle the one correct answer to each question in the test booklet.
- You may write notes in the test booklet.
- Darken the circle on the answer sheet that corresponds to the one correct answer for each question.
- Be cautious with changing answers. If you do change an answer, erase your first mark completely on the answer sheet.
- If you skip a question, make sure to keep your place on the answer sheet.
- Mark any question that you skip in the test booklet so that you can return to it easily.
- Stay in your seat until you receive permission to leave it.
- If you have a question during the test, or if you finish the test before the time is up, raise your hand and a proctor will come to you.
- When the exam is over, put your pencil down and wait for the proctor to collect the test materials from you.
- Sign and print your name on the lines below.

Signature: _____

Print Name: _____

It is also wise to give the students a direction sheet for a computer-administered test. The directions can be printed on a sheet that the students can use as scrap paper, or it can be displayed on the computer screen. **Exhibit 9.5** represents a sample of a computer test directions sheet.

Exhibit 9.5   Sample computer test directions sheet

Exam Number
School of Nursing
Fundamentals of Nursing Care
Examination I
Spring 2017

This is a closed-book, computer-administered test that consists of 50 questions. Each question is worth 2 points. You have 60 minutes to complete the test. Calculators must be checked by the proctor. No other electronic devices are allowed in the testing room.

Select the one option that best answers each question. There is one correct answer for each question. There is no penalty for guessing. Do not waste time on a question that you find difficult. Skip it and return to it when you have reached the end of the test. Click the box in the upper left-hand corner of the screen to mark any question that you want to return to. Avoid wild guessing. Use the knowledge you have to answer every question, even when you are not perfectly sure of your answer. Stay calm and confident, and you will be successful. Good luck!

Follow these directions carefully:

- Use the mouse to click on the one correct answer to each question in the test booklet.
- Be cautious about changing answers.
- If you skip a question, make sure you click the box in the upper left-hand corner of the screen.
- Stay in your seat until you receive permission to leave it.
- If you have a question during the test, or if you finish the test before the time is up, raise your hand and a proctor will come to you.
- When the exam is over, log off the computer and wait for the proctor to collect the test materials from you.
- Sign and print your name in the space below to indicate that you have read these directions.

Signature: _____

Print Name: _____

Answering the questions listed in **Exhibit 9.6** will ensure the thoroughness of your final review of a test.

Reproducing

Reproducing involves yet another time issue, one you can avoid if you administer computerized tests. Most likely your support staff handles the task of reproducing the tests. If your situation is similar to that of most educational institutions, support staff

Exhibit 9.6 Guidelines for a final test review

- Does the test appear professional?
- Are the test directions clear, complete, and accurate?
- Does the test start with easier items?
- Are the difficult items distributed across the blueprint categories?
- Is the key accurate?
- Is the key randomized?
- Does each item stand alone?
- Does any item cue another item?
- Do any of the items overlap in content?
- Does each question test information that is important for a nurse to know?
- Does each question represent the content and instructional outcomes of the course?
- Do the items follow the style guidelines agreed on by the faculty?
- Is the test printed on one side of a page, or is it stapled in book form?
- Is the test free from typographical, spelling, and grammatical errors?
- Is the test formatted correctly, with adequate margins, and with a clear, legible, consistent font?

members have a large number of responsibilities. Plan ahead. You want a professional outcome, so allow staff members enough time to reproduce the tests. Reproduction should be completed several days before the test is scheduled to be administered.

Before you submit a test for copying, be sure that the master is exactly the way you want it. Carefully check that all the items you designated are included, they are numbered consecutively, and the pages are in order. Ask your staff to make a sample copy from the master to check if the contrast is suitable and the quality is acceptable. Set the copier to collate and staple the copies if these features are available. If hand-collating is required, careful checking of the final copies is essential. Remember to make sure your staff members are aware that the test is to be copied on one side only (if this is allowed at your institution) and that enough copies are produced so that there is one for each student and several extras for the examination proctors.

Most paper-and-pencil exams today are scored with a scanner. This frees up a teacher's time and also facilitates the generation of test and item analysis. Students must record their answers to tests that are scanned on a separate sheet, or a scannable form, that is compatible with the scanner. Make sure that the scannable form uses the coding (letters or numbers) for the answer options that correspond to the coding used on the test. Students can become confused if, for example, you labeled the question option letters A through D and the scannable answer form uses number 1 through 4 for the option choices.

Once the tests are reproduced, each test should be numbered and an answer sheet should be marked with the same number. The answer sheet should then be inserted under the cover sheet of each test. This ensures that each answer sheet can be matched to a test booklet and provides a security control for the tests and answer sheets.

Maintaining Security

Safeguarding the security of the test is the teacher's responsibility from the time the items are developed until the test is scored and destroyed. Every faculty member must be responsible for carefully guarding electronic and hard copies of the item bank. Just as you would never leave a copy of your personal bank statement in a lunchroom or fax a copy of it to a public mailroom, the test bank should be treated as a confidential document. If the security of the item bank file is violated, the items are useless.

Electronic test banks must be protected by security measures. Computer files should be encrypted, password-protected, and stored in a securely locked location. If a group of faculty use the same item bank, one member should be designated as being in charge of the bank, and a system should be devised to keep track of the location of and changes made to the bank. Remember, if the security of the bank is violated, the items in the bank cannot be used.

Another important concern is where to store a paper-and-pencil test during the time between reproduction and exam day. A securely locked closet is the simplest solution; just be certain that the exam administrators have access to the closet on exam day (and students or other interested parties do not!). Additional considerations include the security of the copy room and the trash from the copy room. How secure is your test disposal facility? Should you shred exams before disposing of them?

One method for preventing students from taking their scannable sheets and claiming that they handed it in is to provide the students with a $10'' \times 12''$ manila envelope with their names and identification number printed on it. At the end of the exam, each student is reminded to put the test and the scannable form in the envelope before giving it to the proctor. Students are then responsible for what is in the envelope. Although this adds an extra step to the administration process, it increases security and also helps students to remember their identification numbers.

Computer administration of exams solves many of these problems because no paper documents need to be safeguarded. However, access to the computer bank obviously needs to be protected. All test development software programs provide security that restricts access to the test banks and exams. Faculty members must be vigilant about following the directions to maintain security.

Although these questions and concerns may seem extraordinary to some of you, many faculty have been surprised by the extreme measures that desperate students take to obtain copies of exam questions. It is critical that only authorized personnel have access to the test. If a student gains access to the test, the results will lack validity and reliability. By taking a few simple precautions, you can save yourself from a lot of trouble.

Administering a Test

Conditions surrounding the administration of a test are another potential source of measurement error. The main goal of administering a test is to provide students with a fair opportunity to demonstrate their achievement of the learning outcomes. Fair assessment requires that you provide a test-taking environment that is conducive to the students' best efforts while minimizing factors that introduce measurement error. A systematic approach to the administration phase of the testing process limits the problems that can interfere with the reliability and validity of your test results. As with all phases of the test development process, the key factor is to plan ahead.

Computer Test Administration

Because technology is advancing exponentially, it is easy to forecast that classroom testing will be transitioned to computer administration over the next several years. Should you rush to test your students in a computer lab? First, you must assess your resources. What funds are available to implement a computerized testing environment? If you have adequate funding, computerized testing makes sense. If your funds are limited, make sure to keep your priorities in order.

Remember the old adage: garbage in, garbage out. The computer is only a tool; it can facilitate test development and administration, but it cannot compensate for poorly planned tests. The most important aspect of a test is the quality of the items. You can have the most sophisticated computer lab and yet have tests that are inferior to a program that is still administering paper-and-pencil, hand-scored exams. Before you administer tests via any method, you have to develop trustworthy tests. Providing the students with quality exams is the indisputable priority.

However, it behooves every nursing program to prepare for the eventual implementation of computerized testing. The initial phase, whether you are planning to initiate computerized test administration next year or 5 years from now, is to work on developing and organizing a test bank of high-quality items. You will need these items to develop your computerized tests. The best method for organizing a bank is to use test development software. Even if you plan to administer paper-and-pencil tests for the next several years, the time you spend initiating test development software is well invested. The items you develop and refine will form the basis for an effective computerized testing program. Chapter 14, "Instituting Item Banking and Test Development Software," discusses strategies for improving test items based on statistical data produced by software testing programs.

Today many faculty want to implement computerized testing to help prepare students for the NCLEX. In fact, several commercial testing companies who deliver computer-based exams advertise that this format is superior to paper-and-pencil tests because of its ability to prepare students to take computerized exams. Studies conducted by Anna (1998), Rossignol and Scollin (2001), and Killingsworth (2016) identified that students who took computerized exams reported feeling more prepared to take the NCLEX. However, there is no established link between NCLEX success and taking computerized classroom or standardized exams (Killingsworth, 2016; Reising, 2003), Therefore, nurse educators are discouraged from basing their decision to implement computer-based testing on NCLEX success. Instead, Reising suggests basing that decision on the efficiency of computerized testing (p. 329).

Computerized testing has several advantages:

- Exams are easy to assemble, administer, and score.
- Students become familiar with the computer-testing format.
- Scoring is efficient.
- Students can receive immediate feedback.
- Students can review rationales for missed items.

- Multiple-site testing is possible.
- There is no need for paper disposal.
- Test security is built in.

Computerized testing also has several disadvantages:

- Hardware, software, and technical support can be expensive.
- There can be a lengthy learning curve for faculty.
- Frustration can result when technical support is inadequate.
- There is a potential for cheating if there are not enough computers and students have to take a linear test on a computer by appointment.

The main point is that computerized testing is not the key to effective exams: Quality test items are the key to effective exams. Your students are not at a disadvantage for NCLEX success because they take paper-and-pencil exams. While it is important that students are familiar with basic computer operation, the computer is only a tool. In fact, the students can take the computer tutorial as many times as they want on the National Council of State Boards of Nursing (NCSBN) candidate's page at http://www.ncsbn.org. Develop a realistic plan for implementing computerized testing while working diligently on improving the quality of your test items.

Physical Environment

Make sure ahead of time that the environmental conditions of the physical space assigned for the test are appropriate. The room must have sufficient seating, light, and ventilation and be large enough for adequate spacing between desks. Always advise the students to dress in layers. The test environment should also be free from noise and interruptions. If the room is subject to distracting noise, such as from construction work, ask for a room assignment change. Minimize all interruptions by posting a sign on the door to the room stating that a test is in progress. You cannot eliminate all distractions, but planning ahead keeps them to a minimum.

Several days before administering a paper-and-pencil exam, make sure that the tests are ready and do a final count. On the day of the exam, arrive at the testing room at least 30 minutes before the starting time. Arrange the seating to maximize the distance between students. In situations where you are concerned about students sharing information during a test, you may want to assign seats. Assigning seats is one of the most effective deterrents for cheating. If you have a small number in the class, an easy method for seat assignment is to put Post-it notes with student names on each desk or to cut up a student roster and tape each student's name to the assigned seat.

Although seat assignment can be complicated for large lecture groups, it is even more important for deterring cheating than with small groups. One approach is to post the seating diagram outside the classroom and assign seats by number to students. Another suggestion is to seat the students randomly by having them draw their seat number before the test. Whatever method you choose, assigning seats is recommended as the most effective impediment for student cheating.

Seating is also important when administering a computer-based exam. The ideal situation would be to administer the exam to all students at the same time; this would eliminate the possibility of the students sharing the test questions with students who have not yet taken the exam. In this case, seating should be arranged to avoid the same pitfalls that exist with paper-and-pencil tests, which means that seats should be assigned to minimize the ability of students to copy from each other. However, hardware is expensive; many nursing programs do not have the resources to provide every student in a course with a computer for simultaneous test administration. When students take a linear test, meaning that every student receives the same test, by appointment in a computer lab, the risk for cheating is great. Cheating is discussed later in this chapter.

Psychological Environment

When students are excessively anxious during a test, they cannot demonstrate their maximum performance. Miller et al. (2009) identify several teacher behaviors that can increase test anxiety and therefore should be avoided:

- Using tests as a threat or punishment: "If the grades on this test are poor, you can expect the next test to be even more difficult."
- Giving dire warnings: "This is the most important test of the semester."
- Stressing time limits: "You have to work fast to finish this test on time."
- Emphasizing the consequences of failure: "If you fail this exam, you will not proceed in the program."

It is the teacher's responsibility to motivate students to do their best in every testing situation. A positive approach focuses students on their abilities and helps them develop the "I can do it" attitude. You can establish a positive psychological environment for students by preparing them for the test in advance and by using these guidelines to offer them well-developed, fair tests. When students perceive that a test is a fair assessment, test anxiety is reduced.

Clear instructions that are positively focused help to reduce anxiety. Keep the negative words in the directions to a minimum. Emphasize what the students should do, and avoid focusing on what they should not do.

Although both directions in **Exhibit 9.7** convey exactly the same message, which one is more conducive to reducing student anxiety? It is obvious that the negative approach sets up an adversarial student–teacher relationship at the very outset of the test. If you communicate in a positive manner, your students perceive that you consider them to be responsible learners. You thus boost their confidence and reduce test anxiety.

Exhibit 9.7   Positive versus negative directions

Positive
Keep this booklet closed until the proctor tells you to start the test.

Negative
Do not open this booklet until you are told to do so.

While it is important for you to recognize your role in reducing test anxiety, it is just as important for students to recognize that the best antidote for test anxiety is to be well prepared for an exam. Students must be responsible for their own learning. The guidelines presented in this book help you to communicate that message from the outset of a course. When students accept the challenge of attaining the objectives of a course and they are given a fair opportunity to demonstrate that attainment, their anxiety is reduced to a healthy level. Student motivation is enhanced if you clearly communicate to them throughout the semester that, although you are there to facilitate the learning process, they must achieve their own success.

Academic Dishonesty

It is critical that the testing environment not hamper student performance, but preventing the environment from falsely enhancing student performance is equally important. Almost 40 years ago, Ebel (1979) noted, "Cheating on examinations is commonly viewed as a sign of declining ethical standards or as an inevitable consequence of increased emphasis on test scores and grades" (p. 185). Unfortunately, academic dishonesty remains all too common on college campuses today.

McCabe (2009) identified cheating as a major issue in all educational disciplines and the discipline of nursing is not immune from cheating as documented by Krueger (2014). Nurse educators have a particular interest in deterring students from participating in unethical practices. After all, we are preparing future practitioners who are expected to follow a moral and ethical code of professional practice. Academic dishonesty is a violation of a moral code of behavior. Can we feel comfortable that students who violate that code will be safe and honest healthcare professionals?

Cheating   Cheating refers to the use of unauthorized assistance for an academic assignment or exam. Cheating practices include the following:

- Giving or receiving information during a test.
- Using unauthorized notes or information during a test.
- Sharing information for a take-home exam.
- Taking an exam for another student.
- Having another student take an exam for you.
- Obtaining questions before an exam.
- Tampering with an answer sheet after it is corrected.
- Using the same academic work for credit in more than one course.
- Memorizing test items to share with others who will take the test later.

Cheating affects all students. While the dishonest student may receive an inflated grade by cheating, cheating has a negative effect on the honest student. Those who do not cheat are placed at a disadvantage for grades, scholarship awards, graduate school admission, and employment positions (Cizek, 1999). All the effort that goes into developing a measurement instrument is worthless if cheating occurs on an exam because cheating ruins the reliability and the validity of test results. Therefore, teachers have an obligation to discourage cheating and to report it when it does occur. An ounce of prevention is invaluable: Careful planning of classroom tests can counteract the various methods of cheating.

When students perceive testing as a fair opportunity to demonstrate their achievement, the incidence of cheating is reduced. However, it is very naïve to assume that your students will not cheat just because you have painstakingly developed an exam to meet the criteria outlined in this book. The stakes are very high in nursing education, and you are doing a disservice to the honest students if you do not take measures to discourage cheating.

You have to be proactive to counteract cheating. Procedures must be established to maintain test security during the preparation, assembly, reproduction, storage, administration, and scoring of the test. Several procedures specified for choosing and preparing the physical environment for a testing experience also decrease the opportunity for cheating. Having students sign a cover sheet that includes a pledge to uphold the honor code, using identification numbers on the tests and answer sheets, and assigning seating are a few measures that counteract cheating.

Strategies to Prevent Cheating on Classroom Exams   To establish specific strategies to prevent cheating, you must be aware of the methods that students use to cheat on classroom exams. (Cizek, 1999; Faucher & Caves, 2009; Palmer, Bultas, Davis, Schmuke, & Fender, 2016) identify many of the cheating tatics that students use:

- Arranging to sit near friends.
- Looking at another student's paper or computer screen.
- Sharing information stored in cell phones or calculators.
- Using sign language or signals to communicate with other test takers.
- Dropping answer sheets on the floor in view of others.
- Holding answer sheets up so others can see.
- Sharing an eraser with information or answers written on it.
- Leaving one's seat to ask a question of the proctor while surreptitiously observing the answers of others.
- Using a cheat-sheet, written on tissues or hidden in places such as a necktie, skirt hem, pocket, or eyeglass case; taped to the bottom of a shoe or on the back of a water bottle label; or inside a mechanical pencil, to name a few hiding places.
- Writing information on one's body or clothing.
- Having another student take the test.
- Diverting a proctor's attention so that others can cheat.
- Using a microrecorder to record questions for others.
- Photographing questions with a microcamera concealed in a wristwatch, cigarette lighter, or campaign button.
- Storing information in a digital device.
- Accessing the Internet with a digital device.
- Using a virtually invisible earpiece to communicate with other students.
- Removing test materials from the room to share with others.
- Going to the bathroom to review hidden notes.
- Neglecting to turn in an answer sheet and claiming it was lost.

Although computer test administration counteracts some of these cheating strategies, students attempt many of them.

The biggest problem related to cheating on a computerized exam is scheduling. If you have enough computers so that all the students can take the exam simultaneously, you will not have this problem. However, many nursing programs do not have this luxury. The problem arises if students take the same test at different times. How can you be sure that the students are not discussing the exam with those who have not yet taken the test? You cannot. This approach for administering an exam is problematic for several reasons:

- Cheating cannot be prevented.
- Students who take the exam first are at a disadvantage.
- The reliability of the test results will be low.
- The grades on the test are erroneous.

Several strategies have been devised to counteract computer cheating when there are not enough computers to administer a test to an entire group simultaneously:

- Have some of the students take the test on a computer, and have others take the paper-and-pencil form of the same exam at the same time. Depending on how many computers you have, you can rotate the groups for each test in a semester. That way, all students have the opportunity to take a computerized test, and the integrity of the exam is not breached. This is a more secure approach than administering the same exam on a computer to all students by appointment.
- Administer parallel forms of the test at each session. With this approach, all students do not get the same test. However, unless you have a well-developed item bank with the data stored for all the items, you cannot be sure that all the tests are equal. Students would be justified in objecting to the fairness of this approach.
- Ask students to pledge that they will not share information on the test. Educators should be able to expect students, especially nursing students whose honesty is critical in the clinical setting, to be academically honest.

However, there is no way to verify that the students will honor the pledge mentioned above. Therefore, students who are academically dishonest can cheat successfully.

Deterring Cheating Students have devised countless innovative methods to give and receive information before, during, and after a test. These strategies are sometimes impossible to detect or prevent. The best defense is a good offense: The most effective method for preventing cheating is to have an adequate number of vigilant proctors. Two proctors are the minimum for every group-testing situation; it ensures that the students are not left alone if one proctor has to leave the room. Ideally, there should be two proctors for every 20 students. Have additional proctors if you have a reason to be concerned. Once students realize that you are serious about preventing cheating, they will be hesitant to risk the consequences of cheating.

It is your responsibility to make cheating impossible, whether the exam is administered in a paper-and-pencil or computerized format. Consider these strategies, consolidated from the suggestions of several experts (Brown, 2002; Cizek, 1999; DiBartolo & Walsh, 2010; Faucher & Caves, 2009; Hart & Morgan, 2009; Kolanko et al., 2006; Miller et al., 2009; Palmer et al., 2016) to deter cheating:

- Foster a classroom climate that supports honesty.
- Address academic honesty and review policies for dishonesty with students.
- Encourage the "I can do it" attitude by promoting a supportive environment that makes students feel they can succeed.
- Discuss the standards of academic honesty with the students.
- Develop an enforceable and explicit written policy regarding cheating.
- Explain the cheating policy to students, both verbally and in the syllabus.
- State the testing procedure in the syllabus and in the test directions.
- Have the students sign a contract pledging that they will uphold academic integrity.
- Use at least two proctors, who move around the room and are fully aware of the test administration procedure.
- Require that proctors be fully attentive to supervising students, not reading or involved in any other activity.
- Advise proctors to be aware of student gestures and establish eye contact with students as they circulate through the room.
- Use new exams each semester. Develop parallel items, as discussed in Chapter 5, "Selected-Response Format: Developing Multiple-Choice Items."
- Administer more than one form of the same exam, Use the same questions but scramble the options or the items for each version of the test. Even if you have only one form, label the cover sheet as if there are two or more forms. Let the students believe that there is more than one form.
- Arrive early and assign seats before the test. Cheaters try to sit together. Most cheating occurs when students can select their own seats.
- Provide adequate space between seats. Use alternate seats if possible.
- Require students to leave all books, notes, bags, and extraneous clothing at the front of the classroom. Students should not be allowed to wear hats, sunglasses, and so on.
- Do not allow students to bring note paper into the testing room. Provide students with scrap paper if the test is computerized or if they are not allowed to write in the test booklet.
- Prohibit students from sharing materials such as pencils, erasers, or calculators during the test.
- Check all calculators and ban *all* other electronic equipment from the testing room.
- Require students to bring picture identification to the exam if identity is a concern.
- Have students sign the cover sheet of the test.
- Instruct students not to leave their seats but to raise their hands if they have a question.
- Never leave a student alone. Establish a bathroom policy before the test.

- Collect the test materials from students while they remain seated to avoid confusion and distraction at the front of the room.
- Do not allow a latecomer to take the test if someone has finished the test and left the room.
- Use security cameras in the classroom to monitor activities.
- Look carefully at each answer sheet and test booklet as you collect them to make sure they have accurate identifying information, and make sure that there are no stray marks on the answer sheets.
- Use an attendance sheet to check that all test material is collected.
- Shred all scrap paper and exams after a paper-and-pencil test.
- Develop a makeup test policy that discourages students from missing a scheduled exam.
- Provide students with a confidential hotline number to report cheating.

Plagiarism   Plagiarism is a concern when assignments are completed outside class. As Tanner (2004) so succinctly describes, "Regardless of intention, failure to appropriately reference either verbatim or paraphrased work is plagiarism" (p. 291). Plagiarism is stealing the ideas or thoughts of another and presenting them as your own, including:

- quoting someone else without documenting the source;
- paraphrasing someone else's ideas without documenting the source; and
- submitting a paper as your own that you purchased or someone else wrote for you.

Although plagiarism has been a long-standing problem in postsecondary education, the growth of technology and easy access to the Internet has afforded students with the opportunity to obtain papers from a variety of sources. In addition, students can easily access websites for information on a particular topic and cut-and-paste material as they develop their papers (Kiehl, 2006). Often, students do not view this activity as plagiarism. Web-based material is frequently considered to be in the public domain, there for anyone to borrow. Therefore, the first step in enforcing an antiplagiarism program is to develop a policy that clearly defines plagiarism and describes the consequences for violating the policy (Bristol, 2011).

Another important measure for preventing plagiarism is to utilize plagiarism prevention software. The policy related to the use of this software should be communicated clearly to the students, and a mechanism should be established to document that both faculty and students acknowledge the policy. Some schools require the students to add a statement acknowledging that the submitted assignment is the student's original work (Bristol, 2011).

Bassendowski and Salgado (2005) suggest that today's teaching and learning environments need to evolve along with technology. Educators spend significant time detecting plagiarism, time that would be better spent creating assignments that require critical thinking and application to the students' own lives. Bassendowski and Salgado point out that, while considerable literature exists for detecting plagiarism, educators need to focus on designing assessment strategies that have a low potential for plagiarism. Assignments that foster critical thinking and offer real connections to students' professional and personal lives deter plagiarism by requiring original work and encouraging collaboration among students and with faculty.

Academic Integrity Policy   What are the consequences for cheating or plagiarism? This is a question that troubles educators, but it is a question that must be answered. You must understand the policy of your institution. Policies and procedures regarding academic dishonesty can be found on virtually every college campus (Cizek, 1999). Make sure that you are aware of these policies and that the policy established in a nursing department is congruent with the institution's policy.

The consequences for academic dishonesty must be established and documented for both teachers and students before the semester begins. The faculty must agree on the evidence required to establish academic dishonesty and its subsequent consequences. What are the consequences if plagiarism is identified? Do at least two proctors have to agree that students are surreptitiously sharing information? Are there degrees of cheating, ranging from the student who glances across the aisle to see another answer sheet to the student who obtains a copy of the test before the exam? What are the grading consequences? Will students be allowed to finish the test and lose credit? Or will students who cheat receive a zero on the test? Will students who plagiarize fail the course? Whatever the final decisions, it is crucial that you proceed cautiously and make sure that the evidence of academic dishonesty is well documented.

The activities that define academic dishonesty and the punishment associated with that activity must be communicated clearly to the students. However, even when a policy is well defined teachers are often uneasy about accusing a student of dishonesty. You certainly do not want to jump to conclusions and unjustly accuse an honest student of cheating. If you detect that students are attempting to share information or that a student is paying great attention to the answer sheet of a classmate, eye contact and extra vigilance usually discourage the activity. If it does not, quietly change their seats. It is a good policy to keep a seat or two free at the front of the room for this purpose.

If you are certain that a student or students are cheating, you are fully justified in taking the action that has been predetermined by the faculty. Ensure that you have carefully documented the event and that you save any evidence. If you have to remove a student from the classroom, try to keep the disruption to a minimum. In most cases, it will cause less disruption for the rest of the class to remove any violating materials, change the seat assignment, and allow the suspected student to finish the test. To keep the distraction to a minimum, tell the suspected student that you are moving her seat because you suspect that someone is looking at her answers. Follow up after the test if you believe that the suspected student was actually cheating.

Online Testing

The number of online learning courses in higher education has continued to grow. The eighth annual report on online education in the United States found that over 6.1 million students were taking an online course during the fall semester of 2010; this means that 31% of all students in higher education take at least one course online in a semester. Sixty-five percent of the institutions surveyed agreed that online education was critical for the long-term survival of their institution (Allen & Seaman, 2011).

The proliferation of online courses has resulted in the need for faculty to gain expertise in making online courses successful (Allen & Seaman, 2011; Skiba, 2013). This expertise is required for online course preparation, delivery, and assessments. The increasing availability of online courses in nursing education has created a new imperative for nursing faculty to become familiar with using technology for teaching on the Internet.

Online learning environments use a variety of strategies. A course can be offered completely online, or the course can be blended, using both the Internet and traditional face-to-face learning. Online learning requires the instructor to have skills in technology to develop effective learning environments online. Those skills include understanding the strategies for assessing and evaluating learning online (O'Neil, Fisher, & Newbold, 2009).

While there are multiple ways of assessing the online learner, cheating in the online environment is always a potential concern. Technological advances provide many new innovative opportunities for cheating on multiple-choice exams (Garcia & Woo, 2011). Palloff and Pratt (2010) propose using a variety of useful strategies for assessing students that do not involve tests and quizzes. However, nursing education relies heavily on multiple-choice exams to prepare students for initial nursing licensure. The issue that plagues online instructors is how to prevent and detect cheating to ensure the academic integrity of their online student evaluations.

Hart and Morgan (2009) propose several strategies, including the following:

- Create an atmosphere of academic integrity. Identify what you expect from the students and define the consequences of violating the expectations.
- Define the exact conditions under which students must take an exam.
- Avoid using published test banks because students can easily access these on the Internet.
- Add new and original items to the test bank each semester.
- Randomize the questions to create different versions of the test.
- Provide the students with open-book tests. Essays and projects offer the opportunity to demonstrate critical thinking.
- Set time limits for taking the exam.
- Require the student to obtain a proctor based on the instructor's criteria.
- Administer the test at a local testing center if the institution has this resource available.
- Use identification codes and passwords to authenticate the students' identity.
- Require students to use security software that prevents students from copying or referring to additional resources during the exam.
- Employ software products that use digital photographs, web cams, and/or microphones to validate the student's identity during an exam.

While some of these strategies may seem extreme, it is the instructors' responsibility to ensure the integrity of an online examination. Nursing faculty have to decide which strategies are appropriate for their online courses.

Scoring a Test

The main concern with scoring an exam is fairness. The key to fairness is objectivity. Exams that consist of selected-response items have a degree of built-in objectivity because the scorer's opinion cannot influence the score. However, you cannot assume that selected-response exams are inherently objective. Failure to analyze the questions after the test is scored for flaws and adjust the scores accordingly interferes with the fairness of the of the exam results.

While constructed-response items present a high risk for subjective scoring, measures can be used to minimize subjectivity. Chapter 8, "Constructed-Response Format: Developing Short-Answer and Essay Items," reviewed several options. For example, scoring rubrics and answer keys help to maximize objectivity and fairness when scoring constructed-response exams.

Scoring a Classroom Exam

When items on a test are equally weighted, a raw score represents the number of questions that a student answered correctly. After a test is administered, it must be scored, either by hand or by computer, to determine the raw score. Having the students use separate answer sheets facilitates both scoring methods. Obviously, it is important that the students clearly understand the directions for using the answer sheet so that an accurate raw score can be determined.

When tests are computer-based, they can be scored as soon as the student completes the test. This approach provides immediate feedback for the students. However, immediate scoring is not the best policy for a test that contains raw items—items that have never been tested before. It is better for the teacher to review the item analysis data, particularly when the test contains a lot of raw items, before assigning scores to a test to identify any flaws in the test items. Therefore, assigning final grades to a test should be deferred until you have had a chance to examine the test analysis data.

With the wide availability of reasonably priced optical scanning equipment, many schools score objective classroom tests electronically. If the scanner is not interfaced with a test development program, you need to create a key by hand. If you are using a test development software package, it interfaces with the scanning hardware to score the exam; these packages eliminate the need for teacher-generated keys because the tests are scored directly from the item bank where the correct answers are stored. Most of these programs alert you if a student has marked two answers or has omitted an answer. However, it is a good idea to examine each answer sheet for stray marks, incomplete erasures, or omitted answers before you start the scanning process. When implemented properly, electronic scoring is efficient and accurate, and can provide you with detailed analyses of the test results. These analyses offer invaluable information for translating a raw score into a meaningful inference of student achievement.

If you have to score your multiple-choice exams by hand, you can create a scoring template, which is simply an answer sheet with a hole punched out for each of the correct answers. Place the template over a student's answer sheet and fill in each hole that is blank with a red mark. When you remove the template, you can count the number of red marks to determine how many questions were answered incorrectly. Of course, if you are in this situation, you really need to investigate obtaining equipment to score your exams electronically.

An essential detail of scoring is the accuracy of the key. Whatever method you use for scoring, you must make sure that the key is correct before you start the process. First, circle the correct answers on a copy of the test and fill in the answer key based on the keyed copy of the test. Then, have two people double-check the key—one person should read the answers on the key out loud while the other checks that the key corresponds to the answers circled on the test.

Statistical Analysis

Raw scores can be misleading. They are not always an accurate reflection of a student's achievement. Despite all your efforts, mistakes do occur. Errors such as incorrectly keyed items, items that have more than one correct answer, items that are too difficult for the group, or items that mislead students can creep into even the best-planned exam. These are referred to as flawed items, and they should be adjusted before a final score is assigned to a test. Thus, a teacher who simply scores a test and assigns grades without reviewing the results of the test is very misguided.

Once you have determined the raw scores for a test, you need to analyze the results before you can determine the final scores. Using a computer program that provides this information is the most efficient way to approach this analysis. In fact, it is much too time consuming for most teachers to attempt to calculate item data on their own. Teachers who do not obtain computer printouts for their exams are at an extreme disadvantage when trying to determine the accuracy of a raw score. In order to conduct a thorough quantitative review of an exam, teachers should have access to a computer analysis of the test. Chapter 11, "Interpreting Test Results," examines the use of statistical analysis for quantitative review before assigning final scores to an exam and addresses the implications of removing flawed items from a test.

Student Review

In addition to the faculty qualitative review before the test and the statistical review after the test, a student qualitative review, based on the opinions of the test consumers, provides valuable information for determining the final scores of a test. It is best to hold a student review after the test analysis is done but before the grades are assigned. That way you can identify any problem questions before the students have the opportunity to argue during the review.

The purpose of a test review is to help students learn about their reasoning processes and to identify any undetected ambiguities in the test. Allowing students to review the exam before the grades are assigned also provides you with insight when determining what to do with a problem item.

A student review should not be a debate session, where students confront teachers to argue for more points. Nor should it simply consist of a teacher reading the correct answers to the students. Student test reviews can be productive exercises in critical thinking when students are given the opportunity to reflect on their thinking and to examine the process by which they chose their answers.

Because test security is a major concern, student reviews should be held in a strictly controlled setting. Many of the same restrictions that were applied during the test should be enforced during the review session. Students should be required to leave all pencils, pens, notes, texts, electronic devices, hats, sunglasses, and so on, at the front of the room. In addition to the faculty member who is reviewing the test, proctors should also circulate to monitor the room.

It is inadvisable to give students their original answer sheets or test booklets. Many of the test development programs provide individual printouts of students' answers. If these are not available, give students photocopies of their answer sheets. A test that is developed from a software program can be projected to a wall screen from a computer, or overhead transparencies of the test can be made for projection. If students report discrepancies between the score report and their recollection of their answers on the original answer sheet, a faculty member should review the original answer sheets with the students on an individual basis.

It is preferable to hold group review after all students have taken the exam. If students were absent on exam day, the review should be postponed until all students have taken the exam. Even if the makeup test is an alternate form, the students who have not taken the exam have an unfair advantage if a review is held before they take the test. At the very least, students who have not taken the exam should not be allowed to attend the review.

Approach the test review as a learning experience. While exams are given to measure student achievement, structured exam review supports student learning (Wiles, 2015). Provide the students with their raw scores and tell them that you will assign grades after you have their input. Tell the students that the purpose of the review is to help them improve their skills in taking multiple-choice exams that require higher-order thinking. Read each question and ask students to identify the correct answer. Explain why the correct answer is correct and why the distractors are wrong.

Identify questions that have statistical problems. For example, if the data for questions indicate that the higher-end students answered incorrectly, ask, "Would someone who answered B on question two like to discuss their reasoning?" Ask for student volunteers who answered each item incorrectly to explain their thinking and discuss the inconsistencies in their logic. If students have a reasonable argument about the correctness of an option or the clarity of a stem, tell them you will consider their input when determining the final scores. Remember not to make any promises or to take the students' comments personally. Most important, try to keep the atmosphere positive.

To avoid spending an inordinate amount of time in test review, many faculty members allow students to present a written justification for an answer within a certain deadline after the test review. Haladyna (1997) cites the following positive effects that can result from this practice:

- Encourages the students to write persuasively and think critically about their reasoning.
- Recognizes when the students have a correct, creative alternative solution.
- Identifies when lack of learning and/or teaching exists.
- Provides an opportunity for students to vent their feelings.
- Allows students to gain extra points if their justification is accepted.
- Promotes a positive learning environment (p. 235).

If you set a deadline for submission of 1 to 2 days after the class review, you will have time to integrate the students' proposals for alternative solutions with the quantitative analysis of the test (discussed in Chapter 11, "Interpreting Test Results") before you assign grades to the exam.

Many nurse educators find test review sessions to be very unpleasant. However, if you present students with a well-crafted exam that follows the guidelines presented in this book and give the students an opportunity to express their opinions (written or verbal), student contentiousness will be kept to a minimum. You will also find that positive review sessions and the students' written justifications provide ideas for item revision. Pay attention to the students' reasoning processes and note their comments and ideas—they can be very helpful for item analysis as well as for future item development.

Small-group test review is becoming increasingly popular in nursing education. The goal of this exercise is to strengthen students' knowledge base through collaboration and exchange of ideas (Steele, 2006). A variety of approaches are used, but they all include dividing students into small groups immediately after a test and having them review or retake the test as a group. Points are awarded based on the group's performance. The objective is not to inflate the students' grades but rather to provide an opportunity for students to increase their knowledge and improve their test-taking skills. Steele (2006) notes that the group review encourages students to debate, integrate, and synthesize course material, while it decreases challenges to individual items. Steele also identifies that, as long as the test bank is large enough to prevent recirculation of the items more than once every 2 to 3 academic years, a controlled group review process does not compromise the integrity of the item bank.

Wiles (2015) suggests providing the students with an exam review grid. She provides the students with a grid that identifies nursing process, client needs, cognitive levels, and content areas. The students identify their individual weaknesses for each item. The grid helps the students identify their individual pattern of missed questions. The grid can also be used to help students identify their test-taking habits. Did they change answers, read too quickly, or neglect to read an entire question? It is very important for students to understand their own test-taking weaknesses. The grid helps students identify patterns of poor performance and develop strategies for improvement.

Summary

As with all aspects of the assessment process, a systematic approach to assembling, administering, and scoring classroom exams decreases error and safeguards the validity and reliability of your classroom tests. These steps are often overlooked as the clerical aspects of test development, yet they are essential for the integrity of your exams. The practical guidelines offered in this chapter streamline these processes and enable you to put a professional touch on your tests.

The issues of paper-and-pencil versus computer-based test administration, cheating, plagiarism, scoring, and student test review are addressed in this chapter. Cheating and plagiarism affect both the honest and dishonest students by interfering with the reliability of the examination's results, and educators are responsible for taking measures to ensure the integrity of the assessment environment. Strategies for detecting and interfering with student cheating and plagiarism are proposed to assist nursing faculty in developing a plan to ensure the integrity of their assessments. Maintaining the integrity of online student assessment was discussed.

Guidelines for including student assessment through post hoc test review are also suggested. Student comments can be a valuable resource for assigning final test scores and for improving items for future use. Approaches for conducting a productive student test review are offered, with a focus on the positive benefits for both students and teachers.

Learning Activities

1. Describe all the factors that must be considered when arranging items on a test.
2. Create a cover sheet for a real or hypothetical exam. Include all the essential criteria for a complete cover sheet.
3. Compare paper-and-pencil to computer-based administration of a test. What are the advantages and disadvantages of each approach?
4. Develop a plan to deter cheating on a paper-and-pencil or computer-administered exam.
5. Design a grid that students can use to identify their test-taking pattern when reviewing a test.
6. Prepare a plan for student review of an exam. Compare the advantages and disadvantages of large- and small-group test review. Which approach would you implement? Explain your answer.

Web Links

Assessment Systems
http://www.assess.com
Grammarly—Antiplagiarism website
http://www.grammarly.com
The Journal
http://www.thejournal.com
National Council of State Boards of Nursing
http://www.ncsbn.org
Plagiarism dot org
http://www.plagiarism.org
Plagiarism Resources
http://www.park.edu/cetl/quicktips/plagiarism.html
The Sloan Consortium
http://www.sloanconsortium.org/
Turnitin—Antiplagiarism website
http://www.turnitin.com

References

Allen, I. E., & Seaman, J. (2011). *Going the distance: Online education in the United States, 2011.* Retrieved from http://www.onlinelearningsurvey.com/reports/goingthedistance.pdf

Anna, D. J. (1998). Computerized testing in a nursing curriculum: A case study. *Nurse Educator, 23*(4), 22–26.

Bassendowski, S. L., & Salgado, A. J. (2005). Is plagiarism creating an opportunity for the development of new assessment strategies? *International Journal of Nursing Education Scholarship, 2*(1). Retrieved from http://www.bepress.com/ijnes/vol2/iss1/art3

Bristol, T. J. (2011). Plagiarism prevention with technology. *Teaching and Learning in Nursing, 6,* 146–149.

Brookhart, S. M., & Nitko, A. J. (2014). *Educational assessment of students* (7th ed.). Upper Saddle River, NJ: Pearson Education.

Brown, D. L. (2002). Cheating must be okay—Everybody does it! *Nurse Educator, 27*(1), 6–8.

Cizek, G. J. (1999). *Cheating on tests: How to do it, detect it, and prevent it.* Mahwah, NJ: Lawrence Erlbaum Associates.

DiBartolo, M. C., & Walsh, C. M. (2010). Desperate times call for desperate measures: Where are we in addressing academic honesty? *Journal of Nursing Education, 49,* 543–544.

Ebel, R. L. (1979). *Essentials of educational measurement* (3rd ed.). Englewood Cliffs, NJ: Prentice Hall.

Faucher, D. F., & Caves, S. (2009). Academic dishonesty: Innovative cheating techniques and the detection and prevention of them. *Teaching and Learning in Nursing, 4,* 37–41.

Garcia, M., & Woo, A. (2011). The role of security in today's testing programs. *Clear Exam Review, 2,* 16–19.

Haladyna, T. M. (1997). *Writing test items to evaluate higher order thinking.* Needham Heights, MA: Allyn and Bacon.

Hart, L., & Morgan, L. (2009). Strategies for online test security. *Nurse Educator, 34,* 249–253.

Kiehl, E. M. (2006). Using an ethical decision-making model to determine consequences for student plagiarism. *Journal of Nursing Education, 45,* 199–203.

Killingsworth, E. (2016). Use of technology in classroom testing. *Nurse Educator, 41,* 60–61.

Kolanko, K. M., Clark, C., Heinrich, K. T., Olive, D., Serembus, J. F., & Sifford, K. S. (2006). Academic dishonesty, bullying, incivility, and violence: Difficult challenges for nurse educators. *Nursing Education Perspectives, 21,* 34–43.

Krueger, L. (2014). Academic dishonesty among nursing students. *Journal of Nursing Education, 53*(2), 77–87.

McCabe, D. L. (2009). Academic dishonesty in nursing schools: An empirical investigation. *Journal of Nursing Education, 48*(11), 614–623.

Miller, M. D., Linn, R. L., & Gronlund, N. E. (2009). *Measurement and assessment in teaching* (10th ed.). Upper Saddle River, NJ: Pearson Education.

National Council of State Boards of Nursing. (2006). *Computerized adaptive testing (CAT) overview*. Retrieved from http://www.ncsbn.org/1216.htm#why-cat

Nieswiadomy, R. M., Arnold, W. K., & Garza, C. (2001). Changing answers on multiple-choice examinations taken by baccalaureate nursing students. *Journal of Nursing Education, 40*(2), 142–144.

O'Neil, C. A., Fisher, C. A., & Newbold, S. K. (2009). *Developing online learning environments in nursing education*. New York, NY: Springer.

Palloff, R. & Pratt, K. (2010). *Collaborating online: Learning together in community*. San Francisco, CA: John Wiley & Sons.

Palmer, J. L., Bultas, M., Davis, R. L., Schmuke, A. D., & Fender, J. B. (2016). Nursing examinations: Promotion of integrity and prevention of cheating. *Nurse Educator, 41*(4), 180–184.

Reising, D. L. (2003). The relationship between computer testing during a nursing program and NCLEX performance. *Computers in Nursing, 21,* 326–329.

Robinson Kurpius, S. E., & Stafford, M. E. (2006). *Testing and measurement: A user friendly guide*. Thousand Oaks, CA: Sage.

Rossignol, M., & Scollin, P. (2001). Piloting use of computerized practice tests. *Computers in Nursing, 19,* 206–212.

Skiba, D. J. (2013). MOOCs and the future of nursing. *Nursing Education Perspectives, 34,* 202–204.

Steele, S. K. (2006). Group test review and analysis: Learning through examination. *Journal of Nursing Education, 45*(2), 95–96.

Tanner, C. A. (2004). Moral decline or pragmatic decision making? Cheating and plagiarism in perspective. *Journal of Nursing Education, 43*(6), 291–292.

Wiles, L. L. (2015). "Why can't I pass these exams?": Providing individual feedback for nursing students. *Journal of Nursing Education, 54*(1), 55–58.

Establishing Evidence of Reliability and Validity

© Anteromite/Shutterstock

"Facts are stubborn things, but statistics are more pliable."

—MARK TWAIN

The two most important questions to ask about a measurement instrument are:

1. How accurate is the score?
2. How meaningful is the interpretation of the score?

The first question asks about the reliability of the scores obtained with the instrument, while the second examines the validity of the decisions made based on those scores. Just how important are the concepts of reliability and validity to assessment? They are the essential elements for examining a measurement instrument. They form the very basis on which fairness and trustworthiness are established. If teachers are to have confidence in the decisions they make based on the results of their classroom exams, they must be confident that their measurement instruments are providing both valid and reliable results.

There is an additional concern that cannot be overlooked: Students today are becoming more sophisticated. They are starting to question the reliability and validity of the results of the classroom exams on which their futures depend. In today's litigious society, it is not outside the realm of possibility that teachers could be called on to defend their assessment decisions in a court of law. Whether it is to justify the fairness of your grade assignments or to defend yourself in a formal legal proceeding, how well prepared are you to defend your current measurement instruments?

To select, develop, and interpret the results of measurement instruments fairly, it is essential that you have a clear understanding of the concepts related to both reliability and validity. Reliability and validity were introduced in Chapter 2, "The Language of Assessment." This chapter examines how evidence of reliability and validity is established. Review of these concepts is designed to provide you with a foundation for understanding the importance of the reliability and validity of the results of your classroom assessments. You will also find the information useful for selecting, and interpreting the results of, standardized tests.

Reliability

Reliability refers to the consistency of test results, or how constant scores are from one measurement event to another (Miller, Linn, & Gronlund, 2009). Reliability is not about the test itself—it is about the scores that a particular sample obtained on the test. In other words, it is sample dependent. The more consistent measurement results are from one administration of a test to another, the greater the reliability of those test results. A measurement is said to be reliable if it is reproducible—if an independent replication of the same measurement on the same individual would yield the same score. In other words, reliability refers to trustworthy test results.

No test provides results that are 100% reliable: Error is inherent in every type of measurement. Reliability is related to the degree to which test scores are free from measurement error. The lower the error of a measurement is, the more consistent the test scores will be. While error can never be completely eliminated from a measurement instrument, it is important to identify how imperfect the results of an instrument are. Are the results trustworthy enough for your purposes? Or are they so unreliable that you cannot have enough confidence in the results to make a decision based on them?

Measures of Reliability

Several methods are available to help you estimate the reliability of your test scores. Because of measurement error, we can expect a certain amount of variation from one testing episode to another. Reliability measures provide an estimate of the consistency of the test score. The three different approaches for obtaining evidence about reliability are test–retest, parallel forms, and internal consistency. A reliability estimate obtained from one of these approaches is not interchangeable with a value derived by a different technique. These values are not equivalent because each incorporates a unique definition of measurement error (American Educational Research Association [AERA], American Psychological Association, & National Council on Measurement in Education, 1999). Popham (2003) emphasizes that, although all forms of reliability are related to a test's consistency, they are conceptually dissimilar. It is important to recognize that evidence of reliability in one form does not guarantee reliability in another. For example, a test whose results have a high estimate for internal consistency may not yield results that are stable over time (pp. 52–53).

Test–Retest   This method determines the reliability of a test's results by collecting evidence about its stability by giving the identical test to the same individuals on a second occasion and then determining the correlation between the two sets of scores (Brookhart & Nitko, 2014). The time interval between the two administrations can vary from a few days to several years. Longer time periods between testing result in lower reliability estimates because of changes in the students, so it is important to note the time interval when reporting test–retest reliability. The major drawback of this approach is that it requires the exact same test be given to the same individuals on two different occasions, a situation that is not feasible in a classroom setting.

Parallel-Form Reliability   Parallel-form reliability is concerned with the comparability of two alternate forms of a test. With this method, the same person is tested with two different forms of a test, and the reliability of the test's results is represented by the correlation of the scores on the two forms of the test. This method indicates the degree to which the two assessments are measuring the same trait (Miller et al., 2009). Because of the difficulty in constructing two equivalent forms of the same test, this method is not a likely alternative for most classroom teachers. In addition, students most likely would object to duplicate testing for the sake of obtaining reliability. If the parallel forms are administered at different times, then the time interval between testing episodes must be taken into consideration when interpreting the reliability estimate: the shorter the time interval, the higher the reliability estimate will most likely be.

Internal Consistency   Because it is usually not practical or appropriate to repeat a classroom test or to develop an alternative form of the test to determine the reliability of the test results, various statistical methods have been developed to estimate the reliability of test results from a single administration. These methods of analysis estimate the internal consistency of a test and report a reliability coefficient, or an index of the amount of error, for a particular test. Of the three methods for estimating reliability, formulas for determining internal consistency are most appropriate for use with standardized tests. These formulas can also be applied to classroom exams; however, you must use caution when interpreting the results. The factors that affect the interpretation of the reliability coefficient for classroom exams are reviewed later in this chapter.

While correlations for test–retest and parallel-form reliability measures tell us what we can reasonably estimate to be the degree of relationship between two test scores, reliability coefficients give an estimate of internal consistency, or the degree to which the items in one test are measuring the same dimension or construct (Salkind, 2012). While a correlation coefficient ranges between -1.0 and $+1.0$ (with the extremes at both ends indicating perfect correlation), a reliability coefficient falls between 0.0 and 1.0. A reliability coefficient of 1.0 indicates perfect reliability, whereas a reliability coefficient of 0.0 indicates that the test results completely lack reliability (see **Exhibit 10.1**).

Exhibit 10.1   Reliability coefficient

Range 0.0 to $+1.0$
$+1.0$ = PERFECT
0.0 = No Reliability

There are several formulas for obtaining a reliability estimate from a single form of a test. The reliability estimates most frequently reported in today's test analysis computer programs estimate the reliability of the test based on the internal consistency of the test. These formulas rely on the concept that each item in a test can be considered a one-item test (Brookhart & Nitko, 2014). Internal estimates of reliability compare each item in the test with the total score on the test and depend on the variance of the test, the variance of the individual items, and the consistency of the performance of the test takers from item to item (Thorndike, 1997). The higher the variance, or the greater the spread of scores on the test, the higher the reliability coefficient of the test.

Fortunately, you no longer need to be a computational wizard to obtain and interpret test data. With the availability of today's optical scanners and computer hardware and software, valuable test statistics are readily available to the classroom teacher. Therefore, you have easy access to the programs that can help you to efficiently evaluate and improve the quality of your tests. Advanced mathematical skills are not required to use this information.

Although you do not need to actually calculate test statistics, being aware of the factors that influence the reliability coefficient facilitates your ability to interpret test results and improve your classroom assessment instruments. A logical and practical approach for interpreting statistical analysis to improve your tests and to increase your confidence in the judgments you make based on your tests is presented in Chapter 11, "Interpreting Test Results."

Just as students have different learning styles, so do faculty members. Several formulas are included throughout this text for those of you who find the mathematical explanations of statistical analysis helpful. Do not let the complexity of these mathematical formulas baffle you. Only those who are involved in the psychometric analysis of test data need to have a thorough understanding of the calculations involved. Ignore them if you find them confusing; you will never need to perform any of these calculations. However, for many of you, visualizing how the factors associated with reliability affect statistical outcomes helps to demystify the calculations and diminish the intimidating nature of test analysis data.

What is important is that you understand the principles of assessment. The purpose of this discussion is to explain these principles and improve the reliability of the information you obtain from classroom tests. If you are interested in learning more about calculating reliability coefficients and other statistical test data, a clear and comprehensive presentation is provided in Brookhart and Nitko's (2014) *Educational Assessment of Students.*

Reports of reliability calculated from internal consistency include the split-half method, the Kuder–Richardson formula 20 (KR-20), and coefficient alpha. Each of these methods estimates reliability from a single form of a test.

SPLIT-HALF RELIABILITY COEFFICIENT   A split-half procedure arbitrarily splits the test into reasonably equivalent halves so that each individual receives two scores. These two scores are correlated, and a reliability coefficient is determined. This approach yields a correlation coefficient, similar to the test–retest and parallel-form methods; however, only one test is administered. This type of reliability coefficient is referred to as a measure of internal consistency because only one test is administered (Brookhart & Nitko, 2014).

The first step when determining split-half reliability is to decide how to split the test so that the two most equivalent halves are identified. The procedure most often used is to assign the odd-numbered questions to one half-test and the even-numbered questions to the other half-test. Two problems are associated with this method of estimating reliability. The first is that different estimates result from different subdivisions of the test. Second, the correlation only estimates the reliability of the results of half of the test. However, the second problem can be corrected by using the Spearman–Brown prophecy formula, which adjusts the correlation to estimate the reliability of the results for the whole test (Brookhart & Nitko, 2014).

KUDER–RICHARDSON FORMULA 20 AND COEFFICIENT ALPHA RELIABILITY COEFFICIENTS   While the split-half reliability is derived from a planned split of a test;, the reliability coefficients derived from the coefficient alpha and the KR-20 formulas are actually the average of all the split-half coefficients that can be derived from all possible splits of a test (Anastasi & Urbina, 1997). Estimates provided by these formulas are really indications of the degree to which the individual item responses correlate with the total test score or how well a test correlates with itself (Mehrens & Lehmann, 1991). Both estimates of reliability provide information about the degree to which the test items are measuring similar characteristics (Miller et al., 2009).

The KR-20 formula, shown in **Exhibit 10.2**, is used when each item on a test is scored dichotomously—that is, as either correct or incorrect. When the items are not scored dichotomously, the formula for coefficient alpha, shown in **Exhibit 10.3**, is used. The two formulas are essentially the same, except that in coefficient alpha, ΣPQ is replaced by ΣSD_i^2, which is the sum of all the item variances (Anastasi & Urbina, 1997, p. 98). Coefficient alpha is the only commonly available, computer-calculated reliability estimate for instruments whose items can take on a range of values, such as in a personality inventory (Worthen, Borg, & White, 1993, p. 157). It can actually be used to measure the reliability of the results of instruments with either dichotomous or weighted scores because the ΣSD_i^2 is equal to ΣPQ.

Exhibit 10.2   Kuder–Richardson formula

$$KR_{20} = \frac{N}{N-1} \times \frac{SD_t^2 - \Sigma PQ}{SD_t^2}$$

where

N = number of items on the test

SD_t^2 = variance of the test scores

Σ = sum of

P = proportion answering an item correctly

Q = proportion answering an item incorrectly

Exhibit 10.3   Coefficient alpha

$$\alpha = \frac{N}{N-1} \times \frac{SD_t^2 - \Sigma SD_i^2}{SD_t^2}$$

N = number of items on the test

α = coefficient alpha

SD_t^2 = variance of the test scores

Σ = sum of

SD_i^2 = variance of the individual items on the test

The KR-20 and coefficient alpha estimates are used most frequently by test publishers and are reported by most classroom test development software packages. They provide an estimate of the reliability for the total test score based on the consistency with which students respond from one item on a test to the next. Examine the formulas for both the KR-20 and the coefficient alpha (see Exhibits 10.2 and 10.3). They clarify that the higher the variance (SD^2), the higher the reliability of the test results, which means that the more the scores on a test are spread out from the mean, the higher the test reliability coefficient will be. **Exhibit 10.4** demonstrates how the reliability coefficient would be affected if all students obtained the same score on a test. In this case the variability is 0, so the reliability coefficient is 0.

Exhibit 10.4   Coefficient alpha with zero variance

$$\alpha = \frac{N}{N-1} \times \frac{SD_t^2 - \Sigma SD_i^2}{SD_t^2}$$

$$\alpha = \frac{N}{N-1} \times \frac{0-0}{0}$$

$$\alpha = 0$$

where
N = number of items on the test

α = coefficient alpha

SD_t^2 = variance of the test scores

Σ = sum of

SD_i^2 = variance of the individual items on the test

Factors Affecting the Reliability Coefficients of Classroom Exams

Because it can be determined by one test administration, a reliability coefficient is the kind of reliability that is reported by standardized test developers and with test development software packages. Remember, these reliability coefficients are associated with measures of internal consistency and are directly influenced by the spread of scores on the test and the discrimination of the test items (Haladyna, 1997). As the discussion in this chapter has already established, the larger the score variability or spread of scores, the higher the reliability estimate (Miller et al., 2009). Therefore, classroom teachers are immediately faced with the problem that these reliability coefficients do not apply to their classroom exams. In fact, Popham (2003) asks the question, "So, what sorts of reliability evidence should classroom teachers collect for their own tests?" and then responds, "My answer may surprise you. I don't think teachers need to assemble any kind of reliability evidence. There's just too little payoff for the effort involved" (p. 53).

Popham's question and answer illustrate an important consideration for evaluating your classroom exams: "Can you accurately determine the reliability of the results of your classroom exams?" When you depend solely on the reliability coefficient provided by most test development software packages to determine the reliability of the results of your classroom tests, you can easily be misled. The terms *reliability* and *reliability coefficient* may not be synonymous for classroom tests: Your exams may provide consistent results even when the reliability coefficient appears to be less than desirable. The key requirement for teachers is to understand how to interpret the distinct types of test reliability because, as Popham identifies, "An unreliable test will rarely yield scores from which valid inferences can be drawn" (p. 54).

Several factors can introduce error and directly affect the reliability coefficient of your multiple-choice classroom tests. Appropriate measures can be taken to minimize error and maximize the reliability of the results of your classroom tests when you understand these factors. Recognizing the influence of these factors on the reliability coefficient also enables you to make sensible interpretations of your classroom test analysis data.

Quality of the Test Items   The primary requirement for the reliability of test results is that a test has well-constructed items. If the individual test items are clear and focused, they provide reliable information about student ability or achievement. However, poorly constructed items, which are vague and ambiguous, will be open to a variety of student interpretations and provide unreliable test results because they confuse both the high and low achievers on a test. The best way to improve the reliability and validity of classroom test results is to improve the quality of individual test items. Chapter 5, "Selected-Response Format: Developing Multiple-Choice Items," and Chapter 6, "Writing Critical Thinking Multiple-Choice Items," provide extensive guidelines for developing high-quality multiple-choice items, and Chapter 14, "Instituting Item Banking and Test Development Software," examines how to improve the items based on item analysis data.

Item Difficulty (p value)   The item difficulty index (p value) is defined as the percentage of the total group who answered the item correctly on a particular test. The easier a test item is, the higher its p value. An item that is answered correctly by 90 students in a group of 100 students would have a p value of 90% (0.90) for that group on that specific test. It is very important to note that the difficulty index of an item is not a property of the item itself. The p value reflects the ability of the group who answered the item in the context of the set of items that were presented on the test. Ebel and Frisbie (1991) point out that it is more accurate to say,

"'When this test was administered to that particular group, its index of difficulty was 63%,' than to say, 'The index of difficulty for this item is 63%'" (p. 228).

Because the item difficulty index refers to an item as answered by a particular set of students responding to the item as part of a particular set of items on a test, we cannot be dogmatic when applying the past p value history of the item to a subsequent test. Should we expect a group of students to perform as well as a previous group on an individual item? We can expect items to perform similarly with homogenous groups—to give us an estimation of whether or not the p value of an individual item for this new test with a different group of students should have a similar p value as it had on the past test. If there is a discrepancy in the p value of an item between groups, however, we have to look carefully at the groups. Were there differences in the abilities or learning circumstances of the two groups? For example, if an item was administered in a test to a group of senior students, its p value may not be applicable to the item if it was included in a test for a group of first-year students. Or suppose a novice instructor presents a unit of content to a student group, and several of the items have p values that are stored from a test where a seasoned expert presented the content to a previous group.

Tests that are so easy that nearly everyone answers all items correctly or tests that are so difficult that nearly everyone answers all items incorrectly will not identify differences in achievement among students. When the test scores are very similar, there is very little score variability. A test that has low score variability will have a low test reliability coefficient (Mehrens & Lehmann, 1991). Thus, presenting students with challenging items within a moderate difficulty range identifies levels of student achievement and also increases the test's reliability coefficient.

Item Discrimination   Item discrimination is the best indicator of the quality of an item. It identifies the item's ability to differentiate between those who score high and those who score low on a test. If an item is answered correctly by students with high overall test scores and answered incorrectly by students with low overall test scores, the item is said to discriminate, or to differentiate between those who do and those who do not know the material. Highly discriminating items contribute substantially to a test's reliability coefficient because they distinguish between students of different achievement levels (Frisbie, 1988).

A direct relationship exists between the sum of the discrimination indices on a test and the reliability of the test scores—the greater the average of the discrimination indices, the higher the reliability coefficient of the test results (Ebel & Frisbie, 1991). Reliable results are associated with tests that are made up of items with highly positive discrimination indices. Chapter 11, "Interpreting Test Results," provides additional discussion about the relationship between reliability and discrimination indices and methods for identifying, interpreting, and improving item discrimination indices.

Homogeneity of the Test Content   Measurements of internal consistency estimate the reliability of test results by comparing the individual item responses to the total test score. These estimates indicate the extent to which all test items are measuring a single domain (Frisbie, 1988). Therefore, the more consistent the test content, the higher the inter-item consistency and the reliability coefficient will be. A test on content, which is narrowly defined, provides a consistent correlation between individual item responses and the total test score, and enhances the test's reliability coefficient. For example, in a test that focuses solely on medication calculations, every item is directly related to every other item on the test—the knowledge required to answer each item is very consistent, and the total test score directly reflects the student's knowledge of medication calculations (Anastasi & Urbina, 1997).

A test covering a range of content will have heterogeneous items that require different knowledge. For example, in a comprehensive nursing exam, the course objectives are consistent, while areas of content can include clinical knowledge from several areas, including adult health, child health, women's health, and mental health. While all the questions require nursing expertise, the content knowledge required is very broad. Therefore, the total test scores would not necessarily reflect student knowledge of a particular content area, and the test's reliability coefficient will be decreased because the responses to each item will not necessarily correspond to the total test scores.

Some nursing programs have an integrated curriculum, so their exams are built on content areas that vary. It is important when interpreting the reliability coefficient of this test type to keep in mind that the reliability coefficient of a comprehensive test will be lower than a test with a narrowly defined content area. A low reliability coefficient may not reflect the true reliability of the test results; it may only indicate that the test items are measuring a set of skills that are not closely related to each other.

Homogeneity of the Test Group   If the majority of a student group answers most of the items on a test correctly, the scores will have a small spread, and it will be difficult to distinguish the high achievers from the low ones. When a group of students have similar abilities, the spread of scores is diminished. Consider the extreme example (as illustrated in Exhibit 10.4) where everyone receives a score of 100% on a test. There is no variability of their test scores. Because everyone has the same score, it is impossible to determine how the responses to the individual items compare with the total test scores, and the test has a reliability coefficient of 0. Student nurses usually must meet admission criteria; therefore, we should expect a degree of homogeneity in the group. It is important to keep this fact in mind when interpreting the reliability coefficient of a classroom test.

Test Length   A test's reliability coefficient increases as the number of items in the test increases. Increasing the number of items in a test decreases the effect of responses that are correct by chance or guess on the total test score. This is because a longer test provides a more extensive sample of the behavior that is being measured, and it decreases the influence of chance factors, such as guessing (Miller et al., 2009).

For example, suppose that to measure medication calculation ability, you ask students to solve one medication calculation question. The results of this measurement would be highly unreliable. If the question were particularly difficult, most students would fail. If you presented an easy problem, most students would pass. As you add questions to the test, the test results become increasingly more reliable, and you obtain a better estimate of each student's ability. It is important to recognize that the items added to the original test, which increased its length, must have similar statistical properties as the original test. In other words, the additional items must have similar average difficulty and discrimination levels as the items on the original test.

Table 10.1 illustrates how the reliability coefficient of a 10-item test that has an initial reliability coefficient of 0.3 can be increased by adding items. Note that there is a self-limiting point to adding items to a test to increase its reliability coefficient.

Table 10.1 Relation of Test Length to Test Reliability

Number of Items	Test Reliability
10	0.30
20	0.46
40	0.63
80	0.77
160	0.88
320	0.93
640	0.97
∞	1.00

Thus, the higher the reliability coefficient of the original test, the smaller the increase in the reliability coefficient with the added test length.

If time constraints limit the number of items that can be included in a test, you may need to administer tests more frequently. There are many reasons why it would be impossible to administer a test consisting of 250 multiple-choice items. Yet over the course of a semester you probably test your students with at least that many items. The following concept is essential to the meaning of trustworthy grading: Collect enough data so that you can make reliable decisions about students (Haladyna, 1999).

Number of Examinees Sample size affects a test's reliability coefficient. Small samples provide a small spread of scores and therefore low variability. It is obvious that the exam results of five students are not as reliable as the results of 500 students on the same exam. The larger the sample size, the greater the variability of the scores and the higher the reliability coefficient of the test will be.

Speed Speeded tests are performance tests in which speed plays an important role in determining individual scores. In a speeded test, some students do not have time to consider each test item. A power test is one in which there is no time limit or, if there is one, it is so generous that most students are able to finish the test (Lyman, 1998). If a test score depends on speed, the difference in scores depends on the difference in the speed with which the individuals answer the questions. An item's position within a speeded test determines whether an individual even gets the opportunity to answer that item. Internal consistency estimates tend to be falsely high on speeded tests because some of the high-achieving students reach questions that others do not even have the time to answer. This increases the mean inter-item correlation and tends to inflate the reliability estimate when internal consistency procedures are used to analyze a speeded test (Brookhart & Nitko, 2014,).

Speed should not be a factor in determining the scores of a classroom test, unless speed is a critical aspect of the test, such as a typing test. Classroom achievement tests should be power tests. All students should be able to complete the exam comfortably in the allotted time. After all, the purpose of an achievement test is to measure student levels of attainment, not to determine how rapidly they can respond to questions. Speeded tests artificially increase the test's reliability coefficient because the score spread is increased. It is far more preferable to increase the reliability of a test's results by improving the quality of the test items.

Although time constraints are imposed on every classroom assessment, it is important to design your exams to allow sufficient time for all students to attempt every item. Presenting a reasonable number of well-developed questions for the allotted test time is the most effective way to increase the reliability of the results of your classroom exams. A general rule of thumb is to allow 60 minutes for every 50 four-option multiple-choice items on a test, assuming that all items are clear and succinct. Guidelines for developing such items are discussed in Chapter 5, "Selected-Response Format: Developing Multiple-Choice Items," and Chapter 6, "Writing Critical Thinking Multiple-Choice Items."

Test Design, Administration, and Scoring   The design of a test and the conditions under which students take the test can also affect the reliability of the test results. If extraneous factors interfere with or improve students' ability to select the correct responses, their performance on the test will not reflect their true ability. If the scoring of the test is influenced by extraneous factors, such as cheating, the reliability of the test results is questionable. These factors must be taken seriously because they introduce measurement error into the testing situation. Chapter 9, "Assembling, Administering, and Scoring a Test," discusses these factors and also provides practical suggestions for minimizing these sources of error in your classroom exams.

Measurement Error

Measurement error decreases the usefulness of a test. Previous discussion established that no measurement is perfect; all contain error. Some kinds of physical measurement, such as weight and height, have been perfected to the point that, with a good measurement procedure, error is relatively small. In contrast, measurements of behavior contain a larger margin of error. Although we cannot expect tests to provide perfect measurements, there is a limit to how much error we should accept. The greater the confidence that you require when interpreting a test score, the lower the error and the higher the reliability you must require of the test results (see **Figure 10.1**).

Figure 10.1	Lower error results in higher score confidence

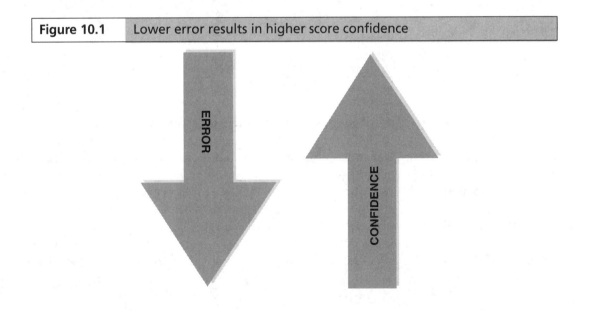

Standard Error of Measurement   The reliability estimates we have examined so far are concerned with the reliability of test scores for a group; the standard error of measurement (SEM) is concerned with the accuracy with which we measure an individual's performance (Brookhart & Nitko, 2014). An individual's true score is one that is free from error and can be obtained only if a test has perfectly reliable results. As we know, perfect reliability is not attainable because error is inherent in every measurement. Although we cannot eliminate measurement error, we can estimate how much error is present in an instrument. This estimation is the SEM: the smaller the SEM, the more reliable the test's score.

Although we can never know an individual's true score, we can estimate the amount by which an obtained score may differ from the hypothetical true score. If we could administer the same test to an individual repeatedly, we would see that the person's scores would vary somewhat from one administration to another and that the distribution of these obtained scores would be normal in shape. The individual's hypothetical true test score would be equal to the average score of this normal distribution of obtained scores, and the SEM would be equal to the standard deviation of the distribution (Lyman, 1998).

The SEM reflects the consistency of an individual's scores if the same test was given to that student again and again. The amount of variation in the scores from one administration to the next is directly related to the reliability of the test results. The higher the reliability of the test results, the less the individual's score would vary from one administration to another (Linn & Gronlund, 2000). Because it is not possible to reassess a student repeatedly, an estimation of an individual's true score is derived from a mathematical equation that combines information about the reliability coefficient and the standard deviation of the test (Worthen et al., 1993, p. 118). As the formula in **Exhibit 10.5** illustrates, the higher the reliability of a test's results and the smaller the standard deviation, the lower the SEM.

Exhibit 10.5   SEM formula

$$SEM = SD\sqrt{1 - r^n}$$

SD $=$ standard deviation

$r^n =$ reliability coefficient of the test

Confidence Bands   The SEM, which is reported as score units, is particularly useful because it is directly applicable to test score interpretations. It provides a safeguard against placing too much emphasis on a single score (Anastasi & Urbina, 1997, p. 109). The SEM tells us how many points should be added to and subtracted from an individual's score to estimate the reasonable limits in which the true score most probably can be found. These reasonable limits provide a confidence band for estimating an individual's true score (Miller et al., 2009).

The SEM demonstrates the imprecision of a single test score. The score report in **Table 10.2** shows that a student has a math score of 500, with an SEM of 10. The SEM of 10 allows you to estimate that this student's true score is likely to be in the

Table 10.2   Score Report with Score Range Illustrating Confidence Band

	Score	SEM	Score Range
Math	500	10	490–510
Verbal	500	50	450–550

Table 10.3   Degree of Confidence Associated with SEM

Degree of Confidence	Number of Standard Errors	Range of Scores or Confidence Band
68%	1	490–510
95%	2	480–520
99.7%	3	470–530

Math score = 500; SEM = 10.

range that is 10 points above or below the student's obtained score of 500. Note that the student has obtained the same verbal score of 500, but that this score has a much larger SEM (50), which means that the student's true verbal score lies somewhere in the range of 450 to 550, a much larger confidence band.

Although you cannot eliminate measurement error, the goal of test construction is to decrease measurement error and increase the reliability of a test's results. As error decreases, confidence increases. A large confidence band indicates large measurement error and decreases the confidence that you can have in the obtained score. With low error, the confidence band decreases, and you can be more confident that the obtained score is a dependable measure. As Table 10.2 illustrates, you can have more confidence in an obtained score of 500, with a score range of 490 to 510, than you can in an obtained score of 500, with a score range of 450 to 550. The message for teachers is clear: Because of measurement error, you must interpret a student's obtained score as an estimate of the true score (Brookhart & Nitko, 2014).

Because the SEM represents the standard deviation of the hypothetical distribution around a student's true score, the SEM can be interpreted in terms of the normal curve. In a normal curve, approximately 68% of the cases fall within one standard deviation of the mean; approximately 95% of the scores fall within two standard deviations; and nearly all scores, greater than 99%, fall within three standard deviations from the mean (Brookhart & Nitko, 2014, p. 76).

How should we interpret the obtained score for a student who has a math score of 500 with an SEM of 10? As **Table 10.3** illustrates, a confidence band of one standard error above and one standard error below the obtained score would allow us 68% confidence that the student's true score falls between 490 and 510, a confidence band of two standard errors above and two standard errors below the obtained score would allow us 95% confidence that the student's true score falls between 480 and 520, and a confidence band of three standard errors above and three standard errors below the obtained score would allow us greater than 99% confidence that the student's true score falls between 470 and 530 (Brookhart & Nitko, 2014, p. 76). Compare Table 10.3 with **Table 10.4**.

Table 10.4 Degree of Confidence Associated with Large SEM

Degree of Confidence	Number of Standard Errors	Range of Scores or Confidence Band
68%	1	450–550
95%	2	400–600
99.7%	3	350–650

Verbal score = 500; SEM = 50.

Although the student has the same obtained score for both math and verbal, the difference in the SEMs for the scores results in much different confidence bands, further illustrating that the smaller the confidence band, the greater confidence you can have in an obtained score. Consider that, with three standard errors of measurement, the student's true verbal score would be in the range of 350 to 650! We can be 99% confident that the student's true score falls within this interval, but with such a large interval, it is difficult to have much confidence in the student's obtained verbal score.

If we interpret a person's obtained score as equivalent to the true score, we make serious misinterpretations. It is important to interpret a student's obtained score in relation to a confidence band and to remember that we do not know where on the interval the student's true score lies. The most accurate way to interpret a student's score is to view it in terms of an interval, not as a single score.

Professionally developed standardized tests are subject to measurement error. Therefore, it is reasonable to assume that classroom tests also contain measurement error. This error makes it impossible to be dogmatic when interpreting test results and clearly illustrates that assigning grades in a course should never be based on the results of one measurement. It is important to collect as much information as possible and consider measurement error when making assessment decisions about students based on classroom exams. Although individual teacher-made assessments may not have established reliability evidence, the total result of many assignments given over the course of a semester can result in a reliable overall judgment of student achievement (McMillan, 2001).

If a test is to be useful, it must provide reliable results; however, reliability alone is not enough. The interpretations that you make about a test's results must have evidence of validity. Validity is the most important aspect of a test; it refers to the degree to which evidence supports your interpretations of the test results, not to the test itself.

Validity

Classroom tests are designed so that teachers can make decisions about a student's achievement. High scores lead to one type of inference, whereas low scores lead to the opposite conclusion. These test-based inferences may or may not be valid. The validity of the inferences made based on classroom assessments is what teachers must be concerned with when making decisions about students. If the inferences are accurate, then the resulting decisions are defensible (Popham, 2003, p. 42).

The *Standards for Educational and Psychological Testing* states, "Validity is a unitary concept. It is the degree to which all the accumulated evidence supports the intended interpretation of test scores for the proposed purpose" (AERA et al., 1999, p. 11). If a test is interpreted in more than one way, each interpretation must be validated. Chapter 2, "The Language of Assessment," provides a detailed discussion related to establishing validity evidence.

Content Validity Index

Although there are no objective empirical methods for obtaining validity evidence based on test content, it is possible to use interrater agreement indices, such as the content validity index (CVI), to rate the relevance of the items on a measurement instrument. With this procedure, a panel of experts is asked to rate the content relevance of each item on a scale of 1 to 4, and the CVI for the total instrument is the percentage of total items that are rated as 3 or 4 by the experts (Waltz, Strickland, & Lenz, 2010). If this procedure is used to rate the items on a multiple-choice exam, it would have to be used during the test development process, and then only items that were rated as highly relevant to the blueprint should be included in the test.

Determining the CVI involves a time commitment that precludes its effectiveness for classroom exams. A group of faculty who are experts in the field but not involved in developing the blueprint or test items would have to serve as the panel of experts to rate each item for relevance to the individual test blueprint and to identify areas of omission before the test is administered. Considering the rigorous nature of the process and the number of exams that are administered each semester, it would not be feasible to carry out this procedure for every classroom exam.

The most important requirement for establishing validity evidence based on test content for a classroom exam is to follow the guidelines presented in this text to build in validity from the beginning of test development. Although it may be helpful to determine the CVI on a few selected exams, be careful not to be misled. Numbers alone do not provide evidence of validity. The most effective and practical approach for establishing validity evidence based on test content of a classroom achievement test is to develop and select items according to a carefully designed test blueprint.

Interpretation of the Validity Coefficient

A validity coefficient is a correlation coefficient that expresses the relationship between two sets of scores. Test developers frequently establish validity evidence by calculating correlation coefficients to measure the relationship between the test and the criterion or construct being measured. While there is no objective numerical value associated with evidence of content-related validity, a validity coefficient can provide evidence that the test is measuring the desired construct or criterion.

The Pearson product-moment correlation coefficient is the most common procedure used for reporting validity. A number ranging between -1 and $+1$ represents the direction (positive or negative) and strength (numerical value) of the relationship between two sets of continuous scores (McMillan, 2001).

A correlation coefficient (r) of $+1$ indicates a perfect positive correlation between the predictor and the criterion, while $r = 1$ indicates a perfect negative correlation. The closer a validity coefficient is to $+1$, the more accurate the test is at predicting the criterion. For example, a validity coefficient of 0.95 applied to the relationship between the scores on a nursing school entrance exam and first-year grade point average is a high positive relationship, and the test would have considerable predictive ability. Because all measurements contain error, however, caution must be taken when interpreting correlations. Test scores should be interpreted as a range when estimating current performance or predicting future performance on a criterion (McMillan, 1997).

Although classroom teachers seldom conduct formal studies to obtain correlation coefficients, the concept is important to understand. As McMillan (1997) explains, "When you have two or more measures of the same thing, and these measures provide similar results, then you have established, albeit informally, criterion-related evidence" (p. 58). For example, if your assessment of a student's critical thinking ability in clinical practice coincides with the student's score on a test that measures critical thinking ability, then you have evidence that your inference about the student's critical thinking ability is valid. This reasoning gives further support to the notion that it is important to obtain several measurements of the same constructs and content to support the validity of your interpretations.

Summary

Reliability is concerned with the consistency of test results. Sound decisions cannot be based on a test that produces inconsistent results. The higher the stakes associated with the use of a test, the more concerned you have to be with the reliability of the test's scores.

The three types of evidence about a test's consistency are test–retest, parallel form, and internal consistency. Although these three kinds of evidence are related, they are not interchangeable. Test–retest and parallel-form evidence of reliability provide correlations between sets of student scores, while internal consistency is concerned with the extent to which the test's items are functioning in a consistent fashion (Brookhart & Nitko, 2014). The measurements produced by these different approaches are not equivalent or interchangeable.

The intended use of test scores affects the type of reliability evidence that is required. When applying internal consistency measures that are designed for interpreting the reliability of the results of standardized exams to a classroom test, you must proceed with caution because several factors influence the value of the reliability coefficient when it is applied to a classroom test. In all cases, when you are concerned with interpreting the score of an individual, the SEM is the best index of consistency.

Validity is the most important aspect of test development. "A sound validity argument integrates various strands of evidence into a coherent account of the degree to which existing evidence and theory support the intended interpretation of test scores for specific uses" (AERA et al., 1999, p. 17). Establishing evidence of validity must begin during the test development process with the establishment of a blueprint, as discussed in Chapter 2, "The Language of Assessment." The blueprint justifies the selected set of items as representing the domain being measured and provides validity evidence for the decisions you make based on the test results.

Reliability and validity form the basis for all assessments. When evidence indicates that a test measures what it intends to measure with a degree of accuracy that can be trusted, the results are considered valid and accurate. Considering the serious decisions made about students based on classroom tests, faculty should have a working knowledge of the concepts of reliability and validity. An understanding of these concepts provides a framework for developing more effective tests and for accurately interpreting and using test results. It also enables you to design methods to collect the evidence of validity and reliability that you must provide when you seek program accreditation.

Learning Activities

1. Define reliability and explain its role when interpreting the results of a classroom exam.
2. Describe the test–retest and parallel-form methods for estimating reliability. Identify the strengths and weaknesses of each.
3. Describe the measures of internal consistency for estimating reliability. Identify the strengths and weaknesses for each of the measures.
4. Identify the factors that affect the calculation of the reliability coefficients when measuring internal consistency. What steps can you take to improve the reliability of your classroom test results?
5. Define the SEM. How can you use the SEM when assigning grades at the end of a semester?
6. Would you use the SEM to adjust scores at the end of a semester? Explain your rationale.
7. Calculate the SEM for an exam that has a KR-20 of 0.76 and a standard deviation of 15.
8. Explain the difference between reliability and validity. How would you establish validity evidence for a classroom exam?
9. Why is validity considered to be the most important factor when interpreting test results?

Web Links

Educational Resources Information Center (ERIC)
http://www.eric.ed.gov
National Council on Measurement in Education (NCME)
http://www.ncme.org
Pathways to School Improvement
http://www.ncrel.org/sdrs/

References

American Educational Research Association, American Psychological Association, & National Council on Measurement in Education. (1999). *Standards for educational and psychological testing*. Washington, DC: American Educational Research Association.

Anastasi, A., & Urbina, S. (1997). *Psychological testing* (7th ed.). Upper Saddle River, NJ: Prentice Hall.

Brookhart, S. M., & Nitko, A. J. (2014). *Educational assessment of students* (7th ed.). Upper Saddle River, NJ: Pearson Education.

Ebel, R. L., & Frisbie, D. A. (1991). *Essentials of educational measurement* (5th ed.). Englewood Cliffs, NJ: Prentice Hall.

Frisbie, D. A. (1988). Reliability of scores from teacher-made tests. *Educational Measurement: Issues and Practice, 7,* 25–35.

Haladyna, T. M. (1997). *Writing test items to evaluate higher order thinking.* Needham Heights, MA: Allyn and Bacon.

Haladyna, T. M. (1999). *A complete guide to student grading.* Needham Heights, MA: Allyn and Bacon.

Linn, R. L., & Gronlund, N. E. (2000). *Measurement and assessment in teaching.* Upper Saddle River, NJ: Prentice Hall.

Lyman, H. L. (1998). Test *scores and what they mean* (6th ed.). Boston, MA: Allyn and Bacon.

McMillan, J. H. (1997). *Classroom assessment: Principles and practice for effective instruction.* Boston, MA: Allyn and Bacon.

McMillan, J. H. (2001). *Essential assessment concepts for teachers and administrators.* Thousand Oaks, CA: Sage.

Mehrens, W. A., & Lehmann, I. J. (1991). *Measurement and evaluation in education and psychology* (4th ed.). New York, NY: Holt, Rinehart, and Winston.

Miller, M. D., Linn, R. L., & Gronlund, N. E. (2009). *Measurement and assessment* (10th ed.). Upper Saddle River, NJ: Pearson Education.

Popham, W. J. (2003). *Test better, teach better: The instructional role of assessment.* Alexandria, VA: Association for Supervision and Curriculum Development.

Salkind, N. J. (2012). *Tests and measurement for people who hate tests and measurement* (2nd ed.). Thousand Oaks, CA: Sage.

Thorndike, R. M. (1997). *Measurement and evaluation in psychology and education* (6th ed.). Upper Saddle River, NJ: Prentice Hall.

Waltz, C. F., Strickland, O. L., & Lenz, E. R. (2010). *Measurement in nursing and health research* (4th ed.). New York, NY: Springer.

Worthen, B. R., Borg, W. R., & White, K. (1993). *Measurement and evaluation in the schools.* White Plains, NY: Longman.

Interpreting Test Results

© Anteromite/Shutterstock

CHAPTER 11

"Statistics is the science of producing unreliable facts from reliable figures."

—Evan Escar

Test development is a process that continues even after a test is administered. In fact, post hoc test analysis is a crucial aspect of the process. One advantage of selected-response exams is that item and test analysis data can be generated from the test results. Multiple-choice questions are particularly amenable to data analysis. These data reports provide valuable information that assists the teacher in assigning fair scores and improving individual items for future use. Test analysis has three goals: to identify whether any of the questions are flawed, to correct any errors and adjust the raw scores, and to improve the items for future use.

Qualitative and quantitative test reviews are equally important; they complement each other. Once you have the statistical data for a test, you can look at the items from a much more objective viewpoint. Inevitably, you and your colleagues who reviewed the exam before it was administered will be surprised by the results of at least 10% of the new items on a test, even though you followed test development guidelines. Sometimes, student responses to even the most expertly written questions are just unpredictable.

Consider the time involved in item writing and revision as an investment. Multiple-choice items can be analyzed, revised, and banked for future use. These items can be polished over time and adapted for reuse on future tests. In fact, the more you refine your items based on data, the better your tests become. Often, the qualitative student review, as discussed in Chapter 9, "Assembling, Administering, and Scoring a Test," explains the statistical results of an item and provides suggestions for revising the item for future use. Reviewing the quantitative data not only provides an invaluable tool for making objective decisions about individual test items and overall test scores, it also guides you to use your time efficiently to improve your questions and develop a valuable testing resource: an item bank. Keep in mind that the more items you analyze, the more proficient you become at writing and identifying high-quality test items that you can bank and use repeatedly. Therefore, the time you invest is time well spent.

Before the advent of reasonably priced testing software, calculating the statistical results of an exam was a task that was impractical for a classroom teacher. Today, many colleges and universities provide machine scoring with statistical reports of tests and item analyses for multiple-choice classroom exams. The aim of this chapter is to demonstrate just how valuable these data reports are as tools for test interpretation and development; without statistical analysis, you have no assurance that your tests are functioning as you intended.

Overall Test Data Analysis

Most test development software packages provide two levels of test analysis data: the overall analysis of the test and a detailed analysis of each item as it relates to the test as a whole. While your first consideration should be to look at the overall picture, both these data sets are essential for a thorough test analysis. Examining test data is well within your purview once you understand the meaning of each of the values. Remember, you do not have to do any actual calculating. Once you use the data, you will appreciate their value to such an extent that I guarantee you will never again assign grades to a multiple-choice exam without reviewing the statistical analysis.

When a test is scored, the initial result is reported as a raw score, or the number of items that a student answered correctly on the test. Statistical analysis assists you with transforming the raw scores into test grades. Appendix B, "Basic Test Statistics," provides an overview of the terminology of statistical analysis. Take the time to review some basic statistical references before examining the example of a statistical test report in **Table 11.1**.

Table 11.1 is a sample test analysis report that contains the typical data you would receive from a testing software program. In fact, this report presents more than enough data to help you make informed decisions about test results. Some

Table 11.1 Sample Test Statistics	
Number of items	100
Number of examinees	92
Mean	75.4
Median	77
Low score	52
High score	93
Alpha	0.754
Standard deviation	7.7
Standard error of measurement (SEM)	3.8
Mean p value	0.754
Mean point biserial index (PBI)	0.36

programs provide even more comprehensive statistics. It is not necessary to make your review too complicated, however; this sample data report is more than sufficient for analysis of a classroom test.

Generally, item statistics for small groups of students are relatively unstable. The stability of test analysis data increases as the number of test takers approaches 100. Therefore, when you have a very small group (50 or fewer), you must consider the relative instability of the data when you interpret the analysis. In fact, test and item analysis should not be interpreted dogmatically, no matter how large the number of students. As this discussion illustrates, analysis of test data requires a variety of interpretations, both qualitative and quantitative. The size of the sample is one of the factors you must consider.

The first step in test analysis is to review the report to make sure that the data report is complete. Check the number of items and examinees, and verify their accuracy. This sample has 100 items, which means the raw score is equal to the percentage correct, and 92 examinees had their answer sheets scored. Once you verify that these figures are correct, you are ready to analyze the results of the test.

Measures of Central Tendency

Measures of central tendency provide a single value that best represents the typical score in a distribution. The mean, the median, and the mode are the three most commonly used measures of central tendency in education. While the mode, which represents the most frequently obtained score in a distribution, has limited usefulness for interpreting classroom test scores, both the mean and the median provide valuable information.

Mean   Most test analysis programs report the mean, or arithmetic average, of the raw scores on the test; in this case (Table 11.1), it is 75.4. The mean percent score is determined by dividing the mean raw score by the total number of items on the test. The mean percent score is equal to the mean raw score in this example because there are 100 items on the test.

One disadvantage of the mean is that it is sensitive to extreme scores. An extreme score, whether very high or very low, can pull the mean toward its direction. This effect is particularly problematic when there is a small group of scores (Reynolds, Livingston, & Wilson, 2008).

For example, let's look at the distributions in **Table 11.2**. Each distribution has an extreme score of 15, yet the smaller number of scores is affected more dramatically than the larger number of scores. The mean of the "A Scores" is 7.4, a score that does not even appear in the distribution, while the score of 15 has a less dramatic effect on the mean of the "B Scores," which is 5.95. It is obvious from these examples that you must consider the effect of extreme scores when interpreting the mean on a test.

It is important to examine the relationship of the mean to the passing standard that you have set. If, for example, your passing standard is 75%, this test has an average score at the passing level. Several factors must be considered when interpreting the mean:

- Were there extreme scores in the distribution?
- What was the quality of teaching, on a range between effective and ineffective?
- What was the students' level of effort to achieve the outcomes, on a range between maximal and minimal?

Table 11.2   Effect of an Extreme Score on the Mean of a Distribution

A Scores	B Scores
5	5
5	5
6	5
6	5
15	5
	5
	5
	5
	5
	5
	6
	6
	6
	6
	6
	6
	6
	6
	6
	15
Mean = 7.4	Mean = 5.95

- Where did the material/objectives fit, on a range between too easy and too difficult?
- How difficult were the items, on a range between too easy and too hard?

If a test has a very low mean, you should investigate whether there is a problem with one of the questions listed above. As Haladyna (1997) points out, if you intentionally give difficult tests, you should adjust your grading policy to ensure that you assign grades fairly in relation to the other courses that students take. Similar consideration should be made if your tests are consistently too easy. The ideal goal is to have a test with a mean that reflects a range of student abilities. A test should be neither too easy nor too difficult, but should reward those students who are high achievers and should identify those who have not met the course objectives. Chapter 13, "Assigning Grades," discusses the issues surrounding grade assignment.

Median   The median in this sample is 77, which represents the middle point in this group of raw scores. In a normal distribution, the mean and the median are the same. If a distribution is positively skewed, meaning that the test is very difficult, with most scores at the low end of the distribution and few very high scores, the mean is pulled to the positive end of the distribution and is higher than the median (Reynolds et al., 2008).

A positively skewed distribution, such as the one depicted in **Figure 11.1**, signals a problem. Why are there so few high scores? What went wrong in the instructional process?

If a distribution is negatively skewed, it means the test was easy for the group, with most scores at the high end of the distribution and few very low scores. The distribution depicted in **Figure 11.2** is one you might expect in a nursing class. After all, all students who are admitted to a nursing program are capable of achieving the objectives.

The mean in a negatively skewed distribution is pulled toward the negative end of the distribution and is lower than the median (Reynolds et al., 2008). Therefore, the mean can give the wrong impression whenever a distribution is seriously skewed. The terms *positively skewed* and *negatively skewed* can seem counterintuitive. Remember this tip: A "positively" skewed distribution has its tail in the positive end of the distribution, while a "negatively" skewed distribution has its tail in the negative end of the distribution. A distribution that is not skewed has the same or very close values for the mean and the median; it resembles a bell and is referred to as a normal distribution or a *bell curve*.

The mean and median in the example of Table 11.1 are close, which means there are probably not many extreme scores in the distribution and the mean is close to the median. The mean in this case can be interpreted as representing a typical score. Of course, you should review the score distribution, which is also included in the test analysis report, before you decide whether the mean actually represents a typical score. Interpretation of graphic and frequency distributions is discussed later in this chapter.

Figure 11.1	A positively skewed distribution

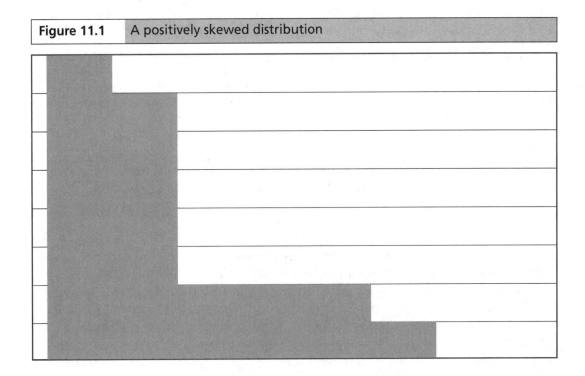

Figure 11.2	A negatively skewed distribution

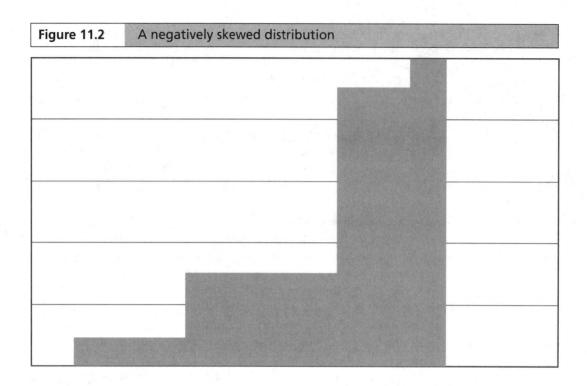

Measures of Variability

Because it is impossible to predict the range of scores for a test based on measures of central tendency alone, it is necessary for us to look further when interpreting a set of scores. In fact, two sets of scores could have the same mean and have a very different spread of scores. We need to examine measures of variability to determine how much the scores spread out from the mean or how much dispersion there is in a distribution.

Range   In the example in Table 11.1, the range of the distribution is 41, the difference between the high (93) and low (52) scores on the test.

$$\text{Range} = \text{highest score} - \text{lowest score}$$

A small range indicates a concentrated distribution of scores, while a large range means that the scores are spread out and that some students have not done well on the test. This value gives us a rough idea of the variability of the test scores.

Standard Deviation   The standard deviation is a more useful measure than the range of the variability of a score distribution. Standard deviation indicates the average distance that scores in a distribution vary from the mean (7.665 in Table 11.1). A large variance indicates that the scores are spread out from the mean, as Chapter 10, "Establishing Evidence of Reliability and Validity," discusses. Conversely, the smaller the variance, the greater the similarity of the scores and the closer they are to the mean. Most software programs report the standard deviation, which is the square root of the variance, in their test analyses reports. The standard deviation tells you the average distance of the scores from the mean, or how much the scores differ, either positively or negatively, from the mean. A small standard deviation means that the scores were bunched together around the mean, while a large standard deviation means that the scores were spread out from the mean.

The standard deviation is most useful for making interpretations about the normal curve, which is a grading method that is discouraged for classroom testing, as Chapter 13, "Assigning Grades," discusses. In the classroom setting, the most useful application of the standard deviation is to help you to understand the reliability coefficient and the standard error of measurement (SEM) for a test.

Reliability Coefficient

Reliability refers to the amount of confidence you can have in a test score, which Chapter 2, "The Language of Assessment," and Chapter 10, "Establishing Evidence of Reliability and Validity," discuss at length The reliability coefficient for our sample in Table 11.1 is reported as alpha, and its value is 0.754.

What reliability coefficient should you expect from the results of your classroom exams? The answer to this question varies, but it relates directly to the level of confidence you must have in the decisions made based on the test results. High-stakes decisions require measurement results with high reliability. In other words, the results of a test that decides whether or not a student graduates from a program of study would require a high level of reliability. For this reason, you should never base such a serious decision on just one classroom exam.

Miller, Linn, and Gronlund (2009) agree that the degree of reliability you must require for the results of a classroom test depends largely on the decision to be made based on the test results. Consider the importance of the decision and whether the decision can be reversed. If the reliability coefficient of a test's results is low, make sure that you make tentative decisions; obtain additional data; and, most important, are willing to reverse your decision.

Miller et al. (2009) report that the reliability coefficients of teacher-made tests usually vary between 0.60 and 0.85. Kehoe (1995) maintains that the results of tests of more than 50 items should have reliability coefficients of greater than 0.80, while Frisbie (1988) asserts that teacher-made test results should yield reliability coefficients that average about 0.50 and that 0.85 is the generally acceptable minimum reliability standard when decisions are being made about individuals based on a single test score. Frisbie also states that reliability coefficients of about 0.50 for the results of teacher-made tests can be tolerated when the scores are combined with other scores to assign a grade. In that case, you should be concerned with the reliability of the score that results from combining the scores.

Our sample's reliability coefficient of 0.754 looks respectable at first glance, according to these standards. This value should not be considered in isolation, however. The factors that affect the reliability coefficient of a test must be taken into account. These factors are discussed in detail in Chapter 10, "Establishing Evidence of Reliability and Validity," and include the following:

- Quality of the test items
- Item difficulty
- Item discrimination

- Homogeneity of the test content
- Homogeneity of the test group
- Test length
- Number of examinees
- Speed
- Test design, administration, and scoring

When reviewing the reliability coefficients of your classroom test results, consider all these factors. If you have a class that consists of a homogeneous group of high-achieving students, you might get a low reliability coefficient on a test of difficult, well-written, heterogeneous items that follow all the guidelines outlined in this text. It is also possible that a low reliability coefficient indicates that the items are either too difficult or too easy for the group of students. On the other hand, you could obtain a high reliability coefficient for a speeded test with a large number of items on narrowly defined content that is administered to a large heterogeneous group of students. Also remember that the testing conditions, quality of teaching, and number of questions and/or examinees are all factors that can affect the reliability of test scores. Low reliability coefficients are most often due to an excess of very easy or very hard items, poorly written items that do not discriminate, or test items that do not represent a unified body of content (Kehoe, 1995).

You must consider all influencing factors when interpreting a reliability coefficient for the results of a test. A test that has a low reliability coefficient could be providing reliable results. Your judgment is a very important part of the equation. As Mark Twain said, "There are three kinds of lies: lies, damned lies, and statistics." Statistical findings are meaningless in themselves, and they can be distorted to fit erroneous interpretations. It is your informed interpretation of the data that adds the ingredient of fairness to your grade assignments. Refer to Chapter 10, "Establishing Evidence of Reliability and Validity," for a detailed discussion related to reliability estimates of classroom exams.

Standard Error of Measurement (SEM)

The SEM enables us to estimate the amount by which a student's obtained score might differ from the student's true score. Chapter 10, "Establishing Evidence of Reliability and Validity," discuss the implications of the SEM on test score interpretation.

The SEM is very important because, if we assume that an obtained score on a test is necessarily the student's true score, we will misinterpret the test results (Reynolds et al., 2008). The SEM for our sample in Table 11.1 is 3.8, which means that the true score for an observed raw score of 72 would range between 68.2 and 75.8. This range is referred to as the confidence band.

Suppose that the passing score on a test was predetermined to be 75. Would you consider adding 4 points to all scores on the test if the SEM was a 4? While it is not advisable to add points, or scale grades, for each individual test, if you are inclined to scale the grades, it is a better practice to wait for the final grade. Suppose you scale up the grades three points for exam one and the scores on exam two are very high. Will you scale down the scores for exam two? You probably would cause a student revolt.

Scaling individual test scores can alter the predetermined weighting of the components of the course grade. The better practice is to wait until the end of the course; look carefully at the means, medians, reliability coefficients, and SEMs for all exams; consider the final score spread; and then add points (if you judge it necessary) to the final grade assignment (refer to the discussion on grading in Chapter 13, "Assigning Grades").

The important lesson to be learned from the SEM is that classroom test scores are not absolute, and they do not represent students' true scores. Measurement error is present in all scores, so you must look at the margin of error in a test and be flexible when translating raw scores into test scores and test scores into course grades. If the statistical analysis provided by your test development software does not provide the SEM, you can calculate it by using the formula in Exhibit 10.5.

Score Distribution

A test score distribution complements the analysis of test data by providing you with a description of how the class as a whole performed on the test. A distribution helps you visualize test results and makes the scores easier to interpret. Score distributions are typically reported in a frequency table or in a graphic format.

Table 11.3 is a grouped frequency distribution associated with the sample data in Table 11.1. This frequency distribution groups the raw scores on the test into four-point intervals. In this distribution, you can see, for example, that six students scored from 84 to 87. This distribution provides a visual representation for interpreting the range of raw scores on a test. It enables you to visualize the significance of test analysis data such as the mean and the median and to identify how the scores on the test are clustered.

Table 11.3 Grouped Frequency Distribution	
92–95	1
88–91	1
84–87	6
80–83	15
76–79	24
72–75	16
68–71	13
64–67	10
60–63	2
56–59	1
52–55	3
N	92

Histogram

For many, a graphic representation of a score distribution provides the clearest visualization of a set of scores. A histogram is a bar graph of a score distribution, with the height of each column indicating the number of students who scored in the interval represented by the horizontal axis. What form should the distribution of a classroom test take? The normal curve is the distribution with which most teachers are familiar. A normal curve is a symmetrical, bell-shaped distribution with the mean and median at the midpoint and scores tapering off toward each extreme, as depicted in **Figure 11.3**. In a normal distribution, more than two-thirds of the scores are located close to the mean—that is, plus or minus one standard deviation (while only a few scores are at the very high or very low extremes of the distribution). Virtually all cases fall within three standard deviations of the mean.

The results of most achievement tests will approximate a normal curve when they are administered to large numbers of people (Reynolds et al., 2008). The key word here is *large*. It is most unlikely that the relatively small number of students in your class represents a normal distribution. You should expect a normal distribution only when you test a large number of people of varying abilities. Chapter 13, "Assigning Grades," discusses why the use of the normal curve is inadvisable for classroom grading.

Refer again to Figure 11.1; it depicts a positively skewed distribution, meaning that most of the test scores are low. The shape of the distribution does not explain the cause of the problem; rather, it is a red flag that indicates that the test needs further analysis. It might mean that the test was too difficult, the items were poorly written or confusing, the teaching/learning activities were inadequate, student motivation was low, or the objectives were unrealistic. This type of distribution alerts you to investigate the cause of the problem and to take corrective action.

| Figure 11.3 | Normal distribution histogram |

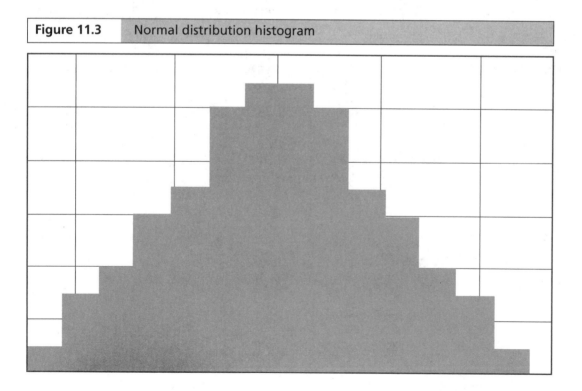

A negatively skewed distribution, such as the one depicted in Figure 11.2, means that most of the scores are high, with only a few students at the low end. There could be several reasons for this distribution, the most desirable one being that the teaching was effective and that the students were highly motivated. It could also mean that the test was too easy or that a copy of the test or the answer key circulated among the students. Whatever the case, further investigation is warranted.

In reality, the histograms that result from your classroom tests will not be as clear cut as the samples provided here. What is important is to examine both the frequency distribution and the histogram that represents the distribution to make sense of the raw scores for the test. Ask yourself what results you expected from the test and then determine what actually happened. A pretest should be positively skewed. A medication calculation test where all students are expected to pass with 90% correct should be negatively skewed. The score distribution for a test is a powerful tool for examining test score results.

Figure 11.4 is a histogram of the frequency distribution from Table 11.3. In the case of our sample, the score interval is four points. Note that the sample histogram illustrates most of the scores clustered between the scores of 64 and 87 and clarifies that the mean of 75.4 represents the average score for this test.

The analysis for this test is not over yet. This histogram should alert the teacher to closely examine the test. Why did 29 students attain scores of 71 or lower? What was the cause for the extremely poor performance of the six students who achieved a raw score between 52 and 63? Answers to these questions can be found in the analysis of the individual items. The analysis of the data, the frequency distribution,

Figure 11.4	Histogram for sample test data

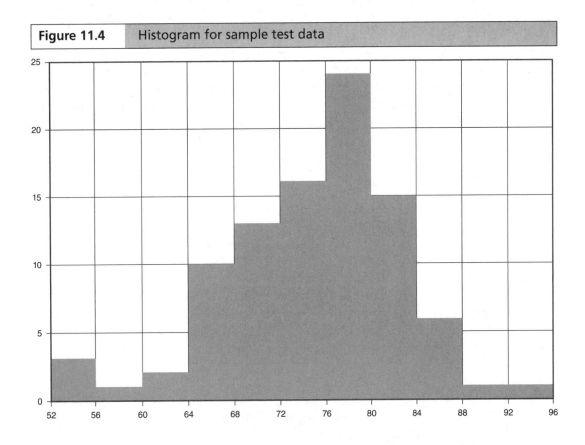

and the histogram (in conjunction with the analysis of the individual items) provide the best approach for determining the grade assignment for a test.

Mean Item Difficulty

The item difficulty index (p value) of an item is the percentage of examinees who answered the item correctly. The mean p value identifies the average p value of the items on a test and tells you how difficult the total test is. The mean p value of a test translates easily into the mean percent correct score on the test (75.4%, in the case of our sample in Table 11.1). It is easy to see that the difficulty of the individual items is what determines the difficulty of the overall test.

Developing an item bank helps to control the difficulty of future exams. Each item should be examined carefully and revised based on the data provided before it is entered into a bank. When you store items with their data, you have an indication of how difficult the items are when you select them for use on future tests. Remember, the difficulty of data associated with an item pertains to its use on a specific exam; it could perform differently in another item set or with a different group of students. You can get a pretty good idea of how an item will work with a similar group from its history, however.

Your ability to write items at particular difficulty levels improves as you develop expertise in item writing. In addition, the more items you analyze, the more proficient you become at recognizing good items and adapting your personal style to write effective test questions. Item analysis is examined in depth later in this chapter.

It is important to note that an item's difficulty level is directly related to its ability to discriminate. If the items on a test are too easy (for example, if the average p value is 100%), there is no discrimination between the high and low scorers because everyone answered every item correctly. According to Kehoe (1995), a good test contains items with p values between 0.30 and 0.80; items that are answered correctly or incorrectly by more than 85% of the examinees have poor discrimination power.

Nursing faculty frequently ask, "How difficult should my classroom test be?" The reason there is no standard response to this important question is because the answer is a very individual one (see Chapter 4, "Implementing Systematic Test Development"). Several factors must be considered. A test is only as hard or as easy as the teacher makes it. First, you have to look at what the passing score is for the course. In many nursing programs, a grade of "C" is the minimum passing score. In fact, most institutions require that students maintain a grade of "C" or better in their major. Because "C" is considered average, you must decide what is considered average performance in relation to your course objectives. Aim to write items to measure student ability in relation to the course content and objectives only. Ask yourself for each item that you design to measure minimal competence (an average-level question), "Should every student be able to answer this question correctly?"

Keeping the p value of your items in the average range of 0.70 to 0.80, for example, yields a test with a mean between 0.70 and 0.80. You will also want to include some easier items (p value above 0.80) to encourage students at the beginning of a test, and you should include some difficult items (p value below 0.70) that are challenging to identify the high-achieving students (Frary, 1995). Reynolds et al. (2008) claim that, for maximum reliability, the optimal mean p value for a 4-option multiple-choice exam is 0.74. Frary recommends limiting the number of items that more than 90%

of the students can answer correctly because these items do not contribute to the reliability of a test's results.

As long as the items relate to the blueprint, having a range of difficulty levels for test items increases the variability of your test scores. Remember, the higher the score variability, the higher the reliability coefficient of the test results will be. Refer again to Chapter 4, "Implementing Systematic Test Development," for additional discussion of this important topic.

Mean Biserial

The point biserial index (PBI) represents the discrimination ability of an item, which is the basic measure of item quality for multiple-choice tests (Kehoe, 1995). It identifies the capability of an item to distinguish between those who scored at the high end on the test and those who scored at the low end.

The PBI is calculated with a complicated statistical formula that determines the correlation between the answers to a particular item on a test (correct or incorrect) and the mean scores on the test. Basically, the formula compares the responses of the students with the highest overall test scores to the students with the lowest overall test scores.

The PBI ranges from -1.0 to $+1.0$; the higher the PBI, the better the item discriminates between the high and low achievers on the test. A positive PBI for an item indicates that students who achieved high scores on the test chose the correct answer for that item more frequently than students who had low scores. If students who achieved low scores on the test chose the correct answer for an item more frequently than students who have high scores, the item will have a negative PBI. When there is little or no difference between the proportion of high-scoring and low-scoring students who select the correct answer, the item will have a low PBI and will contribute nothing to the reliability coefficient of the test because it does not discriminate. The higher the average item discrimination ability, the higher the reliability coefficient of the test results (Ebel, 1979, p. 268).

The PBI is easily available to classroom teachers who have access to test development software. The PBI provides valuable information for refining test items. If you do not have access to test development software to calculate the PBI, it is possible to calculate a similar value that will help you determine the quality of your test items.

The item discrimination index (*D*) of an item is the difference between the percentage of high-scoring students who answered the item correctly and the percentage of low-scoring students who answered the item correctly. While commercial test developers seldom use the *D* value today, it is very useful for classroom teachers who do not have access to the PBI (Brookhart & Nitko, 2014). There are dozens of formulas for calculating the *D* value; Brookhart and Nitko suggest using the formula in **Exhibit 11.1**. The *D* value for the item is the *D* value for the correct answer.

Exhibit 11.1 Formula for calculating *D* for each option

$$D = p_u - p_i$$

p_u = percent (as a decimal) of the upper group selecting the option

p_i = percent (as a decimal) of the lower group selecting the option

Item analysis is the most valuable tool for increasing the fairness of a test and improving the quality of your test items for future use. If you do not have access to this data, **Exbibit 11.2** explains how you can calculate the statistics by hand. While the process may seem tedious, it will provide you with important information that is crucial for examining your test items.

Exhibit 11.2   Hand-calculating item analysis data

1. Arrange the tests in order from the highest to the lowest score.
2. Put the answer sheets of the top-third scorers in a pile.
3. Put the answer sheets of the bottom-third scorers in a pile.
4. For each item on the test, tally how many students from each group selected each option.
5. Compute the difficulty index (p) for each item (this calculation includes only the top and bottom third, but it is sufficient for classroom test analysis).
6. Compute the response frequencies for each option (the percentage of students who selected each option).
7. Compute the discrimination index (D) for the correct answer.
8. Compute the discrimination index (D) for each distractor option.
9. Use the data to analyze the quality of the item (refer to the detailed discussion later in this chapter).

Item 10	A	B	*C	D	Total
Top group	4 (0.13)	3 (0.10)	**21 (0.70)**	2 (0.06)	30
Bottom group	9 (0.30)	6 (0.20)	**10 (0.33)**	5 (0.17)	30
Total	13	9	**31**	7	60
p value of option	0.21	0.15	**0.52**	0.12	
D value of option	−0.17	−0.10	**0.37**	−0.09	

Just as the mean p value represents the average difficulty of the items on the test, the mean PBI represents the average discrimination power of the items on the test. A high mean PBI indicates that the test contains high-quality items (that the items on the test discriminated between the high and low achievers). **Table 11.4** is adapted from Ebel's (1979, p. 267) proposed range for evaluating discrimination indices on the correct answers for items on classroom tests.

Table 11.4   Range for PBI on the Correct Answers in a Classroom Test

>0.40	Very good
0.30–0.39	Good: examine stem and options for clarity
0.20–0.29	Marginal: identify problems with stem and/or options
0.10–0.19	Weak: revise stem and/or options before banking item
0.00–0.10	Very weak: consider rejecting or accepting multiple answers
<0.00	Unacceptable: reject or accept multiple answers for the item

Haladyna (1997) defines a highly discriminating item on a classroom exam as one that has a PBI above 0.20 and a *p* value between 0.60 and 0.90 (p. 240). Kehoe (1995) maintains that items that have a PBI of less than 0.15 should be restructured. The mean PBI for our sample in Table 11.1 is 0.36. According to these criteria, our sample is well within the reasonably good category. For the purposes of overall test analysis, both the mean PBI (0.36) and the mean *p* value (0.754) for our sample are acceptable values, which means that the items on average were challenging and provided distinction between those who scored at the high end on the test and those who scored at the low end. However, you need to examine these values for each individual item before final decisions can be made about the exam.

Individual Item Analysis

Once you have examined the big picture of the test, it is time to analyze each of the pieces. In addition to summary statistics for a test, test development software programs provide statistical analysis of each item on the test. This analysis includes the *p* value and PBI for the correct answer and each of the distractors for every item. Multiple-choice classroom tests can be improved by developing a pool of good items that can be used for future tests. The statistical information from a test item analysis is an invaluable tool for both interpreting test results and improving your items for future use. However, the quality of an item cannot be determined from its statistical data alone. A qualitative review of the actual item alongside the data is the most effective way to determine the need for revision of an item.

General guidelines for using item analysis data to evaluate the items on multiple-choice exams include the following:

- Interpret the data with the size of the sample in mind; the larger the sample, the more dependable the data. Many software programs accumulate item data over time, which increases the overall sample size. However, it is important to note that item analysis data refer to an item's performance on a particular test with a particular group. When the item is included with a different set of items to form a new test or is used in the same test with a different group of students, the data are subject to change. Therefore, accumulated data provide only a general estimate of how an item is performing. Once an item bank is established, however, you will find that most of the items perform consistently over time, particularly those that are edited based on item analysis data.
- Do not use item analysis data dogmatically. The data should be used as a guide for your professional judgment and expertise.
- Do not use item analysis data in isolation. Good data do not guarantee a good item. It is important to review the item to determine its cognitive level.
- Review the data analysis for every option in an item. As the previous discussion of the quantitative test data analysis points out, the *p* value and the PBI for an item correspond to the *p* value and the PBI for the item's correct answer. These data give a picture of how well the item is working. However, it is also important to examine the analysis data for each of the distractors and to examine the question itself before deciding whether or not the question is a valuable one
- Consider potential revisions for every item, but items that have a PBI of less than 0.20 should definitely be restructured. These items are not discriminating

well between the high and low achievers on the test. Frequently, you will find that these items violate the guidelines for item writing. Examine the data for each option and rewrite the items; refer to Chapter 5, "Selected-Response Format: Developing Multiple-Choice Items," for guidelines for item construction.

- Determine the desirability of very difficult items. When an item has a p value of less than 0.30, it usually indicates that the item is too difficult for the group. The general rule is to eliminate an item that fewer than 30% of the group answers correctly. However, it is not wise to set rigid parameters for retaining or eliminating an item; you should use your professional judgment to determine whether an item is appropriately difficult. If a very difficult item discriminates well, it may be a challenging item that should be retained. Each item should be carefully reviewed to determine whether the item difficulty level is desirable or if item revision is indicated. Determine the desirability of very easy items as well; an item that has a difficulty level of greater than 0.90 may be too easy for the group. You cannot remove very easy items from a test (unless you want to cause a student revolt). However, items with very high p values should be examined carefully and revised before they are entered into an item bank.

- Check that every distractor has been selected. Distractors should be distracting. Those that are not chosen by any test taker are not working as you planned. For example, if only the correct answer and one distractor are chosen for a four-option multiple-choice item, then the item is actually a two-option item. Options that are not selected are not contributing to the test and probably should be revised. In many cases, distractors that are not selected may be implausible. Be sure to consider the size of the group when determining why an option was not selected. For example, if your sample is 10 students, you may decide that no one selected an option because there were too few students taking the test. You may decide to try the option on a future test. If no one selects an option after a few administrations of the item, it would be wise to revise the option.

- Look carefully at each option's PBI. An incorrect option that has a positive PBI or a correct option that has a negative PBI usually means that ambiguity in the stem or the option confused the students. If an item's correct option has a negative PBI and one or more distractors have a positive PBI, it means that the students who were the low achievers on the test selected the correct response more frequently than the students who were the high achievers on the test. This finding usually indicates that the high-achieving students were misled by item ambiguity or that the item is a trick item. It may also mean that all the students were so confused by the item they were guessing. One situation that should raise a red flag occurs when an item's correct option has a positive PBI and one of the distractors also has a positive PBI. These results indicate that the distractors were confusing because they attracted some of the high-achieving students. These items require careful examination, both quantitatively and qualitatively, to determine whether to remove them from the test and how to revise them for future use.

Table 11.5 provides a sample of the data printout that would be included in a detailed item analysis of a test. A careful review of these data provides insight into the role that item data can play to assist you in translating how items work on a

Table 11.5   Detailed Item Analysis

	Item Statistics			Options Statistics		
	p Value	PBI	Option	*p* Value for Option	PBI	Key
1.	0.71	0.42	A	0.21	−0.30	
			B	0.03	−0.47	
			C	0.05	−0.29	
			D	**0.71**	**0.42**	**D**
2.	0.70	0.26	A	0.13	−0.19	
			B	0.11	0.02	
			C	**0.70**	**0.26**	**C**
			D	0.06	−0.23	
3.	0.77	0.10	A	0.07	−0.26	
			B	0.04	−0.19	
			C	0.12	0.09	
			D	**0.77**	**0.10**	**D**
4.	0.76	0.27	**A**	**0.76**	**0.27**	**A**
			B	0.00	—	
			C	0.24	−0.27	
			D	0.00	—	
5.	0.258	−0.013	A	0.045	−0.063	
			B	**0.258**	**−0.013**	**B**
			C	0.000	—	
			D	0.697	0.040	
6.	0.32	0.48	**A**	**0.32**	**0.48**	**A**
			B	0.13	−0.24	
			C	0.18	−0.04	
			D	0.38	−0.29	
7.	1.00	—	A	0.00		
			B	0.00		
			C	**0.00**	**—**	**C**
			D	0.00		
8.	0.57	0.168	A	0.04	−0.147	
			B	0.07	−0.147	
			C	0.32	0.14	
			D	**0.57**	**0.168**	**D**
9.	0.352	−0.22	A	0.402	−0.01	
			B	0.183	0.15	
			C	**0.352**	**−0.22**	**C**
			D	0.422	0.10	
10.	0.714	0.43	A	0.159	−0.18	
			B	0.0635	−0.20	
			C	**0.714**	**0.43**	**C**
			D	0.0635	−0.33	

test. You will see how important it is to examine all aspects of data analysis before making scoring decisions on a test.

Note that the p value and the PBI for each item in the Item Statistics category correspond to the p value and PBI of the correct option in the Option Statistics category. For example, item 1 has a p value of 0.71 and a PBI of 0.42—the same data as for option D (the correct answer). The p value figure in the Option Statistics category refers to the percentage of students who chose each option, while the PBI value refers to the biserial for each option. A comprehensive assessment requires that you examine both the difficulty (p value) and the PBI of each item on the test and each distractor for each item.

The difficulty level of the items determines the mean of the test. Your professional judgment is the guide for determining the acceptability of the difficulty level of the items. The suggestions for acceptability of the PBI (see Table 11.4) can be used as a guide to evaluate the discrimination ability of the items. Remember, the high end of this range is a goal for which you should strive. Analysis of these data will not only help you make decisions about the test scores, it will also guide you in improving the items for future use.

Keep in mind that you cannot look at the data in isolation. The data alert you to review the actual item—use the data as a guide. If you have a very small student sample, the data will not be as accurate as they would be with a large sample. You have a dual objective with item analysis review: to help you make scoring decisions about the test at hand and to improve the items in order to bank them for future use. Although your judgment is the key factor, the data are very valuable tools for guiding your judgment. The item analysis data in Table 11.5 is an example of the item analysis data printout many test development software programs provide after a test is scored. The table illustrates how data can be utilized to make informed decisions about test items. Each of the first four items has an acceptable difficulty level. If difficulty was the only available statistical information, you might infer that the items were all operating equally well on the test. Close examination of all the data provides insight into the true functioning of the items and alerts you to examine the items that have questionable data.

Item **1** in **Table 11.6** is an example of an item that worked well statistically. The item has a difficulty level of 0.71 and a PBI of 0.42; these findings indicate that the item discriminated very well between the high achievers and the low achievers on the test. In addition, each of the incorrect options has a negative PBI, which indicates that the low-scoring students chose the distractors more frequently than the high-scoring students. This picture is exactly what you want to have for your items: the correct answer in an acceptable difficulty range with a high positive PBI and all distractors have a negative PBI. Remember, however, that data are not the only parameter for measuring the value of an item. Qualitative review of the item is just as important as the quantitative review: Just because an item has good statistical data does not mean that it is measuring anything of value.

Item **2** in **Table 11.7** has approximately the same p value as item one. Although the PBI of the item is acceptable, this item was not as statistically effective as item one because option B, an incorrect option, has a positive PBI, which means that high-achieving students chose that option. Perhaps the distractor was confusing or tricky. In any event, this information is a red flag for you to take a closer look to determine whether there is a problem with the option. If you looked only at the difficulty level for this item, you would miss the problem with distractor B.

Table 11.6 Item with Very Good Data

Item 1

p Value	PBI	Option	p Value for Option	PBI	Key
0.71	0.42	A	0.21	−0.30	
		B	0.03	−0.47	
		C	0.05	−0.29	
		D	**0.71**	**0.42**	**D**

Table 11.7 Item with Positive PBI on an Incorrect Option

Item 2

p Value	PBI	Option	p Value for Option	PBI	Key
0.70	0.26	A	0.13	−0.19	
		B	0.11	0.02	
		C	**0.70**	**0.26**	**C**
		D	0.06	−0.23	

Table 11.8 Item with Low PBI on Key and Positive PBI on Incorrect Option

Item 3

p Value	PBI	Option	p Value for Option	PBI	Key
0.77	0.10	A	0.07	−0.26	
		B	0.04	−0.19	
		C	0.12	0.09	
		D	**0.77**	**0.10**	**D**

When you examine the actual item and discuss students' reasoning with those students who selected the option, you might decide that the test scores should be adjusted to accept option B as a correct answer. On the other hand, you may decide that it is not appropriate to give credit for option B. You are not obligated to give credit for an incorrect option, only to examine questionable data.

Once you identify what attracted the high achievers to choose option B, you can edit the option so that it is clearly incorrect before you put the item in your item bank. The next time you use the item, it is likely that the high achievers will not be attracted to option B and will choose the correct option, thus increasing the discrimination ability of the item.

Another example of the problems that result from restricting your data review to the difficulty level of the items is exemplified by item **3** in **Table 11.8**. While the item's difficulty level could be considered in the acceptable range the correct answer (D) has very poor discrimination ability, and option C has a positive PBI. This item should be reviewed and option C considered for acceptance as a correct answer on this test.

Once you identify what attracted the high achievers to choose option C, you can edit the option so that it is clearly incorrect before you put the item in your item bank. Doing so will make it more likely that the high achievers will choose the correct option if you use the question in a future test because they will not be distracted by the flawed distractor, and the discrimination ability of the item will increase.

One goal of effective item writing is to develop plausible distractors that are attractive to the uninformed students. For a distractor to contribute to an item, someone must choose it. When no one chooses an option, it is considered a nondistractor. Item 4 in **Table 11.9** has two nondistractors: No one chose either option B or D, and thus it is most likely that these options are not plausible. Although the item has an acceptable difficulty level and it had acceptable discrimination, it was effectively a true–false item. The item should be reviewed and the two options that were not chosen should be revised before the item is banked. You will probably find that when you use the item in a future test, its discrimination power will increase because the low achievers will be attracted to the revised B and D options.

Item 5 in **Table 11.10** is an example of an item where the correct answer has a negative PBI. In addition, option C was not chosen, and item D has a positive PBI and was chosen by most students. These findings indicate that the students were confused and were probably guessing. Perhaps the item is miskeyed, but even if it is miskeyed, option D has very weak discrimination power and needs to be revised. Based on the data of this item, you should review it with the students and consider discarding it from this test and revising it extensively before entering it into your item bank.

Table 11.9 Item with Two Nondistractors

Item 4

p Value	PBI	Option	p Value for Option	PBI	Key
0.76	0.27	A	0.76	0.27	A
		B	0.00	—	
		C	0.24	−0.27	
		D	0.00	—	

Table 11.10 Very Difficult Item with Negative PBI on Key and One Nondistractor

Item 5

p Value	PBI	Option	p Value for Option	PBI	Key
0.258	−0.013	A	0.045	−0.063	
		B	0.258	−0.013	B
		C	0.000	—	
		D	0.697	0.040	

This is a perfect example of why a student review is so important. You want to find out why almost 70% of the students selected the incorrect response. Was the item flawed? Were the learning experiences ineffective? If you can identify the reasons for the flaws in this item, you have a great opportunity to revise the options so the item will provide the information you require the next time you use it in a test.

The results in Table 11.10 wave another red flag. If this question is testing an important concept, the students need another opportunity to master the content. Perhaps you need to offer new learning opportunities and retest the content on a future test.

Look carefully at item **6** in **Table 11.11**. If you were to look only at the difficulty level for this item, you might discard it because it is so difficult. The data indicate, however, that the item has excellent discrimination capability and each of the three distractors have a negative PBI. Perhaps the item is a challenging one that enables the test to identify high-achieving students. Or maybe the item was misleading; even though option D has a negative PBI, 38% of the students selected this incorrect option. To determine the true value of this item, you need to keep the data in mind while you conduct a qualitative review of the item itself.

Item 7 in **Table 11.12** illustrates how an item that is too easy cannot discriminate. Everyone answered this question correctly, and no one chose any of the distractors. This item might be too easy, or maybe it is testing a concept that you want to be certain that the students understand. Be sure you are really honest with yourself when evaluating this item. As was mentioned previously, items that more than 90% of students or fewer than 30% answer correctly lend very little to the quality of a test. Items such as number 7 must be carefully reviewed and revised before they are

Table 11.11   Difficult Item with Acceptable Data

Item 6

p Value	PBI	Option	p Value for Option	PBI	Key
0.32	0.48	A	0.32	0.48	A
		B	0.13	−0.24	
		C	0.18	−0.04	
		D	0.38	−0.29	

Table 11.12   Easy Item

Item 7

p Value	PBI	Option	p Value for Option	PBI	Key
1.00	—	A	0.00	—	
		B	0.00	—	C
		C	1.00	—	
		D	0.00	—	

entered into an item bank. When you have an item that has a very high or very low p value, be especially careful to examine each option to determine its plausibility.

While items 2 and 3 each have positive a positive PBI on an incorrect option, the incorrect options on both items had very low p values. In contrast, item **8** in **Table 11.13** has a positive PBI on distractor C, and distractor C has a substantially high p value: 32% of the students chose option C. This data requires close investigation of the item. Why were so many students attracted to option C? Was there an element of truth in it? If so, option C should be accepted as correct. This finding is another example of the need to have a colleague review your test before you administer it. Remember to ask your colleague to pay special attention to the incorrect options to ensure that they are absolutely incorrect because the incorrect options usually cause the flaws in an item. Better to identify a flawed item before an exam than to have to make adjustments after it is given.

The data for item **9** in **Table 11.14** indicates that the question has serious flaws. First, the correct answer has a negative PBI, which means that the low achievers on the test selected the option more frequently than the high achievers did. In addition, options A and D were chosen more frequently than the correct answer, and options B and D both have a positive PBI. This data is consistent with a very confusing or negative stem. Or perhaps it was keyed incorrectly and option D is the correct answer. This data is typical for an item with a negative stem and underscores how confusing negative stems can be. Obviously, the item must be reviewed and, unless it was keyed incorrectly, the item should be removed from the test.

Table 11.13   Item with Weak PBI on Key and Positive PBI on One Distractor

Item 8

p Value	PBI	Option	p Value for Option	PBI	Key
0.57	0.168	A	0.04	−0.147	
		B	0.07	−0.417	
		C	0.32	0.12	
		D	**0.57**	**0.168**	**D**

Table 11.14   Item with Negative PBI on Key and Positive PBI on Two Distractors

Item 9

p Value	PBI	Option	p Value for Option	PBI	Key
0.352	−0.022	A	0.402	−0.01	
		B	**0.183**	**0.15**	**C**
		C	0.352	−0.22	
		D	0.422	0.10	

Table 11.15   Item with Very Good Data

Item 10

p Value	PBI	Option	p Value for Option	PBI	Key
0.714	0.43	A	0.159	−0.147	
		B	0.0635	−0.217	
		C	**0.714**	**0.43**	C
		D	0.0635	−0.168	

Table 11.16   Examples of Item Data

Item 1	Table 11.6	Item with very good data
Item 2	Table 11.7	Item with positive PBI on incorrect option
Item 3	Table 11.8	Item with low PBI on key and positive PBI on incorrect option
Item 4	Table 11.9	Item with two nondistractors
Item 5	Table 11.10	Difficult item with negative PBI on key and one nondistractor
Item 6	Table 11.11	Difficult item with acceptable data
Item 7	Table 11.12	Easy item
Item 8	Table 11.13	Item with weak PBI on key and positive PBI on one distractor
Item 9	Table 11.14	Item with negative PBI on key and positive PBI on two distractors
Item 10	Table 11.15	Item with very good data

Item **10** in **Table 11.15** is another example of an item that has very good data. Every option was selected, the correct option has a positive PBI, and each of the distractors has a negative PBI. Remember, the data is not the whole story. An item can have very good data and not measure anything of importance. Therefore, it is essential to review the actual item to determine its value.

It is important to examine your very good items carefully. Faculty members often focus on what doesn't work and overlook the items that make a positive contribution to the test. When you identify items that have very good data and that measure important concepts, use them as models to write parallel items. The more exposure you have to what constitutes a good item, the better your item-writing skills will be. **Table 11.16** summarized the item data in Tables 11.6 through 11.15.

It is clear from the sample item analysis review in this chapter that the statistical data provided in most software reports can provide valuable information for making scoring decisions and for improving your items for future use. An understanding of the basic concepts goes a long way toward helping you translate these data. Follow the steps outlined in **Exhibit 11.3** to guide you through the test and item analysis process and review.

Exhibit 11.3 Statistical test analysis

Overall Analysis
- Check data for completeness.
- Assess the relationship of the mean and the median.
- Examine the relationship of the mean to the passing standard.
- Check the score range and standard deviation.
- Examine the reliability coefficient.
- Determine the SEM.
- Examine the mean p value.
- Evaluate the mean PBI.
- Examine the score frequency distribution.
- Assess the test's histogram.

Individual Item Analysis

- Assess each item's p value.
- Examine each item's PBI.
- Identify that the key has a positive PBI.
- Identify whether any distractor has a positive PBI.
- Identify distractors that were not chosen.
- Review items that breach minimum standards.
- Consider discarding or accepting multiple answers on items that are flawed.
- Revise items based on data and student review before entering them into an item bank.

Using Item Analysis to Improve Items

In addition to using item analysis data to analyze the functioning of an item so that decisions can be made about an overall test score, you can also use the data as a powerful vehicle for improving the reliability and validity of classroom test results by guiding the revision and improvement of the individual test items. The revised items can then be included in an item bank, which provides a valuable resource for future test development.

Multiple-choice items lend themselves most effectively to item analysis. The statistics obtained for each item provide information to guide you in improving the item. Remember that there are no dogmatic criteria for revising items; the data should be used as a guide in conjunction with your professional judgment. Item revision should be based on both qualitative and quantitative analyses of the item.

Examine the items in **Exhibits 11.4** through **11.9**. These examples illustrate how qualitative and quantitative analyses can be combined to improve your items for item banking. These specific examples illustrate the potential of item analysis. The combination of statistical data and your professional expertise provides a powerful tool for test development that should not be overlooked.

Exhibit 11.4   Item analysis example 1

Original	Revised
A client has returned to her room from the recovery room S/P Billroth procedure. The nurse's initial assessment includes BP 110/65, pulse 86 and regular, respirations 18, and temperature 100.8. Abdominal dressing is dry and intact. Levin tube is set to low suction draining 25–30 cc/hr; yellow-brown drainage is noted.	A nurse assesses a client who had a Billroth procedure 24 hours ago and identifies the following client findings: blood pressure, 110/65 mmHg; pulse, 87/min and regular; respiration, 18/min; oral temperature, 100.0°F (37.8°C); nasogastric tube to low suction, draining 20–25 mL/hr of yellow-brown drainage. The nurse should recognize that these findings indicate:

Original (continued):

The nurse caring for the client notes the amount and color of the drainage from the Levin tube. The nurse concludes that the color indicates the presence of:

A. normal gastric contents with residual bile.

B. normal gastric contents with old blood.

C. empty stomach with residual fecal matter.

D. empty stomach with residual gastric contents.

Correct answer: B
p value: 0.97
PBI: 0.02

Revised (continued):

A. normal stomach contents with old blood.

B. impending hemorrhage from the stomach.

C. reflux of intestinal contents with old blood.

D. leakage of stomach contents into the peritoneum.

Correct answer: A
p value: 0.72
PBI: 0.29

Choice	Proportion	Response PBI	Choice	Proportion	Response PBI
A	0.00	—	A	0.72	.29
B	0.97	0.02	B	0.18	−0.09
C	0.03	-0.02	C	0.07	−0.22
D	0.00	—	D	0.03	−0.23

Exhibit 11.5   Item analysis example 2

Original	Revised
A young man who has tumbled down a ski slope without one of his skies is lying at the foot of the slope complaining of severe pain in his lower leg. The nurse should:	A high school student falls down a flight of stairs at school and reports severe pain in the right lower leg. Which of these actions should a school nurse take?

Original (continued):

A. elevate his injured leg.

B. cover both legs with a blanket.

C. assess for compartment syndrome.

D. splint his injured leg.

Correct answer: D
p value: 0.87
PBI: 0.14

Revised (continued):

A. Splint the student's right leg.

B. Elevate the student's right leg.

C. Cover the student's right leg with a blanket.

D. Assess the student's right leg for range of motion.

Correct answer: A
p value: 0.71
PBI: 0.37

(continues)

Exhibit 11.5   Item analysis example 2 (*Continued*)

Choice	Proportion	Response PBI	Choice	Proportion	Response PBI
A	0.08	−0.15	A	0.71	0.37
B	0.05	−0.05	B	0.07	−0.20
C	0.00	0.00	C	0.03	−0.10
D	0.87	0.14	D	0.19	−0.48

This item illustrates an easy item; 87% of the students answered it correctly.

The options in the original item are not homogeneous, which probably accounts for the poor biserial (0.14) for the question. While the correct answer has the only positive biserial (0.14) and two of the distractors have a negative biserial, option C was not chosen at all.

The revised item removes extraneous information, eliminates gender, increases the homogeneity of the options, and substitutes an alternative for option C. Note that the item analysis data indicates that the rewritten item was very effective. Because of the improvements, the revised item discriminates much more effectively than the original, it is more difficult, every option was selected, and each of the distractors has a negative biserial.

Exhibit 11.6   Item analysis example 3

Original	Revised
The pharmacological action of antacids such as Mylanta is to:	A nurse should explain to a client that antacids, such as aluminum hydroxide (Mylanta), act to:
A. coat the stomach mucosa.	A. elevate gastric pH.
B. decrease gastric motility.	B. coat the gastric mucosa.
C. elevate gastric pH.	C. inhibit acid production.
D. decrease duodenal pH.	D. neutralize lactose intolerance.
Correct answer: C	Correct answer: A
p value: 0.56	p value: 0.67
PBI: 0.24	PBI: 0.43

Choice	Proportion	Response PBI	Choice	Proportion	Response PBI
A	0.44	−0.24	A	0.67	0.43
B	0.00	—	B	0.10	−0.33
C	0.56	0.24	C	0.18	−0.26
D	0.00	—	D	0.04	−0.29

This item demonstrates how important it is to look at the whole picture. The item was difficult for the group, with a p value of 0.56 and a reasonable point biserial (0.24). If your analysis stopped at this point, you would not see that options B and D were not chosen. You would miss the fact that the item is really a two-option item.

The revised item replaces both distractors that were not selected in the original item. It is evident from the statistical analysis that the revised item is a much more effective item.

Although it is still relatively difficult, it has an excellent point biserial, every option was selected, and all distractors have negative biserials. Option D was the weakest selection.

This is a case where your professional judgment is needed to decide whether to revise the option or retest the item as it is to collect additional data.

Exhibit 11.7   Item analysis example 4

Original	**Revised**
Increasing the flow rate of total parenteral nutrition (TPN) above the prescribed rate is dangerous because it can result in:	A client is receiving total parenteral nutrition (TPN). A nurse should ensure that the TPN does not exceed the prescribed flow rate to prevent:

Original

A. osmotic diuresis and hypoglycemia.

B. hypoglycemia and dumping syndrome.

C. dumping syndrome and electrolyte imbalance.

D. electrolyte imbalance and osmotic diuresis.

Correct answer: D
p value: 0.17
PBI: 0.03

Revised

A. hypoglycemia.

B. pneumothorax.

C. dumping syndrome.

D. electrolyte imbalance.

Correct answer: D
p value: 0.66
PBI: 0.23

Choice	Proportion	Response PBI	Choice	Proportion	Response PBI
A	0.70	−0.13	A	0.09	−0.23
B	0.11	0.17	B	0.09	−0.12
C	0.03	−0.01	C	0.15	−0.10
D	0.17	0.03	D	0.66	−0.23

With a p *value of 0.17 and a point biserial of 0.03, this item would definitely be a candidate for elimination from the test. More than 70% of the students chose distractor A, which has a negative biserial (−0.13), whereas distractor B, which was chosen by almost 11% of the students, has a positive biserial (0.17). The difficulty level of the item and point biserial results indicate that the question is ambiguous, confusing, and in need of revision.*

An examination of the item helps to explain the item analysis. This item violates item-writing guidelines: Options A and C are partially correct, and all the options overlap with at least one other option. This probably accounts for the students' confusion with the question. Should the item simply be discarded? If faculty members believe that the item is testing important information, it is worth it to attempt a rewrite, especially because you can use the item analysis as a guide.

The rewrite of the item presented here simplifies the question and still tests the key concept. The p *value of the revised item (0.66) keeps it in the difficult range. However, the item analysis shows that this version is much more effective than the original. The item has an acceptable point biserial, every option was selected, and every distractor has a negative biserial. Remember, every item should be considered for revision. Would you make any changes before reusing this item on a test?*

Exhibit 11.8   Item analysis example 5

Original	Revised
A nurse caring for a patient with a chest tube connected to a Pleur-Evac system knows that:	A client has a chest tube connected to an underwater-seal drainage system. Which of these observations of the drainage system should the nurse recognize as indicating that the system is functioning properly?
A. bubbling in the water seal should be intermittent.	
B. bubbling should be continuous and constant.	A. Fluctuations in the water-seal chamber
C. there should be no bubbling in the water seal.	B. Fluctuations in the collection chamber
D. bubbling will be seen in the suction regulator.	C. Continuous bubbling in the collection chamber
	D. Continuous bubbling in the water-seal chamber
Correct answer: C	Correct answer: A
p value: 0.84	p value: 0.78
PBI: 0.07	PBI: 0.30

Choice	Proportion	Response PBI	Choice	Proportion	Response PBI
A	0.05	−0.16	A	0.78	0.30
B	0.11	0.03	B	0.05	−0.27
C	0.84	0.07	C	0.03	−0.02
D	0.00	—	D	0.12	−0.16

The original item has a p value of 0.84 and a very weak biserial (0.07). One likely reason that the item is a poor discriminator is because distractor B has a positive biserial and no one chose distractor D. This is another item whose faults would be overlooked without careful item analysis.

The revision is composed of more homogeneous options that increased both the difficulty and discrimination values of the item. The revised item is more difficult than the original, many of the flaws are removed, and the item no longer confuses the high-achieving students. All options are chosen, and all distractors have negative biserials.

Further revision of this item for retesting is a matter of professional judgment.

Incorporating Student Comments   The item analysis examples illustrate that quantitative analysis cannot be used in isolation; your professional judgment is critical to successful item revision. Your qualitative review and the comments that accompany posttest review by both students and your colleagues provide a valuable resource for editing items before they are banked.

When revising items it is most important to write distractors that attract the uninformed students. Student comments during test review often lend themselves to the creation of effective distractors. Be sure to take careful notes of student remarks during review sessions. These remarks provide you with valuable leads for developing effective distractors.

Exhibit 11.9   Item analysis example 6

Original	Revised
A nurse would recognize that a patient is attempting to resist infection when diagnostic laboratory values reveal an elevated:	When assessing a male client, a nurse identifies that the client has the laboratory findings identified in the chart below.

Original

A nurse would recognize that a patient is attempting to resist infection when diagnostic laboratory values reveal an elevated:

A. red blood cell count.

B. white blood cell count.

C. partial thromboplastin time.

D. hematocrit.

Revised

When assessing a male client, a nurse identifies that the client has the laboratory findings identified in the chart below.

	Normal	Client
Red blood cells	4.2–6.9 million/cu mm	4.5 million /cu mm
White blood cells	4,300–10,800 /cu mL	15,000 /cu mL
Hematocrit	45%–62 %	58%

Which of these measures should the nurse include in the client's care plan?

A. Monitor the client's body temperature.

B. Move the client to an isolation room.

C. Observe the client for bleeding.

D. Advise the client to eat iron-rich foods.

Correct answer: B
p value: 1
PBI: 0

Correct answer: A
p value: 0.76
PBI: 0.52

Choice	Proportion	Response PBI	Choice	Proportion	Response PBI
A	0	0.0	A	0.76	0.52
B	1.0		B	0.05	−0.27
C	0		C	0.03	−0.02
D	0		D	0.12	−0.16

The original is an example of an item that is too easy. An item such as this does not contribute to the validity of the test's results. First, it represents recall. All the student has to do is remember that an elevated white blood cell count indicates that the patient has an infection. No interpretation is required. No judgment needs to be made. No action needs to be taken.

However, the question does address an important concept: It is important for the student to recognize the signs of infection. And just as important, the student should know what to do when client has an infection.

The revision addresses the criteria for developing items that assess critical thinking. Instead of telling the student that the client has elevated WBCs, the student is required to interpret a chart of laboratory values. Once the student identifies the problem, the student has to decide which of the actions is appropriate.

The data indicates that the revision is effective. The item's difficulty is increased, and the biserial is an excellent one. In addition, all the options are chosen, and each of the distractors has a negative biserial.

Assigning Test Scores

Once you have collected data from qualitative, statistical, and student review, you can assign scores to an exam. While you might decide to discard an item or accept more than one correct answer for a question, it is usually best not to add points to individual exams. This practice is referred to as scaling scores; see Chapter 13, "Assigning Grades," for more information.

Flawed Items

Items that are seriously flawed should not be counted as part of the final test score. Eliminating poorly functioning items from a test can increase the test's reliability coefficient. Kehoe (1995) provides an example of how eliminating seven items that had PBIs below 0.20 from a test of 30 items with a reliability coefficient of 0.79 resulted in a 23-item test with a reliability coefficient of 0.88.

It is impossible to determine whether an item is seriously flawed based on either quantitative or qualitative analysis alone. To assess the items fairly, you must include the overall test data, item analysis data, student review, and your qualitative review of the items in question. Chapter 14, "Instituting Item Banking and Test Development Software," offers guidelines for using computerized item banking to examine all aspects of an item to determine its quality. If you conclude that an item is flawed based on your comprehensive analysis, you might decide to accept more than one option as the correct answer for the item or to eliminate the item from the test. It is important to note that, because of measurement error, giving the benefit of the doubt to the students is usually the fairest approach.

Adjusting Test Scores to Account for Flawed Items

How do you adjust a test score to account for a flawed item? You could simply add a point to everyone's score, which would obviously increase everyone's score. However, those who answered the flawed item correctly in the first place would actually receive two points for the flawed item. This approach would be considered psychometrically unsound. Two alternate approaches are commonly followed. Let's examine them both so you can decide which one is best suited to your grading philosophy.

The first approach is to discard the flawed item by adjusting the key to accept all the possible answers while keeping the original number of possible points. **Table 11.17** illustrates this approach for a 10-item test with 1 flawed item.

Note that Student A answered the flawed item (number 5) correctly and has a raw score of 7/10. When the key is adjusted to accept all the possible answer options, Student A's score remains at 7/10, or 70%, because the number of possible points is kept at 10.

Table 11.17 illustrates that Student B also had an original raw score of 7/10, or 70%. Because Student B initially answered the flawed item incorrectly, however, Student B's score increases to 8/10 when all the possible options are accepted as correct. Student B's adjusted score is 80%.

Now, let's examine **Table 11.18**, This table illustrates the results of four students on a test of 50 items with three flawed items removed. All four students have a raw score of 76%, which is passing for this course.

Table 11.17 Flawed Item Removed, Key Adjusted, Possible Points Maintained

Student A				Passing = 70%		
Initial Possible Points	**Initial Raw Score**	**Percent Correct**	**Flawed Items Removed**	**Initial Answer on Flawed Item**	**Revised Score**	**Revised Percent Correct**
10	7/10	70%	1	Correct	7/10	70%

Item	Key	Student A Answers	Raw Score*	Adjusted Score*
1.	A	A	c	c
2.	C	C	c	c
3.	B	B	c	c
4.	C	D	x	x
5.	A B C D	D	c	c
6.	B	A	x	x
7.	D	C	x	x
8.	A	A	c	c
9.	C	C	c	c
10.	B	B	c	c
	SCORE		7/10	7/10

Student B				Passing = 70%		
Initial Possible Points	**Initial Raw Score**	**Percentage Correct**	**Flawed Items Removed**	**Initial Answer on Flawed Item**	**Revised Score**	**Revised Percentage Correct**
50	7/10	70%	1	Incorrect	8/10	80%

Item	Key	Student B Answers	Raw Score*	Adjusted Score*
1.	A	A	c	c
2.	C	C	c	c
3.	B	B	c	c
4.	C	C	c	c
5.	A B C D	B	x	c
6.	B	A	c	c
7.	D	C	x	x
8.	A	A	c	c
9.	C	C	c	c
10.	B	A	x	x
	SCORE		7/10	8/10

* c = correct, x = incorrect

Table 11.18 Three Flawed Items Removed from 50-Item Test, Key Adjusted, Possible Points Maintained

Student A Passing = 76%

Possible Points	Raw Score	Percent Correct	Flawed Items	Raw Score Answer	Points Added to Score	Adjusted Score	Adjusted Percent Correct
50	38	76%	1	Correct	0	38/50	76%
			2	Correct	0		
			3	Correct	0		

Student B Passing = 76%

Possible Points	Raw Score	Percent Correct	Flawed Items	Raw Score Answer	Points Added to Score	Adjusted Score	Adjusted Percent Correct
50	38	76%	1	Correct	0	39/50	76%
			2	Correct	0		
			3	Incorrect	1		

Student C Passing = 76%

Possible Points	Raw Score	Percent Correct	Flawed Items	Raw Score Answer	Points Added to Score	Adjusted Score	Adjusted Percent Correct
50	38	76%	1	Correct	0	40/50	80%
			2	Incorrect	1		
			3	Incorrect	1		

Student D Passing = 76%

Possible Points	Raw Score	Percent Correct	Flawed Items	Raw Score Answer	Points Added to Score	Adjusted Score	Adjusted Percent Correct
50	38	76%	1	Incorrect	1	41/50	82%
			2	Incorrect	1		
			3	Incorrect	1		

Student A answered all the flawed items correctly, so Student A's revised score remains at 76% once the flawed items are removed. Student B answered one of the flawed items incorrectly, which means that Student B's adjusted score increases to 78% when all the options on the flawed items are accepted. Similarly, Student C's score increases to 80% and Student D's score increases to 82% when all the options on the flawed items are accepted as correct.

The second approach to accounting for flawed items involves removing the flawed items and adjusting the total number of possible points. **Table 11.19** illustrates this approach for the same 10-item test with one flawed item that was described in Table 11.17. As Table 11.19 illustrates, however, the final results are quite different from the results in Table 11.17.

Let's look first at Student A in Table 11.19. Student A has an initial raw score of 7/10, which is a passing score of 70%. As in Table 11.17, student A answered the flawed item (number 5) correctly. When the flawed item is removed from the test, however, Student A's passing score of 7/10 changes to 6/9, which is 66.7%, a failing score.

On the other hand, Student B, who also has an initial passing score of 7/10, has answered the flawed item (number 5) incorrectly. So, when item number 5 is eliminated from the test, Student B's score becomes 7/9, or 77.7%. As you can see, adjusting the possible number of points has a more dramatic effect on the students' final scores than simply adjusting the key and accepting all the responses as correct.

The effect of adjusting the possible number of points is illustrated even more clearly in **Table 11.20**.

Both Table 11.18 and Table 11.20 illustrate the results for four students on the same 50-item test that has three flawed items. The key-adjusted approach in Table 11.18 results in all four students obtaining a passing grade, while the adjusting-points approach illustrated in Table 11.20 results in Student A receiving a failing grade.

Which approach will you choose to use for flawed items? The choice is up to you. Remember, however, that fairness to students is the pivotal issue here. Students should not be held accountable for defective items in a test. Also keep in mind that the students will have great difficulty accepting that they have gone from a passing to a failing score, which is why I recommend using the key adjusted approach.

However, the choice is a faculty decision. As long as the students are informed of the method that will be implemented, faculty members are justified in implementing whichever method they deem appropriate. The ultimate goal is to remove all defective items from the test bank so you are not caught in this dilemma. This goal can be accomplished by following the guidelines presented in this text.

Whichever approach you decide to use to adjust scores for flawed items, make sure that these items are revised before they are entered into the item bank to ensure they are not reused in their defective condition. Flawed items often have the potential to be revised as very effective items. Careful editing that considers the qualitative and quantitative analysis and that incorporates student comments can assist you with transforming these items into items that contribute to valid and reliable results from your measurement instruments.

Returning Scores to Students

Teachers must carefully consider the issue of confidentiality when returning scores to students. Several test development programs provide individual score reports that

Table 11.19   Flawed Item Removed, Possible Points Adjusted

Student A					Passing = 70%		
Initial Possible Points	Initial Raw Score	Percent Correct	Flawed Items Removed	Adjusted Possible Points	Initial Answer on Flawed Item	Revised Score	Revised Percent Correct
10	7/10	70%	1	9	Correct	6/9	66.7%

Item	Key	Student A Answers	Raw Score*	Adjusted Score*
1.	A	A	c	c
2.	C	C	c	c
3.	B	B	c	c
4.	C	D	x	x
5.	D	D	c	Removed
6.	B	A	x	x
7.	D	C	x	x
8.	A	A	c	c
9.	C	C	c	c
10.	B	B	c	c
	SCORE		7/10	6/9

Student B					Passing = 70%		
Initial Possible Points	Initial Raw Score	Percent Correct	Flawed Items Removed	Adjusted Possible Points	Initial Answer on Flawed Item	Revised Score	Revised Percent Correct
10	7/10	70%	1	9	Correct	6/9	66.7%

Item	Key	Student B Answers	Raw Score*	Adjusted Score*
1.	A	A	c	c
2.	C	C	c	c
3.	B	B	c	c
4.	C	C	c	c
5.	D	B	x	Removed
6.	A	A	c	c
7.	D	C	x	x
8.	A	A	c	c
9.	C	C	c	c
10.	B	B	x	x
	SCORE		7/10	7/9

* c = correct, x = incorrect.

Table 11.20   Three Flawed Items Removed from a 50-Item Test, Possible Points Adjusted

Student A

Passing = 76%

Possible Points	Raw Score	Percent Correct	Flawed Items	Raw Score Answer	Adjusted Possible Points	Adjusted Score	Adjusted Percent Correct
50	38	76%	1	Correct		−1	
			2	Correct		−1	
			3	Correct		−1	
					47	35/47	74.5%

Student B

Passing = 76%

Possible Points	Raw Score	Percent Correct	Flawed Items	Raw Score Answer	Adjusted Possible Points	Adjusted Score	Adjusted Percent Correct
50	38	76%	1	Correct		−1	
			2	Correct		−1	
			3	Incorrect		0	
					47	36/47	76.5%

(continues)

Table 11.20 Three Flawed Items Removed from a 50-Item Test, Possible Points Adjusted (*Continued*)

Student C

Passing = 76%

Possible Points	Raw Score	Percent Correct	Flawed Items	Raw Score Answer	Adjusted Possible Points	Adjusted Score	Adjusted Percent Correct
50	38	76%	1	Correct		−1	
			2	Incorrect Incorrect		0	
			3			0	
					47	37/47	78.7%

Student D

Passing = 76%

Possible Points	Raw Score	Percent Correct	Flawed Items	Raw Score Answer	Adjusted Possible Points	Adjusted Score	Adjusted Percent Correct
50	38	76%	1	Incorrect Incorrect		−1	
			2	Incorrect		0	
			3			0	
					47	38/47	80.9%

can be distributed to students confidentially, and many schools have the ability to distribute scores confidentially on the Internet. If your school's practice is to post student grades, be careful to follow the school's protocol and assign secret identification numbers to each student.

Another important consideration is timeliness. Teachers often assign strict deadlines for assignment submissions, yet they are very lax with returning the same assignments in a timely manner. Although careful consideration of grade assignment requires time, students should not be required to wait so long that the feedback from an exam or written assignment is meaningless.

On the other hand, students often want their test scores before they leave the classroom. It is to the students' advantage to wait. Faculty members need several days to review an exam carefully and examine the data before returning scores to students. For a discussion related to scoring and student test review, refer to Chapter 9, "Assembling, Administering, and Scoring a Test." Keep in mind that, in the interest of fairness, you should set a return deadline with the students and adhere to that deadline.

Summary

Systematic test and item analysis procedures ensure the fairness and accuracy of individual items and the test as a whole. It is impossible to evaluate the effectiveness of an item on a test without examining all the relevant data. Statistical test and item analysis data provide the essential tools for objective review of test results. This chapter provides actual examples of test analysis data to illustrate how these data can be used for objective interpretation of test results. While your first attempt at conducting these analyses will be time consuming, the procedure will become streamlined as you become more proficient and as you incorporate improved items from your item bank in your exams.

Although these data can be very useful for improving your assessments, you must remember that the data are only useful as general indicators, not as precise measures. Data interpretation should be used as only one of the considerations to make when determining the fairness of an assessment; your professional judgment must guide the process.

Learning Activities

1. Define the measures of central tendency included in Table 11.1. Explain how the measures of central tendency would skew a distribution negatively or positively.

2. Define standard deviation. Explain why you would expect a small standard deviation on a test administered to a homogenous group of high-achieving students.

3. Which of these tests would most likely yield a low reliability coefficient?

    A. A test of 50 challenging items administered to a large group of heterogeneous students

    B. A test of 10 easy items administered to a small group of homogeneous students

Explain your answer.

4. Define *p* value. Define discrimination ability. How are the difficulty and discrimination power of an item related? Explain why a high mean PBI indicates that a test contains high-quality items.

5. How would you adjust test scores for flawed items? Explain your rationale for the approach you select.

6. Review and interpret the data from the item analysis in the table below. Discuss your analysis with your colleagues.

	Item Statistics		**Options Statistics**			
	p Value	PBI	Option	*p* Values	PBI	Key
1.	0.737	0.15	A	0.053	−0.21	
			B	0.053	−0.33	
			C	**0.737**	**0.15**	C
			D	0.158	0.15	
2.	0.789	0.02	A	0.105	0.06	
			B	**0.789**	**0.02**	B
			C	0.053	0.16	
			D	0.053	0.21	
3.	0.632	0.44	A	0.053	0.04	
			B	0.056	0.45	
			C	0.263	0.28	
			D	**0.632**	**0.44**	D
4.	0.632	0.01	A	0.211	0.12	
			B	0.00	0.00	
			C	**0.632**	**0.01**	C
			D	0.158	0.15	
5.	0.895	0.57	A	0.053	−0.33	
			B	0.053	0.45	
			C	**0.895**	**0.57**	C
			D	0.00	0.00	

7. Review the items and their data in the tables below. Rewrite the items to improve their performance. Consider both the data and the item analysis for each item. Discuss your revisions with your colleagues.

1. A nurse is assessing a patient who has insulin dependent diabetes mellitus (type 1). The patient has a blood sugar of 60 mg/dL. Which of these additional findings should the nurse expect to identify?
   A. Weakness, diaphoresis, and confusion
   B. Kussmaul's respirations, acetone breath, and headache
   C. Polydypsia, polyuria, and polyphagia
   D. Lethargy, flushed face, and somnolence

	A*	B	C	D
PBI	0.05	−0.06	−0.22	0.17
p value	0.809	0.048	0.067	0.076

2. Which of these measures should a nurse include in the care plan for a patient who had a graft of the femoral artery 8 hours ago?
   A. Keeping the patient's legs elevated above the level of the heart
   B. Encouraging increased fluid intake
   C. Comparing pedal pulses every 2 hours
   D. Assisting the patient to do isometric leg exercises

	A	B	C*	D
PBI	−0.039	0.00	0.31	−0.08
p value	0.144	0.00	0.81	0.046

3. A patient who had a transurethral prostatectomy (TURP) 6 hours ago has a continuous bladder irrigation (CBI). The patient asks a nurse, "Why do I need this irrigation?" Which of these explanations should the nurse offer the patient?
   A. "The irrigation will stop the bleeding in your bladder."
   B. "The irrigation keeps the catheter from being blocked by blood clots."
   C. "The irrigation promotes normal urine production until healing occurs."
   D. "The irrigation provides a route for giving antibiotics directly into the bladder."

	A	B*	C	D
PBI	0.04	−0.18	0.06	0.00
p value	0.095	0.841	0.064	0.00

4. A patient who had abdominal surgery 2 hours ago is in the postanesthesia unit. The patient has an intravenous infusing at 100 mL/hr. A nurse assesses that the patient has dyspnea, moist cough, and an O_2 saturation of 92%. Which of these actions should the nurse take first?
   A. Monitor the patient's heart rate and blood pressure
   B. Assess the patient for peripheral edema
   C. Notify the physician
   D. Slow the patient's intravenous rate to 10 mL/hr

	A	B	C	D*
PBI	0.07	−0.21	0.07	0.14
p value	0.011	0.492	0.064	0.333

5. A patient who had a Billroth II procedure this morning has all of these prescriptions. Which one should the nurse question?
   A. Isotonic leg exercises every 2 hours
   B. Ambulate tomorrow morning
   C. Irrigate the nasogastric tube every 2 hours
   D. Assist the patient to cough and deep breath

	A	B	C*	D
PBI	−0.15	0.28	0.20	−0.23
p value	0.064	0.032	0.571	0.333

Web Links

EXCEL Spreadsheets for Classical Test Analysis
http://languagetesting.info/statistics/excel.html
Introductory Statistics
http://www.psychstat.missouristate.edu/introbook/sbk13m.htm
Schreyer Institute for Teaching Excellence
http://www.schreyerinstitute.psu.edu/Tools/ItemAnalysis/
Test Item Analysis Using an Excel Spreadsheet
http://www.eflclub.com/elvin/publications/2003/itemanalysis.html

References

Brookhart, S. M., & Nitko, A. J. (2014). *Educational assessment of students* (7th ed.). Upper Saddle River, NJ: Pearson Education.

Ebel, R. L. (1979). *Essentials of educational measurement* (3rd ed.). Englewood Cliffs, NJ: Prentice Hall.

Frary, R. (1995). *More multiple-choice item writing do's and don'ts.* Blacksburg, VA: Virginia Polytechnic Institute and State University.

Frisbie, D. A. (1988). Reliability of scores from teacher-made tests. *Educational Measurement: Issues and Practice, 7,* 25–35.

Haladyna, T. M. (1997). *Writing test items to evaluate higher order thinking.* Needham Heights, MA: Allyn and Bacon.

Kehoe, J. (1995). Basic item analysis for multiple-choice tests. *Practical Assessment, Research & Evaluation, 4*(10). Retrieved from http://pareonline.net/getvn.asp?v=4&n=10

Miller, M. D., Linn, R. L., & Gronlund, N. E. (2009). *Measurement and assessment in teaching* (10th ed.). Upper Saddle River, NJ: Pearson Education.

Reynolds, C. R., Livingston, R. B., & Wilson, V. (2008). *Measurement and assessment in education* (2nd ed.). Boston, MA: Allyn & Bacon.

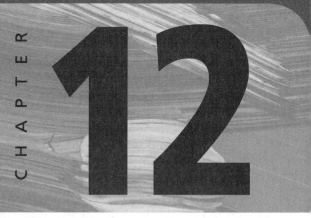

© Anteromite/Shutterstock

Laboratory and Clinical Evaluation

CHAPTER

12

"Information is pretty thin stuff unless mixed with experience."

—CLARENCE DAY

One of the most important goals for nurse educators is to facilitate student transition from the abstractions of the classroom to performance in a reality setting. While classroom and laboratory experiences provide the knowledge base that students must master to practice in the clinical setting, the clinical experience is too often structured as a separate learning experience—as an end in itself. In reality, the classroom, laboratory, and clinical experiences must be integrated to provide realistic opportunities for students to attain the overall course objectives.

Chapter 3, "Developing Instructional Objectives," discussed the importance of providing students with appropriate opportunities to master what they are required to learn in a course. When every learning activity that faculty afford students relates directly to a course objective, the clinical experience becomes the vehicle for students to apply the abstractions of the classroom to real-life nursing practice. This chapter provides guidelines for using the course objectives to design performance evaluation instruments for the laboratory and clinical settings that are student-oriented, user friendly, and developmentally appropriate to the students' level.

Relevance of Objectives

It is not uncommon for educators to focus on developing strategies to facilitate student attainment of course objectives in the theoretical component of a nursing course. A great deal of time is devoted to developing syllabi, lectures, media, case studies, and assessment instruments for the classroom, but planning the means to facilitate student mastery of the course objectives in clinical and laboratory experiences is often neglected. In some cases, faculty assign a separate set of objectives to the clinical component of a course or use a checklist of nursing procedures that students must master at a minimally competent standard as the sole criterion for passing in a skills lab or even in the clinical setting. This practice serves to reduce the experience to a to-do list. The procedures become ends in themselves rather than activities that are part of more complex learning outcomes that facilitate nursing practice.

Laboratory and clinical experiences have the same purpose as classroom learning: to facilitate attainment of the course objectives. When the objectives are realistic and guide all the components of a course, students are able to perceive the course as a unified whole and understand the meaning of the individual activities. When students recognize that the purpose of instruction is relevant to an overall goal, they are more likely to assume responsibility for their own learning.

Students' success in the classroom setting can be directly linked to their understanding of what they must accomplish to attain mastery of the course objectives. So it is logical to expect that students who perceive the clinical experience as an organized learning arena that is related to the classroom experience will be successful in making connections between theory and practice. Therefore, the laboratory and clinical experiences must be designed to afford students the opportunity to attain competency in the course objectives while performing selected nursing skills, acquiring competence in using the nursing process, and developing decision-making ability.

This is not to suggest that clinical instruction should avoid capturing an unplanned learning opportunity. To the contrary, most of what happens in the clinical setting is unpredictable. Within the volatile, and sometimes chaotic, setting of a large medical-surgical unit, for example, instructional objectives and learning outcomes should be designed to provide guidance for the clinical instructor.

Elements of the Clinical/Laboratory Experience

Once the course objectives are established, how do you construct clinical experiences that capture the essence of what you want the student to learn? Although the clinical setting has the potential to afford students the opportunity to apply theories to real problems, O'Connor (2001) points out that "the clinical practice component of nursing education, which has evolved from the apprenticeship model established by Nightingale, remains ill-defined" (p. 177). Tanner (2006) notes that the current clinical placement model is no longer sustainable in today's healthcare environment for several reasons, including the fact that the students' experience is too dependent on events that faculty cannot control. While nurse educators recognize that clinical practice experience is vital to the educational process for nursing students, it can be difficult to keep course objectives as the focal point and rise above the number of tasks that must be accomplished by the students in a continuously changing clinical environment.

Whether the clinical setting is a medical-surgical unit, a skills laboratory, an assisted living facility, or a patient's home, the learning environment must offer opportunities to practice behaviors that address the course objectives. Reilly and Oermann (1992) describe the clinical practice setting as providing "experiences with real clients and real problems [that] enable learners to use knowledge in practice, develop skill in problem-solving and decision-making, learn how to learn, and develop a commitment to be responsible for one's own actions" (p. 115).

In every clinical practice setting, the instructor must recognize that, even though the student may not seem to be connecting with the task at hand, learning is occurring. As Dewey (1938/1997) identified:

> Perhaps the greatest of all pedagogical fallacies is the notion that a person learns only the particular thing he is studying at the time. Collateral learning in the way of formation of enduring attitudes of likes and dislikes, may be and often is much more important than the spelling lesson or lesson in geography or history that is learned. For these attitudes are fundamentally what counts in the future. The most important attitude that can be formed is that of desire to go on learning (p. 48).

Once we recognize that learning is always taking place as the desire to continue learning develops, we can understand why the instructor's role of making sense of the environment to provide objective-based learning opportunities is so critical.

In addition to supporting collateral learning, instructors must facilitate the blending of thought and action for the students. Linking the whys with the hows really does depend on the approach of the instructor, who promotes the students' abilities to make sense of the environment. "The educated man is not just one who knows, but one who gains from his knowledge the power to do" (Cronbach, 1963, p. 42). Cronbach points out that problem solving is not a mere intellectual process: It encompasses impressions, memories of previous similar experiences, the sense of success in problem solving, and the organization of pieces of knowledge into a meaningful body of principles to be applied to new situations.

When students experience the clinical setting, they take in cues and messages from the environment. The instructor assesses their adaptation to the situation and intervenes when the students need assistance to modify or improve their responses to situations. The instructor may use techniques such as comparing the present to situations students have previously encountered. When students are successful, the instructor recognizes that transfer of learning has occurred. "Transfer of ideas and skills occurs if a person understands them and recognizes their relevance to the situation he faces" (Cronbach, 1963, p. 57).

Reflective thinking has also been found to be an important mechanism for blending thought and action. Forneris (2004) identifies the thinking process continuum as one that moves from "knowing what" to "knowing how" and "knowing why." The complex issues that students face in the clinical setting require a reflective process that creates a sense of organization when preparing to take some type of nursing action. The instructor's role is to facilitate this process. Once the student sees the connections, the transfer of principles to real situations takes place. Clinical experiences that are relevant to the instructional objectives help students make the transition from the unknown to the understood—to translate knowledge into action.

Identification of Clinical Action Elements

A student in the laboratory setting is exposed to principles related to typical basic nursing skills and the practice of those skills. Generally, this is a low-stress learning environment, except during evaluation or return demonstration events. Most evaluation tools in this setting leave some room for interpretation and instructor judgment.

Sometimes, however, the constriction on the students' movements or explanations are so severe that one misstep may lead to increased student stress and failure. A first-semester student demonstrating the sequences of taking vital signs, for example, may be able to describe how to take an apical pulse and compare it with the radial pulse, but he or she may not place the stethoscope exactly on the point of maximum impulse (PMI). If the evaluation tool stipulates, "Places the bell of the stethoscope on the patient's PMI" as a step in the evaluation process, should the instructor mark the student's overall performance as pass or fail? When teachers expect perfect performance from a novice student, the level of stress only increases the student's chance for failure. The instructor's role is to support the student's self-confidence—to facilitate learning and acquisition of new skills while promoting the desire to go on learning.

Gaberson and Oermann (1999) identify five steps in the process of clinical teaching:

1. Identifying outcomes
2. Assessing learning needs
3. Planning clinical learning activities
4. Instructing students in clinical practice
5. Evaluating student learning and performance (p. 88)

Identifying Outcomes

Because the clinical experience is an integral part of a nursing course and not a separate entity, the course objectives and outcomes should guide the design of the clinical experiences. Therefore, the course objectives must be developed before you can plan any learning activities, including the clinical experience.

The course objectives identify where the students should be at the end of the course. They provide students with a map that identifies the starting and ending points, while the outcomes identify the behaviors that must be accomplished along the way. Although the course objectives guide the journey, they should not provide every minute detail of a clinical experience, just as outcomes cannot spell out every patient encounter and task to accomplish. If we expect students to succeed, they must understand where they are going; the course objectives must be relevant to the clinical setting and explained to students so that they provide a clear guide.

Assessing Learning Needs

Assessment of learning needs implies that students do have different learning needs. It would be counterproductive to overinvest in a student who glides through the clinical experience with little instructor intervention at the expense of a student who cannot seem to get organized. For example, consider a group of students where one or two are outperforming their peers in the clinical setting. Most of the students are performing adequately for their level, making missteps along the way, but one or two students need additional instructor guidance and intervention. During the clinical experience, it would be sound educational practice for the clinical instructor to implement unique instructional approaches to help each individual learner accomplish the course objectives. This approach requires that flexibility of learning activities be incorporated during the planning phase of the clinical experiences.

Planning Clinical Learning Experiences

How can we ensure that clinical learning activities are related to course objectives and student performance outcomes? If students are expected to care for patients who have complex health issues by the end of the semester, for example, then the learning activities should include opportunities for students to intervene with a variety of patients who have complex health issues.

Consider a course objective in an introductory nursing course that focuses on using the nursing process when providing patient care. A beginning student could be expected to assess the patient; provide morning care; and identify the patient's healthcare issues, laboratory values, and medications. In an advanced course, the more experienced student would be expected to perform at a level requiring more complex nursing actions. An intense instructor-guided approach should challenge the student to meet the same course objective of using the nursing process when providing patient care; however, the learning opportunities would require the student to perform at a higher level. For example, the student may be expected to conduct an in-depth patient assessment, perform complex wound care, initiate discharge teaching, and administer intravenous medication.

Students build on what they know to accomplish a clinical assignment. They rely on previous experience to carry out activities they have performed successfully in prior semesters, and they build on these experiences to develop their abilities. Nursing programs usually strive to increase the complexity of students' clinical assignments as they progress through the course sequence. When complexity is viewed as caring for an increasing number of patients using the same skills that were accomplished in previous semesters without further acquisition of applied knowledge, students are not being provided with experiences that address the course objectives.

It would be unreasonable to expect the beginning student to complete discharge teaching adequately or to make swift connections between a patient's blood urea nitrogen level and the prescribed nutritional therapy, for example. It would also be shortsighted for an instructor to be satisfied with the advanced student's ability to assess and provide morning care efficiently for three patients without consideration of the course objectives. Psychomotor efficiency is not the hallmark of professional practice. Worthwhile learning experiences are based on the course objectives.

Instructing and Evaluating

Instructing and evaluating students in the clinical setting occur hand in hand. To individualize the process, the instructor must consider that each student is unique and that each clinical group includes individuals with a variety of abilities. For example, a nursing instructor might encounter a situation where one student can accurately discuss a disease process yet is unable to hang the intravenous medication safely to treat it; another student cannot explain why a patient who is in congestive heart failure needs a Foley catheter but can insert it flawlessly. Several questions arise:

- Which one is the superior student?
- Why do these differences occur?
- What do these discrepancies mean?

How can we effectively teach each student so that the theoretically adept student can apply knowledge to action and the technically capable student can make the connections to nursing knowledge? One effective instructional and assessment strategy is to use the Socratic method: question, question, question the students. Stretch each student's thought processes so that the smaller pieces of information begin to create a picture of the patient. Ask questions, such as:

- Why?
- How?
- What would happen if . . . ?
- What patient outcome do you want to see?

Tell students that they can ask themselves the following questions when they are faced with a decision:

- What would the prudent nurse do?
- What action best protects the patient?

These questions nudge students out of the concrete black-and-white world of skill performance into the gray areas of clinical decision making and critical thinking, or decision discrimination.

Questioning also serves to focus the attention of the student who needs additional guidance. During the planning phase of clinical instruction, it is not possible to discern the individual learning styles and needs of each student in a clinical group. These needs surface during the instructional process and can sometimes frustrate even the most patient clinical instructor. Students who perform marginally in the clinical arena often display similar behaviors: distraction from the main concerns, avoidance, and forgetfulness. Consistent refocusing and questioning are tools that the instructor can use to reduce student anxiety, encourage independence, and instill a measure of instructional vitamin C (i.e., confidence) with each satisfactory response to a question. This approach also serves to help focus students who unwittingly fall prey to the sometimes overwhelming sensory stimulation of a busy acute care unit and find themselves caught up in trivia or in another student's learning needs.

Evaluation of a student's performance should be an ongoing process that is integrated with instruction. The student's responses to questioning, decision-making processes, clinical judgments, and demonstration of skills help to inform the instructor about the student's day-to-day and long-term progress toward fulfilling course objectives.

A valuable asset for an instructor who, for example, must evaluate a group of 10 students in a clinical group is a comprehensive, user-friendly, clinical performance evaluation tool. Such a tool helps the instructor organize information about the students' progress in an objective fashion, assists in avoiding subjective biases, and provides a record of performance. Development of tools that are based on course objectives, identify student growth, and are level appropriate is critical to student success. Without continuous informal feedback and formal evaluation midway and at the end of the semester, students may as well be tossed out to sea without a compass.

Thus, program and course objectives are truly the cornerstone of student clinical learning and practice. These objectives must make sense to the instructor, who in turn interprets them for students. When a syllabus has a list of objectives that are merely read through at the beginning of a course and are not closely connected to the clinical performance evaluation, then the instructor has no reference point, and students may be misguided or inadequately challenged and informed. Before you begin to develop a clinical or laboratory evaluation tool, ask yourself at what level should students be able to apply and integrate knowledge, make decisions, use information and data, implement procedures, and behave in the practice setting in relation to each of the course objectives at the end of the clinical experience.

The Professional Role

In addition to the performance of procedural skills and the development and exercise of sound clinical decision making, the evolution of student to professional requires behaviors in the affective domain that involve interactions with patients, families, and healthcare team members. The instructor's ability to role-model, set the professional tone, practice culturally sensitive nursing, and exemplify values that support the American Nurses Association's *Code of Ethics* guides the student to the refinement of a professional personae.

A student who demonstrates flawless psychomotor technique, accurately recites normal complete blood count ranges, and recalls side effects of a patient's cardiac medication, for example, may not correctly interpret communication cues, display appropriate responses to human behavior, interact therapeutically with patients, or act in a manner that reflects professional values such as honesty and fairness. Affective behaviors are often difficult to articulate and assess, which is why objectives for each clinical course must include the progression of professional role development. The final nursing course, which focuses on the transition from student to practicing nurse, cannot be the only time professional development is addressed. Becoming a professional is an ongoing process. Activities and evaluations to address that process should be included each and every time the student practices in the clinical setting.

Designing and Using a Performance Tool

Student evaluation strategies should be designed to provide feedback to both students and teachers about what the students really know and understand and their ability to examine nursing situations from multiple perspectives (Ironside & Valiga, 2006). An important advantage of having cogent assessment strategies and performance evaluation tools for the laboratory and clinical settings is that they serve to remove ambiguity and excessive subjectivity from the process. For example, while the classroom instructor may have a clear idea of the criteria for student performance on an oncology unit, that criteria must be communicated to the clinical (frequently adjunct) instructors. If the criteria are not communicated, the clinical instructors may design the experience around their own expertise and preferences, without due consideration of the course objectives. This would be a particular problem if a clinical instructor did not appreciate the relevance of the course objectives and outcomes or did not consider them meaningful enough to make educational sense in an active learning environment.

A major pitfall of approaching clinical instruction and evaluation without considering course objectives is a tendency to rely on the students' successful repetition of tasks to signal a pass in clinical performance. It becomes easy to confuse clinical competency with task competency when clinical instruction is not framed consistently by learning objectives that address both the cognitive and psychomotor abilities of the student.

Using a Taxonomy

Nursing educators have collectively spent countless hours attempting to design the perfect performance evaluation tool to capture a snapshot of student behavior in the clinical and/or laboratory settings. One way to design a tool that is logical and user friendly is to refer to an educational taxonomy. Bloom's taxonomy is a time-honored guide that has recently undergone revision and continues to provide a helpful approach for guiding the instruction and evaluation of students who are learning in unpredictable situations (for a more detailed discussion of this taxonomy, refer to Chapter 3, "Developing Instructional Objectives"). The advantage of using Bloom's taxonomy is that it deconstructs the complexity of the learning process, making evaluation more logical for the clinical instructor who is trying to manage multiple priorities.

Bloom, Englehart, Furst, Hill, and Krathwohl (1956) identify three domains of behavior for classifying objectives:

1. Cognitive
2. Psychomotor
3. Affective

Consideration of these learning domains is very useful for clinical evaluation. Rather than viewing the three domains separately, you can strengthen your clinical performance evaluation by finding creative ways to blend them into a multidimensional learning experience. It is important to recognize that students learn from simple units to complex processes, and although students are all unique, learning experiences are perceived and influenced in similar ways. Therefore, when designing a clinical performance evaluation tool, integration of behaviors from all three domains should be considered so that one domain informs rather than obscures the others.

The cognitive domain is focused on thought processes that draw on memory, acquired knowledge, abstractions, application of abstract material to real situations, analysis of relationships and principles, synthesis of parts into a transformed whole, and evaluation of information based on criteria. How is this domain addressed in the clinical setting? O'Connor (2001) states that, in the clinical setting, "the clinical instructor's skilled questioning of students should reflect this focus" (p. 36). Just as evidence-based practice relies on research findings, objectives in this domain should reflect sound decision making that is derived from the rational use of the critical thinking process.

The psychomotor domain encompasses the student's coordinated ability to execute a task requiring gross or fine motor skills. This domain requires the cognitive structure for purposes of framing the student's ability to understand the why of the action being taken. The psychomotor domain is used primarily in the college laboratory setting, where skill mastery is the main concern. Many students are heavily focused on success in this domain, spending hours of time memorizing procedural steps rather than developing a rationale for how a procedure should unfold.

The affective domain completes the triad and involves feelings, attitudes, and values. The affective domain is related to student motivation and readiness to learn, the value placed on the learning situation, the attitudes the student brings into the learning situation, and the student's overall perception of the learning situation. This domain, which is not easily quantified, is often assessed with anecdotal information rather than measurable data. It can be difficult to interpret emotions and feelings from a student's overt behavior; therefore, there is a potential for misinterpretation of anecdotal student data. For example, an instructor could perceive a student interaction as uncaring when the student was experiencing apprehension. Clearly enunciated objectives are essential for fair evaluation in the affective domain.

O'Connor (2001, pp. 148–149) suggests using techniques that encourage students to engage in reflection to access behaviors in the affective domain. Encouraging students to explore their feelings related to real-life clinical situations helps them to clarify values and resolve ethical dilemmas. This approach also provides a stimulus for the development of caring behaviors. Students must learn how to act in response to the caring impulses they feel when responding to the needs of patients. Using trigger questions to prompt discussions that focus on the caring behaviors of nurses is an effective method to facilitate learning caring behaviors.

Assessment of Mastery Learning

Instructional objectives should not be constrained to become merely a to-do list. However, it is almost conventional practice to evaluate laboratory and clinical skills by signing off on students' abilities to perform specific tasks. We can deconstruct the skills laboratory by posing several questions:

- What activity in the laboratory setting will assist the student to attain a specific course objective?
- What defines a clinical skill?
- Why do we want the student to learn the skill?
- What determines that it is performed well or poorly?
- How often must the student perform the skill to fulfill instructor expectations?
- How does skills acquisition in a laboratory setting integrate with theoretical knowledge?

The final question links the role of skills acquisition in clinical nursing courses to theory and compels us to think of creative ways to break out of the comfort zone of the traditional cookbook method of skills instruction and checklist evaluation.

One way to compromise between broad course objectives and specific procedure checklists is to develop a rubric for the objectives that encompasses and links the domains of learning to produce a holistic view of what students' performance should be when the course concludes. Refer again to the mastery-level general course objective in Exhibit 3.4. Under this objective, several learning outcomes define the behaviors that are accepted as demonstrating safe behavior. Note that the outcomes are not merely related to the psychomotor performance of a procedure but also include several behaviors related to the cognitive domain, such as "Discusses the rationale for the procedure," and the affective domain, "Identifies the impact of the procedure on the client."

Table 12.1 translates the general objective with its defining learning outcomes from Exhibit 3.4 into a pass/fail evaluation tool that can be used for all procedures in a nursing course. This tool takes the procedure beyond the mere rote performance of a skill because students are required to think about the procedure as well as perform it with a predetermined degree of accuracy. A companion procedure checklist that would simply require a pass/fail or observed/not observed would accompany the outcome, "Completes procedure."

When a procedure checklist that simply requires a pass/fail or observed/not observed is the only method used to evaluate psychomotor skills, student abilities are not assessed adequately. In other words, this approach, though efficient, does little to provide cogent feedback to students and reduces skills to rote memorization. The key is to identify the learning outcomes that define the objective ("Safely performs basic nursing procedures," in this case) and use those outcomes to design both clinical and classroom evaluation instruments.

An important issue to address is the criteria for passing a course. In some nursing programs, a student's failure to pass any of the learning outcomes results in failure for the procedure and ultimately the course itself. Caution should be exercised

Table 12.1   Sample Pass/Fail Skills Lab Evaluation Form

NU 101 Foundations of Nursing Practice
Objective I: Safely Performs Basic Nursing Procedures

Outcomes	Blood Pressure		Oral Medications		IM Injections		Urinary Catheterization	
	Pass	Fail	Pass	Fail	Pass	Fail	Pass	Fail
Discusses rationale								
Identifies impact on the client								
Explains procedure to the client								
Selects equipment								
Completes procedure (refer to specific checklist)								
Uses appropriate aseptic technique								
Interprets client response								
Reports and documents results								
Provides appropriate follow-up								

when using this approach. For example, would a single breach of sterile technique result in failure of a learning outcome? At first glance, it would. However, when placed within the context of the entire course objective, what exactly constituted the student's failure? Was the failure in meeting this learning outcome due to blatant carelessness and neglect, overwhelming anxiety, or lack of knowledge? Does failure to meet the standards of a learning outcome lend itself to remediation or course failure? How many times can a student fail to meet the requirements of a learning outcome? Twice? Three times? Does a student's inability to perform a skill or make a prudent priority judgment reflect flaws in the student's reasoning process, in the educational approach, or both? In other words, perhaps a fresh look at the evaluative process and the use of tools that can pinpoint problems can assist the instructor in making an informed decision about whether failure or remediation is the best option for the student.

In addition to pass/fail, another approach is to discriminate levels of performance by using a rating scale for each of the learning outcomes; for example, a 4 or 5 means an excellent performance, a 2 or 3 is a typically average or acceptable performance, and a 0 or 1 is unacceptable. The faculty must designate what total score is required for passing the objective and clearly communicate this requirement to the students before the evaluation takes place. Because we must guard against subjectivity in all student evaluations, this approach is an improvement over the strict pass/fail method. **Table 12.2** illustrates an evaluation tool that uses a rating scale to evaluate student performance.

Assessment of Developmental Learning

Because the main focus of nursing education is developmental learning, as described in Chapter 3, "Developing Instructional Objectives," we are looking for student progress toward an ultimate goal when we develop a clinical evaluation tool. The ideal tool should be based on the course objectives, lend itself to daily use in a continuously changing clinical setting, and allow for leeway in the instructional and evaluation process to account for individual differences among students.

The purpose of evaluation of student progress in the clinical setting is both formative and summative, as reviewed in Chapter 2, "The Language of Assessment." Therefore, clinical evaluation should ascertain whether the student is meeting the course criteria during the clinical experience and should provide guidance for the student to be ultimately successful in meeting the course objectives in the performance of clinical work. At the same time, the course objectives need to be broad enough to incorporate clinical outcomes that address students' abilities to apply knowledge, problem-solve and evaluate, communicate, interact, and perform nursing actions.

One approach for assessing developmental learning is to use critical thinking as an evaluative focal point. This approach opens up a variety of avenues for evaluating student performance. Forneris (2004) identifies four core attributes of critical thinking:

1. Reflection
2. Context
3. Dialogue
4. Time

As an instructor interacts with a student in the clinical area, these attributes can be evaluated within the framework of course objectives. For example, reflection indicates

Table 12.2 Sample Rating Scale Skills Laboratory Evaluation Form

NU 101 Foundations of Nursing Practice
Objective I: Safely Performs Basic Nursing Procedures

Outcomes	Blood Pressure Score 1–5*	Oral Medications Score 1–5*	IM Injections Score 1–5*	Urinary Catheterization Score 1–5*
Discusses rationale				
Identifies impact on the client				
Explains procedure to the client				
Selects equipment				
Completes procedure (refer to specific checklist)				
Uses appropriate aseptic technique				
Interprets client response				
Reports and documents results				
Provides appropriate follow-up				
Total Score				

*Scores:

1 = Unable to accurately demonstrate outcome behavior

2 = Incomplete performance, with 1 or 2 safety errors

3 = Safe performance, with 1 or 2 nonsafety errors

4 = Accurate performance, with no errors

5 = Thorough, complete, and in-depth performance

how the student solves problems and evaluates outcomes. Context addresses the student's ability to discern and work within cultural and situational circumstances. Dialogue requires active student participation to answer the why questions in clinical setting. Time refers to both the student's application of past, present, and future when planning, implementing, and evaluating and the time frames within which nursing actions should be reasonably performed.

Focusing on the four core attributes of critical thinking encourages a variety of methods for student instruction and evaluation. Context can be addressed through the use of student narratives. One example would require students to identify and discuss a real situation that reflects the cultural impact on health care. Reflection can be addressed through student journals; writing in a journal is useful because it provides the opportunity to highlight critical incidents and allows students to express feelings about a care experience (Forneris, 2004). Dialogue can be accomplished either in a one-to-one interaction with the instructor or in conferences or seminars. Critical dialogue helps the students focus on the important aspects of a care situation to interpret actions and events (Forneris, 2004).

Temporal requirements must also be addressed in a clinical situation. Timeliness in giving care, medications, and treatments should be considered. In addition, educational strategies should be used to engage the learner in analyzing past and present actions when planning future actions. Helping students to analyze thinking over time leads to the ability to refine anticipatory planning (Forneris, 2004). The ability to set priorities and use short- and long-term goals help students to identify patterns related to time that can be transferred to other learning situations.

Portfolio Assessment

The developmental nature of learning in nursing practice requires faculty members to consider more nontraditional evaluative designs, such as use of a student portfolio, when facilitating and evaluating clinical performance. The portfolio process offers the opportunity to "more accurately assess a range of abilities, such as critical thinking, problem-solving, and clinical decision-making" (Forker & McDonald, 1996, p. 9). With less focus on textbook content and more on thought processes, including discrimination and creativity, use of the student portfolio can demonstrate a wide range of student abilities that can easily complement the student's actual, real-time clinical performance. Portfolio content can include a variety of requirements, such as concept maps, journals, narratives, and self-evaluation. Senior students can be required to design their own portfolio to demonstrate accomplishment of the course objectives. The portfolio can reflect progress over a semester and, if carried to the next semester, can reflect growth throughout a nursing program. This process helps both the student and the teacher assess learning issues and evaluate overall progress. Several authors offer specific suggestions to promote the use of portfolio development for clinical evaluation (Ramey & Hay, 2003; Robertson, Elster, & Kruse, 2004; Schaffer, Nelson, & Litt, 2005; Tracy, Marino, Richo, & Daly, 2000). The general consensus is that the portfolio acknowledges progress and helps students take ownership of their own learning.

Implementing a Clinical Evaluation Tool

The clinical setting offers the students a range of experiences that challenge all domains of learning and behavioral performance. The challenge for the clinical instructor is to evaluate student performance against objective standards. When we evaluate student performance using tried and true clinical evaluation tools, sacred cows that have evolved over time and are based on tradition, we may be judging students using instruments that may no longer reflect:

- What it is we want students to achieve in the clinical setting
- How we want students to think, prioritize, make decisions, and act in the clinical setting
- The changing nature, scope, and management of the healthcare structures within which the students perform

Organizing a clinical evaluation tool that is relevant to the course objectives, user friendly, and comprehensive is a challenging task. Three goals must be considered:

1. The clinical evaluation tool must reflect the essence of the course objectives so that the clinical experience and the theoretical classes are unified.
2. It must reflect the developmental progress of the student from the beginning to graduation.
3. It must reflect all domains of learning within the framework of the course objectives.

An important issue that often arises when constructing a clinical evaluation tool is the specificity of behaviors required to ensure that students are ready to progress in the course sequence. Global statements can be too vague to address behaviors, whereas very specific statements can be so exhaustive that the tool becomes unwieldy. If you design your objectives carefully, according to the framework suggested in Chapter 3, "Developing Instructional Objectives," you will solve this problem. While the same general objectives are used in each course, the learning outcomes increase in complexity as students progress through the course sequence. When students reach the final course, they are required to demonstrate behaviors that indicate successful attainment of the program outcomes. This framework offers evidence of logical student progression toward an ultimate goal and also offers the foundation for a meaningful clinical evaluation tool.

The evaluation tool must contain language that is clear, concise, and unambiguous. While the course objectives guide the outcomes and competencies that are required for the semester, the evaluation tool is the vehicle for documenting student progress toward meeting those outcomes and competencies. Therefore, the tool should provide for at least midterm and end-of-semester feedback. This is especially important for students who are having difficulty meeting clinical expectations. Specific comments regarding unmet expectations must be documented in the clinical evaluation tool.

The design of the rating portion of clinical evaluation tools varies widely from program to program. Some programs use a simple pass/fail or satisfactory/ unsatisfactory system, while others add a "needs improvement" advisory. A more informative approach is to base the clinical evaluation tool on a scoring rubric that differentiates between levels of performance. This approach provides a framework for the development of a logical clinical evaluation tool that relates directly to the course objectives, supplies a method of outcome measurement, and yields substantially more information than the pass/fail system. Moskal (2003) suggests that rubrics should reflect clear differences between achievement levels and offers six recommendations for developing scoring rubrics:

1. The criteria for the task should be clearly aligned with the stated goals and objectives.
2. The criteria should be stated in terms of observable behaviors.
3. The language of the rubric should be clear and easily understood by the students.
4. The number of points assigned to each level of the scoring rubric should make sense.
5. The separation between scoring levels should be clear.
6. The statement of the criteria should be bias free (pp. 4–5).

One method for evaluating a student's ability to meet course objectives is to use a rubric designed to differentiate the student who has a set of skills that is superior to those of the typical student and to differentiate the typical or average student from the student who consistently does not meet course expectations. Rubrics can be designed to differentiate several levels of performance, depending on the degree of distinction desired by the nursing program.

A scale of 1 to 4 is a manageable yet informative rubric scheme that can be designed to reflect several levels of performance. Refer to the objectives from Exhibit 3.10 The outcomes listed under the fourth-semester communication objective are used to develop the clinical evaluation tool in the rubric in **Table 12.3**. This rubric is based on the outcomes and demonstrates how course objectives can be

Table 12.3 Sample Clinical Evaluation Tool

NU 425 Advanced Nursing Practice
Objective I: Facilitates Effective Communication in HealthCare Settings

	Midterm Score	Midterm Comments and Suggestions	Final Score	Final Comments
Uses appropriate therapeutic communication skills				
Adapts communication approach				
Minimizes barriers to communication				
Interprets effectiveness of communication				
Reports significant information promptly				
Documents relevant information				
Maintains working relationships				
Maintains confidentiality				
Uses appropriate channels of communication				
Uses information technology to support patient care				
Total Score				

Rating scale:

4 = Demonstrates a thorough and in-depth understanding of concepts and applies them to patient care. Utilizes creative, confident, and proficient approaches to nursing practice. Shows insight when analyzing and evaluating patient care situations. Consistently excels in demonstrating outcome behavior.

3 = Demonstrates adequate understanding of concepts and applies them to patient care. Utilizes effective approaches to nursing practice. Analyzes and evaluates patient care situations accurately. Consistently demonstrates outcome behavior.

2 = Needs some assistance to apply concepts to nursing practice. Performs inconsistently but safely with guidance. Contributes to group discussion when analyzing and evaluating patient care situations. Demonstrates outcome behavior with assistance.

1 = Requires consistent guidance to apply concepts to patient care situations. Analysis and evaluation of patient care situations consistently requires verbal cues. Unable to demonstrate outcome behavior independently.

evaluated directly. The rubric uses a Likert scale to distinguish the superior student (4) from the average student (3). It also differentiates the student who may be able to succeed with intensive intervention (2) from the student who most likely will not meet the course objective (1). The faculty must designate what total score is required for passing the objective. This requirement must be clearly communicated to the students at the outset of the clinical experience.

Sander and Trible (2009) report success with implementing a virtual clinical evaluation tool, which is a rubric based on measurable outcomes and uses a Likert scale for grading. It was developed for online use with an Excel spreadsheet. Both students and faculty have secure online access to the spreadsheets; daily evaluation is optional, but both formative and summative evaluation is required. Both faculty and students report having positive experiences with the tool, and the online process has been especially well received by the computer-savvy generation of students.

Summary

The clinical experience in nursing education cannot be considered a separate entity when it is linked to a theory component. Therefore, the objectives of the overall course must guide the learning experiences and evaluative measures for both the theory and clinical components of a course. The clinical and theoretical experiences are both means for students to achieve the course objectives.

This chapter expands on the general premise of the text: that the course objectives provide the framework for instruction, learning, and evaluation in all aspects of a course, including clinical experiences. Sample evaluative tools, which are based on the course objectives and use scoring rubrics, are presented as examples that illustrate how to unify all the components of a nursing course. The chapter demonstrates that the clinical component of a course should provide students with individualized opportunities to meet the overall course objectives.

Learning Activities

1. Select an objective from a course you have taught or plan to teach. Develop four or five learning outcomes that define the behavior the students must demonstrate to show evidence of meeting the objective.

2. Identify two or three clinical experiences that will provide opportunities for students to develop proficiency in the learning outcomes.

3. Use the learning outcomes to develop a clinical assessment tool for the course objective you identified in Learning Activity 1. Include opportunities for both formative and summative evaluation.

Web Links

American Nurses Association—Professional Nursing Standards
http://www.nursingworld.org/nursingstandards
International Nursing Association for Clinical Simulation and Learning
http://www.inacsl.org/INACSL_2010/
Internet Resources for Assessment in Higher Education
http://www2.acs.ncsu.edu/upa/assmt/resource.htm

National Center for Research on Evaluation Standards and Student Testing (CRESST)

http://www.crest.org

National Council of State Boards of Nursing (NCSBN)—Position Paper on Clinical Instruction in Prelicensure Nursing Programs

http://www.ncsbn.org/Final_Clinical_Instr_Pre_Nsg_programs.pdf

National Council on Measurement in Education (NCME)

http://www.ncme.org

References

Bloom, B. S. (Ed.), Englehart, M. D., Furst, E. J., Hill, W. H., & Krathwohl, D. R. (1956). *Taxonomy of educational objectives: The classification of educational goals.* New York, NY: Longmans, Green and Co.

Cronbach, L. J. (1963). *Educational psychology* (2nd ed.). New York, NY: Harcourt, Brace, & World.

Dewey, J. (1938/1997). *Experience and education.* New York, NY: Touchstone.

Forker, J. E., & McDonald, M. E. (1996). Methodologic trends in the healthcare professions: Portfolio assessment. *Nurse Educator, 21,* 9–10.

Forneris, S. G. (2004). Exploring the attributes of critical thinking: A conceptual basis. *International Journal of Nursing Education Scholarship, 1*(1). Retrieved from http://www.bepress.com/ijnes/vol1/iss1/art9

Gaberson, K. B., & Oermann, M. H. (1999). *Clinical teaching strategies in nursing.* New York, NY: Springer.

Ironside, P. M., & Valiga, T. M. (2006). Creating a vision for the future of nursing education. *Nursing Education Perspectives, 27,* 120–121.

Moskal, B. M. (2003). Recommendations for developing classroom assessments and scoring rubrics. *Practical Assessment, Research & Evaluation, 8*(14). Retrieved from http://PAREonline.net/getvn.asp?v=8&n=14

O'Connor, A. B. (2001). *Clinical instruction and evaluation: A teaching resource.* Sudbury, MA: Jones and Bartlett and National League for Nursing.

Ramey, S. L., & Hay, M. L. (2003). Using electronic portfolios to measure student achievement and assess curricular integrity. *Nurse Educator, 28,* 31–36.

Reilly, D. E., & Oermann, M. H. (1992). *Clinical teaching in nursing education* (2nd ed.). New York, NY: National League for Nursing.

Robertson, J. F., Elster, S., & Kruse, G. (2004). Portfolio outcome assessment: Lessons learned. *Nurse Educator, 29,* 52–53.

Sander, R., & Trible, K. A. (2009). The virtual clinical evaluation tool. *Journal of Nursing Education, 47*(1), 33–36.

Schaffer, M. A., Nelson, P., & Litt, E. (2005). Using portfolios to evaluate achievement of population-based public health nursing competencies in baccalaureate nursing students. *Nursing Education Perspectives, 26,* 104–112.

Tanner, C. A. (2006). The next transformation: Clinical education. *Journal of Nursing Education, 45,* 99–100.

Tracy, S. M., Marino, G. J., Richo, K. M., & Daly, E. M. (2000). The clinical achievement portfolio: An outcomes-based assessment project in nursing education. *Nurse Educator, 25,* 241.

Assigning Grades

CHAPTER 13

© Anteromite/Shutterstock

"What a mark means is determined not only by how it was defined when the marking system was adopted, but also, and perhaps more importantly, by the way it is actually used."

—ROBERT EBEL

Grades matter. Classroom grades represent a high-stakes situation for many reasons. They are the basis for decisions about progression in a program. They determine who graduates. They send an authoritative message about the quality of a student's work to employers and graduate schools. Because of the powerful influence that classroom grades have on the lives of students, it is imperative that the assignment of grades is based on high-quality information (Brookhart & Nitko, 2014).

A grade is a label that represents a summary of a student's achievement of the course content and instructional objectives. There is no simple grading system. Grading is a complex process that is subject to error because course grades are derived from a combination of scores from instruments that are all subject to measurement error. Because grades have such serious implications, every assignment that has a direct impact on a student's course grade must have evidence of validity and reliability and must be interpreted with extreme objectivity. Only with a clear understanding of the factors that influence grading you can reduce error and develop a fair and objective system for assigning grades.

Grading Principles

Grades represent the culmination of the assessment process. They symbolize the quality of a student's performance. The principles of grading incorporate the elements of the assessment process presented in this book. These elements are links

307

in the processes; they contribute individually and as a whole to quality assessment practices. The process of grading is only as strong as the weakest link in the process.

No grading system is perfect. It is important to acknowledge that grades are influenced by subjectivity and measurement error. Only by following a systematic assessment plan you can have confidence that your instructional process is valid and that the grades you assign represent a fair evaluation of student performance.

Experts agree that a grading plan must be based on the principles of grading (Brookhart & Nitko, 2014; Miller, Linn, & Gronlund, 2009; Russell & Airasian, 2011). These principles include the following:

- Grades are important. Grades send powerful messages that have significant impact on the lives of students.

- Grades should be based only on the course objectives and content that guides instruction. It is unfair to assign grades based on comparing a student's performance with others in the class. If you follow the assessment guidelines presented in this book, your classroom tests will be based on the content and instructional objectives of your course.

- Grades should be assigned fairly. While subjective grading depends on a teacher's judgment, objective grading leads to the same result no matter who assigns the grade. Every measurement instrument that contributes to a grade must meet this standard for fairness. To meet the fairness criterion, teachers have to be willing to admit when they have made a mistake. They must recognize, for example, when an item on a test might have misled students or might have had two feasible answers.

- Grades should be based on credible assessment. Validity and reliability provide the foundation for trustworthy assessment and fair grading. The more confidence you have in the results of the measurements you use, the more confidence you have in the grades you assign. At the same time, objective grades require adequate evidence—you cannot make valid decisions based on insufficient evidence.

- Grades must be confidential. Teachers are prevented by law from discussing or divulging the grades of students who are 18 years old or older without the written permission of the student. Care must be taken to protect student privacy during all phases of the grading process. Even the posting of grades can pose a threat to confidentiality if a system is used that enables students to decode each other's grades.

- Grading policies should be clearly written in the course syllabus and discussed on the first day of class. You should review the policy with the students and clarify any misconceptions. These practices are essential to enable students to plan strategies for success.

- Grades influence students' incentive to learn, and grades are intended to reflect what a student has learned. Haladyna (1997) asserts that, although grades are extrinsic motivators, a well-defined grading method increases student motivation and propels the student toward more learning, eventually leading to intrinsic motivation.

While high grades motivate students, lower-than-expected grades or grades that are perceived as unfair can diminish student motivation. Instead of prompting greater effort, low grades, especially those perceived as unfair, might cause students to withdraw from learning. Most importantly, teachers have a responsibility to be objective with grading. Grades should never be used as a form of punishment for student behavior that is not related to the course objectives.

Although you want to provide incentives for students, fairness does not require that you assign high grades to all students. In fact, lowering standards to ensure high grades decreases student motivation and effort and reduces the validity of your grade assignments. Fairness in grading requires that you set standards that can be realistically achieved by students if they work hard (Russell & Airasian, 2011).

Philosophy of Grading

The process of grading requires teachers to develop a plan that is in harmony with their personal grading philosophy. Grading decisions are based not only on established principles but also on a teacher's beliefs about the teaching–learning process (Frisbe & Waltman, 1992). These principles and beliefs are incorporated into a grading philosophy, which guides a teacher's grading plan.

Before you can develop a plan, you need to identify your grading philosophy. Frisbe and Waltman (1992, p. 36) present a series of nine "should" questions for teachers to answer when examining their beliefs about grading. These questions have no right or wrong answers; reasonable people disagree. However, these questions must be answered to help you to articulate your grading philosophy. Your answers must be consistent with one another if you are to form a solid basis for your grading plan.

1. What Meaning Should Each Grade Symbol Carry?

The meaning of each grade must be clearly understood by both students and the teacher. This question has two components: "What areas of student achievement are included in the grade?" and "How do the symbols reflect the degree of student achievement?"

Although some institutions use numerical grades, letters are used most frequently to represent the degree of student performance on a scale that ranges from excellent to failing. Pluses and/or minuses are often used with the letters to further delineate the level of student performance. The parent institution usually determines the letters that can be used for grade assignment and the definition of each letter assignment. **Table 13.1** presents a sample of an institution's grading scale.

The parent institution usually mandates how these letter grades are translated into numerical values so that a grade point average (GPA) can be calculated for each student. The numerical values associated with each letter are frequently referred to as quality points, as **Table 13.2** illustrates. It is important that the grading symbols and quality point equivalents are consistent across departments in a college or university so that students' GPAs are consistent.

The GPA is computed by multiplying the credit value for each course by the number of points associated with the grade earned to obtain the total quality points for each course. The total quality points for each course are then added together,

Table 13.1 Sample Grading Scale	
A	Outstanding
A−	Superior
B+	Very good
B	Good
B−	Above average
C+	Upper level of average
C	Average
C−	Poor
D	Minimal pass
F	Fail
P	Pass
W	Withdraw

Table 13.2 Sample Quality Point Index	
Grade	Quality Points
A	4.0
A−	3.7
B+	3.5
B	3.0
B−	2.7
C+	2.5
C	2.0
C−	1.7
D	1.0
F	0

and this sum is divided by the total number of credit hours to obtain the scholastic average, or GPA, for each student. **Table 13.3** provides an example of how grades are translated into quality points to calculate a student's GPA. The GPA is used to set a standard for retention and graduation. It is also used to rank students and is an important factor for employment and graduate school admission.

Every college or university publishes a course catalog in which the description of the letter grades and their associated quality points are clearly described, along with the school's academic policies. The school's catalog constitutes a contract with the students: It spells out the academic requirements for receiving a degree from the institution. While your parent institution might determine what grading symbol to use, individual departments or faculty members are usually responsible for determining

Table 13.3   Sample GPA Calculation

Course	Grade	Points	Total Credit Hours	Total Quality Points
Hist 101	A	4.0	3	12.0
Soc 101	C+	2.5	3	7.5
Eng 101	B	3.0	3	9.0
Art 101	B+	3.5	3	10.5
Total			12	39
GPA				**= 3.25**

The GPA is determined by dividing the total quality points by the total credit hours (39 ÷ 12 = 3.25).

the achievement components to be considered and the level of performance that is required for translation of student achievement into a specific grade symbol.

Will your grade assignment include only achievement of the defined content and instructional objectives, or will you consider class participation and effort as part of the grade? What level of understanding does a grade of B represent? What does "good" mean? Before you can assign a grade, you must determine what the grading symbols mean. Your grading plan should incorporate your answers to these nine questions.

2. What Should Failure Mean?

It is a difficult task to assign a failing grade to a student. The negative consequences of the F grade create an emotional atmosphere that most teachers would prefer to avoid (Frisbe & Waltman, 1992). Other grades can also have negative significance. For example, a grade of D might be unsatisfactory for progression in a program or might not count toward graduation. Brookhart and Nitko (2014) point out that your answer to this question should be consistent with your perception of the meaning of all grades. They suggest establishing minimum standards of performance on the curriculum and learning outcomes and assigning a failing grade to those students who consistently perform below those minimum standards.

3. What Elements of Performance Should Be Incorporated in a Grade?

Grades should be assigned objectively. Once you decide what a grade symbolizes, all extraneous information should be kept out of the grading decision. In other words, if grades are designed to reflect achievement levels of the course content and objectives, only achievement activities should be included in the grade decision.

Components such as effort and class participation should thus be excluded from grading criteria. These factors are far too arbitrary and subjective to be included in an objective grade. It is unfair to grade a student on what could very well be a personality issue. Also, how can you objectively assign a grade to effort? Is an unassertive student necessarily uninvolved in the class presentation? Unless constructs such as effort and assertiveness are operationally defined and included in your course objectives, it is unfair to include these factors in your grade assignments. It is particularly unfair to use a subjective evaluation of a student's class participation to decrease a student's overall grade.

If you want students to participate in class, an assignment such as an oral presentation that is graded with objective criteria and that are shared with the students is one fair way to assign a grade. An objective grade is one that a student can figure out based on the course syllabus, without additional subjective input from the teacher (Haladyna, 1997).

4. How Should the Grades in a Class Be Distributed?

Is there a limit to the number of A grades you will assign? Will C be the average grade? What percentage of failing grades is acceptable? Although it is unusual, some institutions do have policies about grade distribution that influences the grades you assign. Even when there is no written policy, professors who assign a large number of high or low grades might be questioned by school administrators about their grading policy. If your grade distribution is consistent with your answers to the first three questions, you can justify your grade assignments.

The final grade for a course should represent a comparison of the students' performance to the course objectives. A discussion on norm- versus criterion-related grading methods is included in this chapter.

5. What Components Should Go Into a Final Grade?

Your grading plan specifies the components that determine the final grade for a course. Frisbe and Waltman (1992) explain that the separate scores that are combined to determine the final course grade must reflect the meaning that you have assigned for the grade symbols. Each assessment task that contributes to a grade must reflect the elements of performance you designated in question three. If your definition of the grade components includes only achievement in the areas of course content and instructional objectives, then components such as class participation and effort should be excluded from the final grade.

6. How Should the Components of the Grade Be Combined?

Once the components of a grade are determined, you must decide how to weight the scores derived from each of these measurements to determine a composite grade. Will each component be worth an equal percentage of the grade, or should some be counted more heavily? The answer to this question determines how you calculate the composite grade.

7. What Method Should Be Used to Assign Grades?

After you combine the measurement scores, you must assign final grades to the students. Frisbe and Waltman (1992) remind us that your method of grade assignment must reflect your definition of the meaning of the grade symbols. If your answer to question one indicates that grades reflect degrees of student achievement of the content and instructional objectives of the course, it would be illogical to assign grades based on a curve. Methods for assigning grades are discussed later in this chapter.

8. Should Borderline Cases Be Reviewed?

How will you handle the situation where a composite grade puts a student right on the borderline between passing and failing? How close to passing must a student's composite score be before it is rounded up? Will you allow students to submit work for extra credit to raise a borderline grade? If all grades are particularly low, will you add points or scale the scores?

Previous discussion has established that all measurements contain error. Therefore, will you look only at a student's observed score, or will you take the standard error of measurement (SEM) into account when considering what the student's true score might be? Many experts, including Brookhart and Nitko (2014), recommend giving the student the benefit of the doubt by collecting additional information to help you decide whether the student's true score is greater than the observed score. In fact, Brookhart and Nitko recommend that educators give the higher grade when there is serious doubt about whether a student is above or below the boundary for passing.

9. What Other Factors Should Influence the Grading Policy?

The parent institution for your nursing program has considerable authority in determining the academic policies that you must follow when assigning grades. Issues such as grade distribution, course credit, and degree requirements have an impact on your grading philosophy. You have to be cognizant of these issues when you develop your plan.

Some nursing programs use a uniform system of grading. This approach makes sense as long as it allows for differences in instructional approaches. Teachers should always have flexibility when deciding on the components of a grade. When a uniform system is devised, faculty members must come to a consensus on all the issues surrounding the development of a grading philosophy. Each of these nine questions must be addressed as a group. Agreeing on a grading policy is not an easy task for a faculty group, but it is essential for ensuring fairness—particularly for courses that consist of several sections.

Another issue that faculty must face when assigning grades is to consider the criteria applied in other departments. It is unfair to punish nursing students with a stringent grading policy or reward them with a very lenient grading policy that diminishes their standing in the greater college community. While it is very important to maintain your academic standards, you should consider the implications of your grade assignments on the GPAs of nursing students compared with other students in your college or university.

Developing a Grading Plan

Calculating course grades is not just a mathematical exercise; it is an expression of your philosophy. A sound grading plan incorporates your philosophy with the principles of grading to assign grades. The model you use for weighting the components of the final grade communicates to your students what you believe is important; it tells them where they should put their efforts (Walvoord & Anderson, 1998). Regardless of which model you use to establish your grading system, the standard should be established before the plan is initiated. In fact, the plan should be communicated to the students at the outset of the course so they know how to focus their efforts.

Weighting Components of a Grade

The first step in the grading process is to determine what components will be included in the grade and how the components will be combined to produce a composite grade. Every assessment of achievement is not necessarily of equal importance in the determination of a grade; you need to develop a system to assign weights to the various components. The amount of weight you allot for each component will be based on your judgment of the significance of the component in the grading scheme. Brookhart and Nitko (2014) suggest that you make a list of all the assessment tasks for the semester, decide how each task relates to the course content and objectives, and then assign a weight based on how important each task is in relation to the composite grade.

A grade represents a judgment about a student's achievement. To judge that achievement, a standard must be identified against which to compare student performance. Once you have decided how your grading components will be weighted, you must determine which framework to use to serve as the basis for assigning student grades. The two most commonly used are the absolute standard, or criterion-referenced grading, and the relative standard, or norm-referenced grading.

Criterion-Referenced Grading   An absolute standard, or criterion-referenced grading, compares a student's performance to a predetermined standard of performance and assigns grades based on the student's attainment of the objectives and mastery of the content (Russell & Airasian, 2011). With this model, grades are based solely on the standards. Students who demonstrate a high level of achievement receive high grades without regard to how well other students perform (Brookhart & Nitko, 2014). When this standard is applied, all students could theoretically receive a grade of A. Of course, it is also theoretically possible that every student could receive a grade of F. Remember, however, that all aspects of the assessment process work in concert. Careful design of your measurement instruments ensures that the items discriminate and that you have a range of scores that reflect levels of student achievement. It also ensures that you have a valid and reliable basis for determining grade assignments based on your predetermined set of criteria.

Criterion-referenced grading methods require that the performance standards be clearly described and that the measurement instruments that comprise the composite score yield valid and reliable information about student achievement in relation to the standards. The content and instructional objectives that are established at the outset of the course include the standards that are used to determine student grades. If you follow the guidelines described in this book to establish a systematic assessment plan, your classroom exams will provide trustworthy information about student performance related to those standards.

The model you use to translate the scores into a letter grade is a matter of personal choice, although the choice should be consistent for all sections of the same course. Whichever model you choose, the criteria must be explained to students and should be included in the course syllabus.

FIXED PERCENTAGE SCALE   The formula for the fixed percentage method includes the weighting you have assigned to each assessment task. An explanation of how you weight the grades, such as that in **Table 13.4**, should be included in the course syllabus.

Table 13.4   Sample Grade Weighting

Item	Percent
Pharmacology quiz	10
Unit I exam	20
Unit II exam	20
Nursing process paper	0
Final exam	30

Table 13.5   Calculation of Grades Using the Fixed Percentage Method

SCORES	Pharmacology Quiz		Unit I Exam		Unit II Exam		Nursing Process Paper		Final Exam		Grade
Weights	10% (.1)		20% (.2)		20% (.2)		20% (.2)		30% (.3)		
	CS	WS	CS	WS	CS	WS	CS	WS	CS	WS	
T. Bass	85	**8.5**	80	**16**	90	**18**	75	**15**	85	**25.5**	83%
A. Crew	90	**9.0**	88	**17.6**	84	**16.8**	90	**18**	86	**25.8**	87.2%
G. Lamb	95	**9.5**	90	**18**	82	**16.4**	80	**16**	90	**27**	86.9%

Multiply each component percent score (CS) by its percentage weighting to obtain the weighted score (WS) for each component. Add the WS for each component to obtain the composite grade.

With this method, a percent correct score is determined for every component of the assessment composite, including exams, term papers, and presentations. Each component is given a percent correct, which represents the percentage of the maximum score that the student received on the component (Brookhart & Nitko, 2014). For example, a student who earns a score of 46 of 50 possible points on an exam would receive a score of 92%. **Table 13.5** illustrates how the percent score for each component is multiplied by the weight assigned to it and how the products for all components are summed to determine the final score.

Note that in Table 13.5 a letter grade is not assigned until the final grade is calculated. It is important not to assign letter grades to each component of the final grade; rather, enter those grades as percent scores and translate the average of the percent scores for all the components into the final letter grade for the course.

By using a gradebook that has a column for calculating the weight of each grade as the semester progresses, the calculation of the composite grade will be less tedious at the end of the course. If you keep your grades by hand, it is a good idea to keep the weighted grade figure in red or in some color that contrasts with the percent score. Table 13.5 indicates the weighted grade in a bold font.

You can also enter your grades into an electronic spreadsheet and have the program do the calculations for you. A simple spreadsheet is easy to develop, and most schools have resources to help you gain expertise in using the computer software programs that produce spreadsheets. Several electronic gradebook programs are also available that facilitate the process of calculating grades. The better ones offer several options for specifying rules for assigning grades and also provide the ability to maintain class rosters, keep track of attendance, and prepare summary grade reports for groups and individual students. Several of the test development software programs discussed in Chapter 14, "Instituting Item Banking and Test Development Software," link to gradebooks that interface with the testing program to import scores automatically and calculate grades based on your grading plan.

It is important to recognize that the relationship between the percent composite score and the scale for determining a grade is a subjective process. Assigning grades requires synthesizing a great deal of information into a single symbol, and the cutoff between grade categories is always arbitrary (Brookhart & Nitko, 2014). The more systematic your grading plan is, the more objective your grade assignments will be.

Although the parent institution defines the symbols—usually a letter—to be used for grading and the quality points assigned to each letter, the translation of the percent composite score to a letter is usually left to the individual department or faculty members. In these situations, faculty determines the achievement levels that correspond to the letters identified by the parent institution. While faculty should always have the authority to determine the components of a composite score, they must sometimes follow the guidelines of the college or university for translating a composite percent correct score to a letter grade, as is shown in **Table 13.6**. Whatever the case, it is important that students are fully aware of how to interpret the grading scale.

Total Points Scale   With the total points scale, the composite grade for the student is the total of the points that the student receives. Each assessment task is assigned a number of points based on the weight assigned to it, and the point total at the end of the course is translated into a composite grade based on the number of points required for the grade.

A maximum number of points of 100 or 1,000 make this system easier for the student to understand. **Table 13.7** illustrates how the sample grade weighting from Table 13.4 would translate to a total points scale.

Table 13.6 Sample Translation of a Composite Percent Correct Score to a Letter Grade	
Grade Assignment	
Composite Percent Score	**Grade**
90–100	A
80–89	B
70–79	C
60–69	D
<60	F

Table 13.7   Sample Total Points Scale

Pharmacology quiz	100
Unit I exam	200
Unit II exam	200
Nursing process paper	200
Final exam	300
Maximum points	1,000

Table 13.8   Sample Calculation of Grades Using the Total Points Method

SCORES	Pharmacology Quiz		Unit I Exam		Unit II Exam		Nursing Process Paper		Final Exam		Total Points
Points	100		200		200		200		300		
	CS	WS	CS	WS	CS	WS	CS	WS	CS	WS	
T. Bass	85	85	80	160	90	180	75	150	85	255	830
A. Crew	90	90	88	176	84	168	90	180	86	258	872
G. Lamb	95	95	90	180	82	164	80	160	90	270	869

Multiply each component percent score (CS) by its number of points to obtain the weighted score (WS) for each component. Add the WS for each component to obtain the total number of points.

Table 13.9   Sample Translation of Total Points Composite to a Letter Grade

Grade Assignment

Total Points Composite Score	Grade
900–1,000	A
800–899	B
700–799	C
600–699	D
<600	F

Table 13.8 illustrates how grades can be calculated by using a total points scale. The relationship between the composite score derived from a total points scale score and the scale for determining a letter grade is just as arbitrary as the fixed percent scale, as shown in **Table 13.9**.

The grade symbols determined by the parent institution define the grade range and the quality points assigned to each grade. The question you must answer is, "How many total points correspond to each letter grade?"

Norm-Referenced Grading   A relative standard, or norm-referenced grading, assigns student grades based on their ranking compared with other students in the class regarding a combination of assessment results. With this approach to grading, students are ranked in order of performance or are graded on a curve whereby the teacher predetermines the percentage of students who will receive each grade. The curve is meant to represent a normal distribution.

Grading on the normal curve yields a percentage of As and Fs and Bs and Ds, so the number of high grades is balanced by an equal number of low grades. Worthen, Borg, and White (1993) say that the most common method used to determine letter grades based on the normal curve is based on the mean and standard deviation of the test. They explain that if the test results yield a normal curve, then grades would be distributed as follows:

> A = approximately 7% (1.5 standard deviations above the mean)
> B = approximately 24% (0.5 to 1.5 standard deviations above the mean)
> C = approximately 38% (0.5 standard deviations above the mean to 0.5 standard deviations below the mean)
> D = approximately 24% (0.5 to 1.5 standard deviations below the mean)
> F = approximately 7% (1.5 standard deviations below the mean) (p. 385)

This method presents several problems for assigning classroom grades. First, classroom measurements are unlikely to yield a normal distribution of scores. When teachers who want to use a relative standard for grading recognize that classroom groups are too small for assessment results to resemble a normal curve, they sometimes use their judgment to establish a grading curve that ensures a distribution of grades. These judgments arbitrarily establish quotas for each grade to be given, as shown in **Table 13.10**.

Second, the normative group is the students in a given class; in other words, the standard is totally dependent on the composition of the class with no indication of actual student achievement. Therefore, a student's grade depends more on the other students in the class than on how well the student has mastered the material (Worthen et al., 1993).

In the example illustrated in Table 13.10, the teacher predetermined that only 10% of the class will receive a grade of A, while 5% will be destined for failure. With this plan, in a class of 30 students, only three would receive an A regardless of the

Table 13.10   Example of Arbitrary Assignment of Grade Quotas

Grade	Percent of Students
A	10
B	25
C	50
D	10
F	5

Table 13.11 Comparison of Absolute and Referenced Grading

Absolute Standard	Reference Standard
Predetermines criteria for grade assignment	Predetermines quotas for each grade assignment
Bases grade on student achievement	Bases grade on comparison of students
Depends on achievement of standard	Depends on composition of class
Can be designed to foster student cooperation	Establishes unhealthy student competition
Enables all students to pass	Ensures that some students fail

mastery level of the individual students. If the best student in this group had a composite score of only 40 of a possible 100 points, the student would receive a grade of A. On the other hand, if the lowest achieving student in a group of high-achieving students received 85 of a possible 100 points, that student would necessarily receive a grade of F. Walvoord and Anderson (1998) associate grading on the curve with focusing the teacher's role on awarding grades by formula rather than on rewarding student learning with earned and deserved grades. When setting a distribution of scores, the teacher should allow for the possibility that no one will fail the course. If students have mastered the objectives and content of the course, they should pass despite their ranking in the class. As Miller and colleagues (2009) state, "Thus, even when grading is done on a relative basis, the pass–fail decision must be based on an absolute standard of achievement if it is to be educationally sound" (p. 382).

Most experts agree that educationally sound grading should be based on a student's level of achievement, not on some relative ranking in a group. Haladyna (1997) maintains that the relative standard should never be used for classroom grading because it is associated with so many negative consequences, such as:

- Establishing unhealthy competition among the top students for the limited number of A grades
- Reducing cooperation among students at all levels who recognize that their success depends on the performance of their classmates
- Ensuring that some students will fail no matter what their level of mastery
- Demoralizing those students who are ranked at the bottom of the group and undermining their learning efforts

Refer to **Table 13.11** for a comparison of absolute and reference standard grading.

Pass/Fail Grading

Most colleges and universities enable students to take courses on a pass/fail basis. Usually, the number of times a student can opt for the pass/fail grade is limited, and the pass/fail grade is not included in the calculation of the student's GPA. Some experts maintain that pass/fail grading encourages students to experiment, to take courses that they otherwise would avoid for fear of decreasing their GPA. Others argue that the pass/fail option discourages high achievement and encourages students to direct their study efforts at merely passing. Usually, this option is not offered for courses in the student's major. The policy for pass/fail grading, which varies widely among schools, is always stated in the official course catalog.

Many nursing programs use the pass/fail option for grading clinical practice. When nursing students are expected to demonstrate achievement of all objectives measured in a practice setting, pass/fail is an appropriate grade assignment. In addition, clinical evaluation is prone to subjectivity. Even with the most objective assessment instrument, it can be very difficult to distinguish between different levels of proficiency among students in the clinical practice setting. It is essential that the clinical evaluation instrument be congruent with the objectives and content of the overall course. In fact, assessment of several of your learning outcomes might be conducive only to clinical evaluation (as Tables 3.4 and 3.5 illustrate). Refer to Chapter 12, "Laboratory and Clinical Evaluation," for further discussion and examples of evaluation tools for assessment in the clinical setting.

The critical concern with the pass/fail grading option is that the course follows all the assessment guidelines. When a student elects the pass/fail option, the professor does not necessarily know of this selection, so the student is graded on the same basis as other students in the class who elect to receive a grade; it is the registrar who converts the grade to pass/fail. When a course is given on a pass/fail basis to an entire class, the instructor must be careful to ensure that the grading criteria are as precise as the criteria for a graded course. A grade plan should be developed, and the student's composite grade should reflect a score above the passing level based on the standard in order to receive a passing score.

Adjusting Grades

In an attempt to increase the fairness of classroom grade assignments and to give students the maximum opportunity to demonstrate achievement, teachers have devised a variety of methods to enhance classroom grades. You might want to increase the grade assignments if, for example, the semester exams were more difficult than you intended. Although you do not want to make grade changes frivolously, it is better to make changes than to assign grades that are unfair (Russell & Airasian, 2011).

Scaling Grades

When grades are scaled, a certain number of set points are added to each student's score. Although the number of failures might be a reasonable impetus for increasing grades, the shape of the grade curve is not. Reviewing test and item analysis and examining the appropriateness of the expected performance standard determine whether—and how many—points should be added to the scores.

Most teachers are very concerned with grade inflation. Assigning grades requires a balancing act. A careful analysis of each assessment component of your grades will help you determine whether the final grades need to be adjusted. The best approach is to wait until the end of the course to make grade changes (see Chapter 11, "Interpreting Test Results"). If, for example, you added points to the first exam, that exam would have a greater weight in the final course grade. To maintain the designated weighting of the components, determine the grades based on the predetermined weighting and adjust the final composite grade.

The SEM should be considered when assigning a grade, as Chapter 11 also suggests. Remember, students' obtained scores are not necessarily their true scores. The SEM requires that you be flexible when translating raw scores into grades. The best practice is not to add points for the SEM on individual exams but to wait until the end of the course and consider the average of the SEMs for the semester when deciding whether to add points to all of the students' final grades.

Keep in mind that adjusting grades is a subjective process and that fairness does not mean that everyone gets a high grade. Remember, lowering standards to assign higher grades discourages student effort and decreases the validity of the grades. Your discretion is essential. Before you alter the grades, carefully examine the qualitative and quantitative analyses of all exams to determine how well they measure the course objectives and learning outcomes and then apply the adjustment equally for all students (Russell & Airasian, 2011).

Giving Extra Credit

Extra-credit assignments can motivate students to pursue an area of particular interest to them. They also provide an opportunity to delve into a topic in depth and to experience the satisfaction that accompanies an accomplishment.

The practice of giving extra credit is widespread at all levels of education. Extra credit can assume forms such as allowing students to redo a paper or write a report for a unit on which they performed poorly. Extra-credit items can also be included on an exam as either constructed- or selected-response items to allow all students the opportunity to increase their grades. As long as the extra-credit assignment addresses the content and objectives of the course, it is an acceptable method for assessing student achievement.

Remember, assessment procedures should be designed to give students every opportunity to demonstrate attainment of the course objectives. Just be certain that extra-credit activities do not unfairly alter the weighting of the course components and that they are equally available to all students. Some programs allow students to complete a project for extra credit that is only included in the final grade for students who pass the major components of the course—for example, students must have a passing average on the multiple-choice exams before extra credit is added to the final grade.

Dropping the Lowest Grade

Discounting the students' lowest test grade when determining the final composite score has advantages and disadvantages. Although the practice enables students to have a bad day, Trice (2000) points out that it disconnects assessment from the course objectives because, when teachers drop a grade, they are saying that the students do not need to meet some of the course objectives. It also alters the weighting of the course content and objectives. Trice proposes that a better practice is to allow students to take a makeup exam on the content on which they performed poorly. A good application for extra credit is to allow students to complete one extra-credit assignment in the area of their weakest test score.

Usually, extra-credit opportunities and the option for dropping the lowest grade are clearly spelled out in the course syllabus. The instructional process is not one that you should set in stone, however. If a grading standard or criterion turns out to be inappropriate or unfair, it should be changed (Russell & Airasian, 2011). While you cannot make your grading criteria more stringent at the end of a course than what you have designated in the syllabus, students will never object to having an added opportunity to demonstrate their attainment of objectives. Grades are important to students. Failing students are not the only ones who are concerned with extra-credit assignments; high-achieving students have bad days too. The key concern is to apply all criteria fairly and equally to all students.

Summary

An equitable grading plan is based on grading principles and the teacher's philosophy of grading. Classroom grades have serious implications for students; teachers must be aware of these implications and the variables that affect grading to determine what grading system best suits the needs of their students. Although the selection of a grading framework is up to the teacher, experts generally agree that a norm-referenced system is inappropriate for classroom grading. It is important that teachers maintain flexibility, give thoughtful consideration to each of the decisions that must be made when developing a scheme for classroom grading, and share the final plan with the students at the outset of the course.

A grade is only as fair as the instructional process on which it is based. The ultimate goal of a systematic assessment plan is the assignment of grades that fairly reflect student mastery of the content and objectives of a course. Each component of the assessment plan plays an important role in achieving this outcome. The guidelines presented in this text build on each other and work together in the assessment process to create an overall plan that ultimately results in fair grade assignment. Appendix A, "Steps for Implementing a Systematic Assessment Plan," delineates the steps for implementing a systematic assessment plan.

Learning Activities

1. Answer the nine questions proposed by Frisbe and Waltman (1992).
2. Describe your personal grading philosophy.
3. Calculate grades for a hypothetical or actual course you are teaching using both the fixed percent method and the total points method. Which method do you prefer? Explain your selection.
4. Describe two different approaches for adjusting grades. Which one do you prefer? Explain your selection.
5. What is your opinion on considering SEM when assigning grades? How would you incorporate SEM into your grade assignments?

Web Links

American Educational Research Association
http://www.aera.net
American Federation of Teachers
http://www.aft.org
Educational Resources Information Canter
http://www.eric.ed.gov
Internet Resources for Assessment in Higher Education
http://www2.acs.ncsu.edu/upa/assmt/resource.htm
National Council on Measurement in Education
http://www.ncme.org
Nurse Educator Assessment Continuing Education
http://www.nurseeducatorace.com
Park University: Effective Grading Strategies
http://www.park.edu/cetl/quicktips/grading.html

References

Brookhart, S. M., & Nitko, A. J. (2014). *Educational assessment of students* (7th ed.). Upper Saddle River, NJ: Pearson Education.

Frisbe, D. A., & Waltman, K. K. (1992). Developing a personal grading plan. *Educational Measurement: Issues and Practice, 11,* 35–42.

Haladyna, T. M. (1997). *Writing test items to evaluate higher-order thinking.* Needham Heights, MA: Allyn and Bacon.

Miller, M. D., Linn, R. L., & Gronlund, N. E. (2009). *Measurement and assessment in teaching* (10th ed.). Upper Saddle River, NJ: Pearson Education.

Russell, M. K., & Airasian, P. W. (2011). *Classroom assessment* (7th ed.). New York, NY: McGraw Hill.

Trice, A. D. (2000). *A handbook of classroom assessment.* New York, NY: Longman.

Walvoord, B. E., & Anderson, V. J. (1998). *Effective grading.* San Francisco, CA: Jossey-Bass.

Worthen, B. R., Borg, W. R., & White, K. (1993). *Measurement and evaluation in the schools.* White Plains, NY: Longman.

© Anteromite/Shutterstock

Instituting Item Banking and Test Development Software

14

"Change is not made without inconvenience, even from worse to better."

—RICHARD HOOKER

Computer technology is rapidly changing the face of educational assessment at every level. Several years ago, very few educators could afford to take advantage of computerized testing. Fortunately, the current widespread availability of personal computers, coupled with the proliferation of sophisticated test development software that is designed to be user friendly, has made electronic item banking a workable reality. The potential for streamlining the process of preparing trustworthy selected-response classroom exams is now readily available to classroom teachers (McDonald, 2008). The software, which is reasonably priced, offers educators the best possible approach for ensuring the quality and objective fairness of their classroom assessments.

The time has arrived for every educator who uses selected-response classroom exams to institute item banking and test development software. If you are having difficulty convincing your administration to fund the purchase of the hardware and software required to initiate computer-assisted test development, this chapter should help you to argue the case.

Even if you are fully funded and have administration's support, you may meet with some faculty resistance when you introduce a computerized testing program. Resistance accompanies all change. Those who are not comfortable with computer technology will be the most resistant. The important thing to remember is that these programs are only tools; in fact, most programs are designed to require a minimum level of computer expertise. Think of the technology as simply replacing your pen, index card, calculator, and file cabinet. The software does not create the test; it facilitates your work and allows you to create the best possible assessment

325

instrument. Although there is a learning curve associated with acquiring computer skills, the payoff is well worth the effort.

The key to a smooth transition from manual test development to a computerized testing program is careful planning. The goals of this chapter are to demonstrate that developing an item bank and implementing test development software is the most efficient means for actualizing a systematic assessment plan, to improve your skills at editing and updating items based on analysis data, and to help you identify your priorities when selecting test development software. This information provides the basis for developing a plan to streamline the process of implementing a computerized testing program. Today's software programs offer such advantages for test development that educators can no longer afford to ignore the potential of technology.

Establishing an Item Bank

An item bank, as defined in Chapter 2, "The Language of Assessment," is an organized collection of accessible test items designed to facilitate the preparation of future exams. Item banking is an essential tool for the development of trustworthy selected-response classroom exams. An item bank allows you to deposit items that can be withdrawn as needed (Rudner, 1998), thereby eliminating the need to write all new items for every exam. It is also a valuable tool for developing makeup exams and a helpful asset for junior and adjunct faculty. A well-developed item bank supplies new faculty with a valuable resource for developing tests and also provides a working example of quality item writing.

As the previous chapters illustrate, test development is a time-consuming process that requires considerable effort, a time commitment that you certainly would rather not expend every semester. While most teachers recycle their selected-response test items, a well-planned item bank provides a systematic approach for using item analysis data to improve your items, particularly multiple-choice items, when you save them and, as a result, improve your classroom assessments. The effort that you invest in developing items can be banked in an organized manner for future use.

Before the advent of the personal computer, experts who advocated item banking for classroom multiple-choice test development usually advised writing each item on an individual index card with codes for categories such as course content and objective. Once the item was administered, it was edited, and item analysis data was calculated and hand-entered on each card. The cards were then manually filed, ready to be edited and sorted for use on future tests.

This process was daunting by its very nature. Obtaining item analysis data required complex calculations that were tedious and time consuming, even with the help of a calculator. Electronic scoring and data analysis improved the process somewhat, but each statistic still had to be hand-entered on the index cards, and teachers still had to hand-sort the items to meet the blueprint specifications and have the items retyped for each new test. Another option was to photocopy the individual items to produce the test, which resulted in an unprofessional test appearance at best. In either case, even when data were obtained by scanning the answer sheets, the process was so time consuming that the data were often lost before the items were reused.

This process also required that the item analysis be recalculated and entered on the index cards after each test administration. Although these procedures benefited the students of those enterprising teachers who undertook the arduous task of manually creating item banks, the effort required for developing and maintaining an up-to-date manual item bank required a nearly impossible time commitment for most teachers. As a result, the use of item banking for selected-response classroom testing was confined to those programs seriously committed to the concept and willing to devote the time to establishing a bank and, more important, to keeping it current.

The software programs available today have completely changed this process. They electronically manage the filing, sorting, storing, retrieval, statistical calculation, and updating of items for classroom testing, thereby freeing the teacher to commit the necessary time to ensuring the quality of the items in the bank.

Editing Items

While technology has the capacity for managing the administrative aspects of test development, the challenge for faculty is the quality enhancement of the items that comprise the bank. Quality is the most important issue in item banking; in fact, it is the central issue. The purpose of an item bank is to improve the items over time so that you eventually have a collection of high-quality items that lighten the clerical burden of test construction and facilitate the development of classroom tests that provide valid and reliable results.

To have an item bank that is a viable force for improving the quality of classroom examinations, each item that is entered into the bank must be carefully edited. The first time an item is used in an exam, there is no way to predict with any degree of certainty how the item will work, no matter how carefully it is constructed. The ambiguities and technical defects that were missed during test construction are revealed with item analysis, and this information can be used to revise and improve the items for future use (Miller, Linn, & Gronlund, 2009). The statistical data for each item that is an outcome of test administration provide a powerful tool for teachers to improve test items. Considering the important role that tests play in education, it is essential that teachers use item analysis to improve the items they use in their classroom tests. Refer to Chapter 11, "Interpreting Test Results," for in-depth discussion on interpreting and using item analysis data.

In addition to improving test items, item analysis also improves your item-writing skills. The more experience you have reviewing statistical analysis of test items, the more proficient you will become at recognizing the qualities that contribute to item difficulty and make them discriminate effectively. Practice with identifying defective items helps you to avoid flaws when you create items. Experience with rewording and modifying items based on item analysis helps you develop expertise with writing original items and critiquing textbook item banks. The ultimate effect of experience with item analysis is an improvement of your general test construction skills (Miller et al., 2009).

Selecting a Test Development Software Program

Test development/item banking software offers the most efficient means for streamlining the test development process. In fact, today's technology is so powerful it cannot be ignored by anyone who is involved in creating and improving tests. The decision today is not whether to implement a test development software program but which program to implement. To make an informed decision, you need to be aware of the capabilities offered by the available software programs and prioritize your needs to decide which options are most important for you. It is also crucial that you consult with the information technology department of your school because its staff members can provide you with assistance for determining the compatibility of the available test development software with the hardware and software programs in your institution.

Hardware Requirements

Your first concern is to identify your current hardware capabilities. It is essential that your computer system and electronic scanner are compatible with and capable of running the program that you purchase. Your hardware capacity limits your choice of software. On the other hand, if you are fortunate enough to have the funding to purchase a new computer and scanning system, you can select the software program of your dreams and purchase the hardware to suit the software. Computer administration of classroom exams is only one reason to purchase computer hardware and software. As we have established, quality items are the backbone for high-quality exams.

If your budget is limited, your priority should be to purchase hardware and software that facilitates test development and item banking. You do not need to wait until you can afford a computer for each student. Purchase a program that transitions into computer administration, but keep in mind that the most important purchase is to obtain a user-friendly program that facilitates the development of quality test items.

Item Banking Facility

When reviewing software programs, it is important for you to identify what capability is essential for your particular needs and then match those needs to a program that is as simple to operate as possible (Ward & Murray-Ward, 1994). Your initial review should answer these questions:

- How many items can the bank hold?
- What item formats does the bank support?
- Is the manual clearly written and easy to understand?
- Is online support available?
- How is the security of the program maintained?
- Does the bank store items with their item analysis data?
- Does the bank store accumulated data for each item?
- What information can be included in a printout of the item bank?
- Does the program include p values and point biserials for all the options?
- Is the software compatible with the server in your institution?
- Is the program compatible with computer administration of classroom exams?

Once you have this basic information, closely examine the features of the program, several of which are described in the discussion that follows. Take careful notes as you review each software program to select the program that is best suited to your needs; also, be sure to consult with the information technology department at your institution before making your final decision. It is also helpful to ask the software publisher for referrals from institutions that are using the software. Follow-up with these institutions to determine what their experience has been with using the software.

Sample Test and Item Analysis Data

Table 14.1 provides an example of the item analysis data that you should require from test development software. Note that the p value (0.68) and the point biserial index (PBI) (0.36) of the item correspond with the p value and PBI of choice B, the correct answer. This example also provides the p values and the PBIs of the distractors, information that is critical for thorough item analysis.

Table 14.2 provides an example of the data that is required for a complete analysis of the results of a test. Refer to Chapter 11, "Interpreting Test Results," for an in-depth discussion and guides for reviewing both test and item analysis data.

Table 14.1   Sample Item Analysis Data

Correct answer = **B**
p value (difficulty): **0.68**
PBI (point biserial index): **0.36**

Choice	p Value	PBI
A	0.09	−0.08
B	0.68	**0.36**
C	0.12	−0.21
D	0.11	−0.25

Table 14.2   Sample Test Analysis Data

Number of items	100
Number of examinees	92
Mean	75.4
Median	77
Low score	52
High score	93
Alpha	0.754
Standard deviation	7.7
Standard error of measurement (SEM)	3.8
Mean p value	0.754
Mean PBI	0.36

Item Importing and Exporting

This is an essential timesaving feature. If you have items stored in exams in electronic word processing files or if you plan to use a commercially prepared item bank, make sure the software program you purchase allows you to import these items easily into the item bank. If the program does not provide this function, you will need to type in the items manually. Carefully check this feature to make sure that the importing facility does not require complicated formatting of your current items. The most user-friendly programs allow you to save your word processing file as a .txt file, which is then automatically imported into an existing item bank. Once the items are in the bank, they can be edited, revised, and coded.

Item importing is also important for future item development. As you are certainly aware, only one person should work on an electronic file at one time. This is also true for item banking files. To avoid confusion and overwriting of the files when a group teaches a course, one faculty member must be responsible for administering and maintaining the item bank files. Faculty members in the group should be able to develop items in a word processing program, and the item banking program should have the capability of easily importing these items into the bank. A smooth importing facility allows faculty who do not have the test-authoring software on their home computers to develop items in a word processing program for importing into the item bank.

Exporting is another important feature. There are several reasons why you may want to export your items into a word processing file. Most important, you may decide to change software programs in the future, so you do not want your items to be accessible only through the item bank. The export feature should be as seamless as the import feature. Make sure you see a demonstration of both features before you purchase a software program.

Word Processing

Word processing capability is an essential feature that you should carefully consider. Because items will be continuously edited and revised over time, the word processing capability of the software program is very important. Features such as cutting, pasting, font selection, and spell checking are important for word processing capability because they help to streamline the item development process. Consider also whether the program provides use of special characters and how it handles graphics. Some programs cannot handle graphics in the item file, so they must be kept in a separate file or even pasted into a hard copy of the test and photocopied. Make sure the word processing capabilities are user friendly; an awkward program becomes very frustrating over time and may interfere with continued faculty receptivity to the test development program.

Item Classification

To query an item bank to retrieve items, the items must be classified. The best scheme for organizing your banks is to have a bank for each course and to classify the items in the course. Look for an item banking program that provides coding for at least 8 to 10 classification areas. A drop-down box for entering codes is a valuable

Table 14.3 Suggested Item Classification Codes	
Nursing process	Topic
Client need	Subtopic
Course objective	Key words
Learning outcome	Cognitive level
Content area	Author

tool. This feature stores the codes and drops them down for you to mouse-click so that you do not have to repeatedly type the codes into the program. Determine the maximum number of classification areas you require. Suggestions for coding are presented in **Table 14.3**.

Do not make your comprehensive coding plan too complicated. Simplicity is best when you are beginning this process. The five categories in the first column in Table 14.3 are a good starting point. You can always add codes as your expertise develops. One word of caution: Although you can add codes, it can be very complicated to change codes, particularly on a large bank of items. Determining a classification scheme is another stage in the test development process where planning is crucial.

Item codes allow you to query the bank to select items for inclusion on a test. For example, you could query the bank to see all items that have not yet been used this semester in a particular content area and objective, and the program would allow you to view all items that meet those criteria. You could then select items from that group to meet the specific blueprint specifications for a test. Once the test is assembled, many programs print a cross-reference table or blueprint grid that specifies how many items are included on the test for each criterion.

When planning your classification scheme, it is important to be consistent across courses that may share item banks. The best approach is to obtain a consensus among the faculty for classification areas. It is a good idea to leave one or two fields blank for use by an individual course or faculty member. Just be sure to consider the implications of having different fields if banks need to be combined or divided in the future.

Supplemental Fields

The item bank should have at least two supplemental fields for storing documentation information. When items are carefully documented, the validity of your tests is increased. Having fields such as item rationales and references readily accessible facilitates the process of editing and revising items. Most programs allow for these fields to be projected for group viewing, which is a great asset for student test review and also for faculty group review of items. Ease of availability encourages faculty to use these fields to increase the quality of their items. One advantage of having supplemental fields for each item is that the effort of documenting the item is never lost because the information in the field is permanently attached to the item. Be sure to document your items as they are written, as Chapter 5, "Selected-Response Format: Developing Multiple-Choice Items," suggests. Documenting old items can be a daunting task that should be approached gradually. Be realistic. If you set impossible goals, you will not succeed. The ultimate objective is to have a working item bank.

Test Assembly

Ease of test assembly is an important feature of test development software. Most programs provide for operator assembly or random selection of items by the computer within query parameters defined by the teacher. When you initially use the software, you may want to select the items from a hard copy, but you will soon find that selecting the items from the computer screen expedites the test assembly process. However, when a test contains items from several different teachers, it is usually preferable to have the teachers select their items from a hard copy of the item bank and have the bank administrator assemble the test on the computer.

Test assembly features vary among programs. Some allow on-screen viewing and selection of items; others require that you first select the items and then enter the item identification numbers into the program to assemble the test on the computer screen. Programs also vary in the number of variables that can be entered into a query for selecting items. To facilitate the selection of items to meet a test blueprint, choose a program that allows you to enter at least three categories (content area, objective, and date last used) into a query for item selection.

It is also wise to choose a program that allows you to print out a blueprint. This feature can also be used to generate cross-reference tables such as those illustrated in Tables 15.5, 15.6, and 15.7. The blueprint generated by the software is a precise picture of the criteria covered on the test, documenting content-related evidence of validity. Keep in mind that the more reports you want to generate, the more carefully your items must be coded and the more categories the software must allow you to include in a cross-reference.

Ward and Murray-Ward (1994) point out the desirability of several features for test-authoring software. These include the ability to do the following:

- Produce an item map that indicates the key and the codes for each item on a test
- Store and print general test directions
- Number pages and items automatically
- Print tests in a two-column format
- Avoid inserting a page break in the middle of an item

Additional features that enhance the quality of a software program include the ability to:

- Construct tests from multiple item banks
- Indicate the date last used for each item
- Estimate the difficulty of the test based on the histories of the stored items
- Create multiple versions of a test by scrambling items and/or options
- Code items to prevent them from being scrambled
- Code items that should not be included on the same exam
- Print out a test blueprint or a cross-reference table

Note that if the program has the ability to create multiple versions by scrambling items or item options, it is important that you can block an item from having its options scrambled. The options for certain items, such as those that have numerical answers, should be kept as they are written. In addition, some items should not be included on the same test. The software should have the ability to code items so that items that cue each other are not used on the same exam.

You should select a test-authoring program that allows you to develop and administer online tests; however, you should not purchase a program that is exclusively for online testing, particularly if you are new to computerized-test development. Whether you administer tests online or in a pencil-and-paper format, it is the quality of the items that matters most. Do not be misled by the bells and whistles of online testing programs. Online testing requires a very large bank of items, and it probably will take you several years before you can accumulate a large bank of high-quality items. In the meantime, it is important to have the ability to administer pencil-and-paper tests to generate that large bank of items.

However, when making your selection, remember that online test administration is becoming more prevalent. Even if you are using paper-and-pencil tests now, the capacity to deliver online tests should certainly be one factor in your selection of a test-authoring program. It makes sense to have the capability to administer tests online in the future no matter what your current capacity. Your goal with software selection should be to obtain the program that has the capabilities that you most want and need to enable you to efficiently produce tests that are developed with high-quality items (Ward & Murray-Ward, 1994).

Scoring and Reporting

Although tests administered online are automatically scored, printed tests require a separate scoring process, usually through an electronic scanning machine. Some programs require that you produce a key by hand; others score the test through the item bank where the correct answer is stored. When the need for a key is eliminated, the chance of error decreases, so a program that scores through the bank is preferable. Another essential feature for a scoring facility is the ability to adjust the scores based on posttest analysis.

A major concern when selecting a program is the type of score report produced by the program. The report should provide test statistics, such as those that are included in Table 14.2, because these statistics, discussed in Chapter 11, "Interpreting Test Results," are essential for score interpretation. Also, if the report does not include the item analysis data as illustrated in Table 14.1, you will be handicapped in determining whether an item should be eliminated from a test as well as with revising and improving your items.

In addition to creating reports for the teachers, many software programs provide individual student test reports. The reports give students individual feedback, including the total test score and rationales for each item. When the report provides a printout of each student's individual item responses, the need to return answer sheets to the students during test review is eliminated. Some reports track the students' progress by providing them with their cumulative test average in a course.

Storage of Item Data History

Item analysis capability is an essential feature of a test-authoring software program. You cannot improve your items without the data on which to base your revisions. Some programs include a scoring and analysis program, while others interface with a separate analysis program. The important concern is that the item bank, scoring, and test analysis functions work smoothly together and that the item analysis data are imported electronically into the item bank. Manual entry of data is so tedious and time consuming that it eventually will be neglected; therefore, electronic import and accumulation of analysis data are essential criteria when you are considering the purchase of test-authoring software.

A software program should save an item's data analysis history, including the p value and point biserial for the items as well as for each distractor. Refer again to Table 14.1; it illustrates the minimum item data information that you should require of a test-authoring program. Look for a program that accumulates data in the item history because accumulated data provide a much better estimate of how an item is working than the data results from a small sample. Some programs store important data, such as date modified and date last used. Date modified is important when evaluating stored item analysis, and date last used is essential when assembling a test to ensure that items are not reused in the same semester and are rotated from year to year.

Gradebook Facility

Programs that do not have an internal gradebook usually have the ability to interface with an external gradebook program. These programs streamline the clerical aspects of tracking and calculating student grades. Exam scores are entered electronically into the grading program, and course grades, based on the instructor input of grading criteria, are calculated and stored for each student.

It is important to maintain confidentiality when posting student grades. The ability to transmit grades securely to students is an important feature to obtain in a gradebook program. Some programs generate an anonymous identification number for each student and create a list for posting grades. Others have the ability to create an individual report for each student or transfer the grades to a secure website for student access. Be sure to select a gradebook that allows you to post grades according to the policy of your institution.

Cost

Some may argue that cost should be your first concern. A better approach is to look at several programs in various price ranges to provide you with a comprehensive basis for comparison so that you can carefully determine your needs and find a reasonable compromise between what you can afford and what you really want. When considering cost, remember to factor in the cost of new hardware if it is needed. Hardware includes your computer, monitor, printer, and scanner and may also include a new copier. The ideal copier collates and staples your exams. Sometimes, the cost of new hardware is money well spent; it actually could save you money. Honestly assess your current hardware capabilities and, if you are severely limited by them, consider the feasibility of gradually purchasing new equipment.

An obvious cost concern is the price of the software. Examine the user agreements carefully. How many users are allowed to access the software? Are you purchasing or leasing the program? Will you be entitled to free upgrades? Is there a fee for technical support? All these issues affect the ultimate cost of the program.

Hidden costs are also associated with computerized-test administration. How expensive are the scannable sheets that are required for the program? Will you need to hire additional staff to maintain the bank? Will word processors be needed to key in current questions?

Computerized-test development software is a long-term cost saver. However, you need to take a close look at your startup costs so that you do not derail your project before it is begun. Carefully consider each of the questions in **Exhibit 14.1** before you purchase a test development software program.

Exhibit 14.1   Questions to ask when assessing test development software

What are your hardware capabilities?
Is the program compatible with the current technology in use at your institution?
How is the security of the program maintained?
How many items can the bank hold?
What information can be included in a printout of the item bank?
What item formats does the bank support?
Is the manual clearly written and easy to understand?
Is online support available?
Is there a charge for technical support?
How does the program import and export items?
Are you satisfied with the demonstration of the import and export functions?
Does the word processing program provide easy access to the following features?

• Spell checking

• Font selection

• Cutting and pasting

Does the number of classification areas meet your needs?
Does the program have drop-down boxes to facilitate item classification?
Does the number of supplemental fields meet your needs?
Can the program print a cross-reference table for the test?
Examine the case in which the program assembles a test:

• How many classification areas can be entered in a query for selecting items for a test?

• What is the procedure for entering test specifications into the program, on screen and/or hard copy?

• Can the software create a test based on the test blueprint?

• Does the test assembly have the capacity to access more than one bank?

• Can the user view items by user-specified criteria?

• Can more than one version of the test be created?

• If item options can be scrambled, can an item be coded to prevent scrambling of its options?

Can items that should not be used together on an exam be coded?

(continues)

Exhibit 14.1 Questions to ask when assessing test development software (*Continued*)

Does the test developer function estimate the difficulty of the test based on stored item histories?

Does the software have the following features?

- Produces print copies of the test
- Administers tests online
- Maps items with keys and codes
- Stores and prints test direction
- Numbers pages automatically
- Has the ability to print tests in one- or two-column format

How are the tests scored: both online and pencil and paper?

Does a key need to be entered manually?

What is the availability and cost of required scannable forms?

How does the program adjust the scores based on post test analysis?

Examine the adequacy of the score report:

- What test statistics are included in the test analysis?
- What statistical data are included in the individual item analysis?

What item data are automatically stored in the item history?

Are the item data accumulated in the item history?

Are date last used and date last edited stored with the item?

If a student report is available, what information does it provide?

Does the program have, or interface with, a gradebook program?

How user friendly are the gradebook functions?

How flexible is the input of the grading criteria?

Does the gradebook keep running calculations of each student's grades?

How does the gradebook facilitate the posting of student grades?

What is the cost of hardware replacement or upgrade?

What does the software cost?

Are current customers entitled to discounted upgrades?

Are there any hidden costs associated with computerized testing?

Implementing Test Development Software

Planning is the most important step for developing an item bank (Rudner, 1998). To ensure that your decision to institute electronic test development will be actualized, a team of committed individuals must take the initiative to generate a plan of action and lay the groundwork for successful implementation of the software. When developing the plan, it is crucial to acknowledge that purchase and application of test development software is not an end in itself; the software is a tool that is only as good as the information it manipulates. The axiom "garbage in, garbage out" applies here. The critical first step is to follow the guidelines presented in this text to formulate a plan for the systematic assessment of learning outcomes across the curriculum. Only then you can evaluate the available software to determine which program best facilitates the ongoing implementation of your systematic assessment plan.

You may have the impression from the discussion in the previous section that test development software is extremely complex. If you think about it, you probably agree that this is a typical reaction to any new software program, particularly when you are reading about it without having the program to manipulate. Working with the actual program gives you a much better feel for how it operates. Be sure to obtain demo disks for each of the programs you want to evaluate. It is important that the program you purchase be user friendly because the faculty who use the program will have a wide range of computer ability.

Appointing Test Bank Administrators

Once you have developed your plan, purchased your software, and created your item classification scheme, you are ready to use the software to create your item bank. At this point, it is essential that one or more item bank administrators be appointed if they are not already in place. Although item banking software streamlines the process of test development, it is a complex process that involves a wide cast of participants. When everyone is in charge, no one is in charge. Successful implementation of an item bank requires management and coordination.

The responsibility for making the decision for how to manage the program lies with the faculty as a group. A variety of factors will enter into the decision, including whether courses are taught by a group or individual faculty, the size of the program, the number of faculty members, the computer expertise of the faculty, the availability of technical support on the campus, and the willingness of faculty to participate as coordinators of the item bank. Administering an item bank, especially when it is being developed, is a sizable responsibility that requires well-organized individuals who have at least basic computer skills and who are willing to devote the time and face the challenges of implementing change. A practical approach is to assign one bank administrator for each course, with these administrators forming the item bank committee that oversees the entire bank. Some programs choose to use the services of a consultant to facilitate the initiation of the bank. Although this approach is expensive initially, a consultant who is experienced at setting up test development software for a nursing program will save you time, and could save you money, in the long run.

Faculty who commit to instituting and administering the item bank are making a very worthwhile contribution to the quality of student education. Directing the operation of an item bank should not be considered an extra assignment. It is a time-consuming responsibility, particularly during the initiation of the bank, that should be acknowledged in terms of faculty workload. This may be a hard sell to school administrators, but the burden of this responsibility could easily overwhelm faculty volunteers if they are expected to carry a full workload in addition to item banking coordination. Considering item bank administration as part of a faculty member's workload ensures that the faculty who volunteer to administer the bank will be able to devote the time necessary to ensure the successful implementation of the software.

The work of the faculty administrators can be greatly facilitated if a member of the support staff develops expertise in managing the clerical aspects of the item bank. Duties such as scanning, entering rosters, importing and exporting items, importing item data, printing hard copies of tests and item banks, and even assembling tests based on faculty selection are responsibilities that can be assumed by a knowledgeable support staff member under the direction of the bank administrator. Do not be misled into believing that clerical staff can assume sole responsibility for the item bank. Remember, the biggest concern with item banking is the quality of the questions. Coding, item editing, and interpreting item analysis are among the roles of the administrator that can be assumed only by a faculty member.

Establishing Procedures

To expedite item banking, implementation procedures must be established to direct the process. It is very important that the entire faculty take ownership of the item bank. Therefore, although the bank administrators may draft the procedures, the entire faculty should have input into making the final decision for the processes that direct the item bank. Consult with other schools that are using the software. Keep the procedures as simple as possible and have written guidelines to avoid confusion. Remember, your plan does not have to be perfect: Keep it flexible and open to change as your test development process evolves.

Item Editing and Revision Testing companies subject their items to rigorous review by content experts; in addition, they employ a professional editor to ensure that the items on their tests adhere to their style guides. Although schools cannot be held to these standards, it is important that a system be developed to edit and revise all items based on both content and style before they are entered into the bank. Every item that is proposed for bank entry should be subjected to the same process. This is a task that is very time consuming when a bank is initiated, but it becomes more manageable once the bank is established. The process can be handled by the individual bank administrators or by the item bank committee. Whichever system is used, it is essential that an edited item be returned to the faculty author for final approval before it is entered into the bank.

Selecting Exam Items The procedure for selecting items for inclusion in a test is largely determined by the software program you select. However, you need to set up a logistical plan. To create a test from a software bank, all test items must be in the bank. If you have established a process for entering items into the bank, all items in the bank will meet the faculty's standards for item quality. Therefore, junior faculty or adjunct instructors can use the bank and be assured of the quality of the items that they select for a test.

While having an item bank improves item quality, it is essential that faculty members have the freedom and ability to compose new items. In fact, faculty item-writing efforts should be encouraged because the larger the bank, the more useful it is. All items should go through the same process for entry into the bank. One very important note: Editing is always easier than writing the original. The item-editing process should be a helpful and congenial one.

If one person composes exams, the selection process is simple. The faculty member can choose items to meet the blueprint from either a hard copy of the bank or on the computer screen. When a faculty group is involved in the selection process, it is usually best to provide each member with the test blueprint and a hard copy of the items that relate to their piece of the course. Make sure that the hard copy includes the stored difficulty and discrimination values, the classifications, and the date last used for each item. This information assists faculty in selecting items and ensures that items are not reused in a semester. In fact, if your bank is large enough, it is wise to use as few of the same items as possible in consecutive years.

Once the items are selected, the bank administrator should collect the selections of each faculty member and assemble the exam as discussed in Chapter 9, "Assembling, Administering, and Scoring a Test." During pretest review, faculty members should ensure that their item selections have been entered accurately on the test.

Posttest Item Revision   The first section of this chapter addresses the procedure for posttest item revision. When the item data are automatically entered into the item bank, item revision is facilitated—your task is to determine how to implement the revision. The bank administrator, the item bank committee, or the faculty author of the item can make revisions. When you are new to this process, it is probably best to work on revisions as a group or to circulate hard copies of the items for faculty input. It is essential that you do not overlook this step in the test development process: Item revision based on analysis data is the key to quality test items. Maintaining a system ensures that revision does not get put off and eventually forgotten.

Exhibit 14.2 is an example of an item bank screen. Note that it includes fields for all the requirements identified for quality test development software. Solution, reference, classification, item analysis data, date last used, and date modified are all available to facilitate test development, item analysis, and item revision. **Exhibit 14.3** summarizes the steps for implementing a test development software program.

Exhibit 14.2   Sample item bank screen

Cardiovascular 101
A client who is receiving intravenous heparin has an activated partial thromboplastin time (APTT) of two and one-half times the control. In addition to documenting the finding, which of these actions would be appropriate for a nurse to take?

A. Call the lab for a stat repeat of the test.
B. Discontinue the client's heparin infusion immediately.
C. Continue to monitor the client.*
D. Alert the blood bank to have a unit of packed cells available.

Solution
This question asks the student to recognize that the APTT should be between 1.5 and 2.5 times the control for a client who is receiving heparin. It requires the student to apply that information. In this question, although the client's APTT is within the range, it is at the top of the range. The nurse could also check the client's vital signs or observe for adverse effects, such as hematuria. However, the question asks the student to discriminate among the options offered, and only one of these is correct.

Reference
Shannon, M. T., & Wilson, B. A. (1992). *Govoni & Hayes: Drugs and nursing implications.* Norwalk, CT: Appleton and Lange, p. 645.

(continues)

Exhibit 14.2   Sample item bank screen (*Continued*)

Nsg Process	Client Need	Objective*	L Outcome*	Content	Cog Level	Author
Implement	Pharm therapy	Crit Think/3	3/11	Anticoag.	App	Smith

Cumulative Item Analysis

p(Diff) Value	PBI
0.74	0.65

Response Frequencies (%)

A	B	C	D	E
13	3	10	74	NA

Date Last Used	Date Modified
1/25/2015	2/15/2015

* Objectives and Learning Outcomes are assigned a number to facilitate entry into a classification scheme.

Exhibit 14.3   Implementing test development software

- Assemble a team of committed faculty members.
- Develop a plan for systematic assessment of outcomes.
- Review and select test development software.
- Create item classification scheme.
- Appoint item bank administrators.
- Establish process for item editing, revision, and inclusion in the bank.
- Establish a procedure for selecting items for exams.
- Determine a procedure for revising items based on posttest analysis

Incorporating Textbook Item Banks

Most current nursing textbooks provide faculty with a test bank of items that complement the text. Do not assume that these items are of high quality simply because they have been published. In fact, the quality of these banks varies widely. Very few banks contain items that have been pilot-tested on students, so there are no assurances that these items will function well on a test.

While textbook items can be helpful, they should be used with caution. Many faculty members are under the erroneous impression that the items in these banks are of superior quality. Although items in a textbook test bank should be subjected to the same rigorous standards that you require of your own items, most textbook test banks violate item-writing guidelines (Masters et al., 2001). In addition, faculty members often assume that textbook banks contain items that have a proven statistical history, but publishers seldom pretest these items. The items are raw items; they have no data associated with them.

In many cases, when you examine the items, the concept being tested is worthwhile but the item is not constructed in accordance with the guidelines presented in previous chapters, which means that most of the items require revision. Chapter 5, "Selected-Response Format: Developing Multiple-Choice Items," and Chapter 6, "Writing Critical Thinking Multiple-Choice Items," are helpful guides for revising these items. Pay close attention to the distractors; they often need work. Take advantage of these banks as a valuable resource for finding items to revise and incorporate into your item bank.

Summary

While test-authoring software provides nursing faculty with an invaluable tool for facilitating the test development process, it can fulfill its potential only if it is part of a carefully developed plan for systematic assessment. As with all technology, the quality of the final product is related to the human input. Before you can successfully use a testing software program to implement an overall assessment plan, you must be conversant with the principles of assessment.

Item analysis data are valuable tools provided by test development software. The data provided for each item must be combined with your professional expertise to enhance the quality of your test items. General guidelines and specific examples are combined in this chapter to provide faculty with direction for implementing test revision based on item analysis.

Having a clear idea of your assessment needs is a prerequisite for making an informed decision about which software program to purchase. Several software programs are currently available that provide item banking and test development capabilities with the capacity for online test administration. Making your selection undoubtedly requires that you make some compromises, but the potential of test development software requires that you make a decision. There is no reason to put off your purchase. The available software is fully capable of handling the needs of a school-based testing program. Consult with your colleagues, contact schools that are using the software successfully, follow the guidelines provided in this chapter to make a decision, and take the initiative to move your assessment program into the 21st century. The longer you wait, the more time is wasted.

Learning Activities

1. Identify five advantages of item development software.
2. List the features you would require in a test development software program.
3. Review the questions in Exhibit 14.1. Select a test development program from the options listed in the Web Links section and ask the questions of your selected program.
4. Review the classification codes from Table 14.3. Which codes would you include if your program allowed only six codes?
5. Use the table to classify 10 items from a test you have administered.
6. Request a trial copy of the program from one of the websites from the list in "Web Links" below. Enter five items into the program and create a sample test.

Web Links

Test Development Software
http://www.classmarker.com
http://www.exambuilder.com
http://www.examsoft.com
http://www.LXR.com
http://www.questionmark.com
http://www.scantron.com/parsystem/

References

Masters, J. C., Hulsmeyer, B. S., Pike, M. E., Leichty, K., Miller, M. T., & Verset, A. L. (2001). Assessment of multiple-choice questions in selected test banks accompanying textbooks used in nursing education. *Journal of Nursing Education, 40,* 25–31.

McDonald, M. E. (2008). Developing trustworthy classroom tests. In B. K. Penn (Ed.), *Mastering the teaching role: A guide for nurse educators.* Philadelphia, PA: F. A. Davis.

Miller, M. D., Linn, R. L., & Gronlund, N. E. (2009). *Measurement and assessment in teaching* (10th ed.). Upper Saddle River, NJ: Pearson Education.

Rudner, L. M. (1998). Item banking. *Practical Assessment, Research & Evaluation, 6*(4). Retrieved from http://PAREonline.net/getvn.asp?v=6&n=4

Ward, A. W., & Murray-Ward, M. (1994). Guidelines for the development of item banks. *Educational Measurement: Issues and Practice, 13,* 34–39.

Preparing Students for the Licensure Exam: The Importance of NCLEX

CHAPTER 15

© Anteromite/Shutterstock

"Whether you believe that you can, or you believe that you cannot, you are correct."

—HENRY FORD

The National Council Licensure Exam (NCLEX) has a powerful impact on nursing education; it determines which graduates will be allowed to practice nursing. Not only does it affect the future of the graduates of nursing programs, it has an enormous influence on the future of the nursing programs that prepare the graduates for nursing practice. For better or sometimes for worse, the impact of the NCLEX pass rate influences the way in which nursing students prepare to enter their chosen profession.

Although nurse educators are well aware of the impact of NCLEX on nursing education, many are not conversant with every aspect of the process for licensure. This chapter is designed to familiarize nurse educators with the NCLEX process and to address the concerns of both students and educators. This chapter examines the NCLEX issues that every nurse educator should be aware of. Even if you are familiar with the NCLEX process, you will find this chapter to be a valuable resource for guiding students.

The NCLEX Application Process

The National Council of State Boards of Nursing (NCSBN) is a nonprofit organization that is responsible for developing and administering the NCLEX. The NCLEX-RN is administered to candidates seeking to obtain registered nurse licensure, and the NCLEX-PN is administered to candidates seeking to be licensed as practical or vocational nurses. Pearson Professional Testing (Pearson VUE) currently provides test administration services for the NCSBN. Before graduates of nursing programs can schedule an appointment to take the NCLEX, they must apply for licensure to the board of nursing in the state or territory in which they want to be licensed. The individual boards have varying requirements for licensure, but the NCLEX is required by the state boards of nursing in all 50 states, the District of Columbia, and 4 U.S. territories (NCSBN, 2016c).

In addition, the NCSBN opened registration for Canadian applicants to take the NCLEX-RN for licensure to practice nursing in Canada starting in 2015. While the NCLEX is currently offered in 10 foreign countries for licensure in the United States, the partnership with the 10 Canadian RN regulatory bodies is the first time that the NCLEX is administered as a requirement for licensure in another country (NCSBN, 2014b)

Once the graduates register with Pearson VUE to take the exam and meet the pretesting requirements of their individual states, their state board of nursing will certify that they are eligible to take the NCLEX and they will receive an Authorization to Test from Pearson VUE. At that point, the students can schedule an appointment with Pearson VUE to take the NCLEX (NCSBN, 2016e). Nursing faculty should advise students to carefully review the Candidate's Bulletin, which is published each year on the National Council's website at http://www.ncsbn.org. This is the primary source for determining the current requirements for taking the NCLEX exams.

Development of the NCLEX

The NCLEX is designed to measure the nursing abilities of new graduates who are entering the profession to ensure that healthcare consumers receive safe nursing care. Both the NCLEX-RN and the NCLEX-PN are developed using the same procedure; they are constructed according to exacting psychometric standards to measure the competencies that are required for safe entry-level nursing practice (NCSBN, 2015, 2016a). The NCSBN defines *entry level* as the nursing practice that novice nurses engage in during the first few months after graduation. During this period, newly licensed nurses are expected to depend on skills acquired during their nursing education to provide safe client care (Smith & Crawford, 2002).

The NCLEX Practice Analyses

The purpose of a practice analysis is to define a professional practice in terms of the actual activities that a new practitioner must be able to perform competently and safely. This description forms the foundation for a licensing exam that relates to the actual practice of the profession. In fact, a practice analysis is essential for validating that the content included in a high-stakes exam, such as a licensing exam, actually relates to the profession's practice (Chinn & Hertz, 2010). The NCSBN performs RN and PN practice analyses to link the NCLEX exams to nursing practice.

The NCSBN practice analyses are nonexperimental descriptive studies that guide content distribution on the NCLEX licensure exams and provide content-related evidence of validity (Wendt, Kenny, & Brown, 2010). The practice analyses are surveys that contain statements describing the activities that nurses perform in their practice. Representative samples of nurses (RNs for the NCLEX-RN and LPNs/LVNs for the NCLEX-PN) are selected to respond to the surveys. The responders indicate whether each of the nursing activities on the survey is applicable to their work setting. They are asked to identify how often they performed each activity on the last day that they worked and what level of priority they would assign to the activity (NCSBN, 2015, 2016a). While the same format is used for both, the RN practice analysis identifies the activities that relate to the practice of registered nurses and the PN practice analysis identifies the activities that relate to the practice of practical nurses. Both surveys identify nursing care activity statements that are developed by a panel of experts.

The ratings of the activities, both for priority and frequency of performance, determine how they are represented proportionately on the NCLEX exams. This representation is the framework for the NCLEX test plan or blueprint (NCSBN, 2015, 2016a). Thus, the RN and PN practice analyses link the NCLEX examinations to nursing practice.

The NCLEX Test Plan

The practice analysis is conducted for each exam on a 3-year cycle, and the test plans are changed based on the findings identified in the practice analyses. The 2016 NCLEX-RN test plan was developed from a 2014 practice analysis study of newly licensed registered nurses (NCSBN, 2015), while the 2017 NCLEX-PN test plan was developed from a 2015 practice analysis study of newly licensed practical/vocational nurses (NCSBN, 2016c, 2017a). The analysis of the responses related to the activities in the surveys identifies the knowledge, skills, and abilities that are essential to meet the needs of clients when providing nursing care and are the basis for the content of the tests. The best source for tracking current changes in the test plan is to monitor the NCSBN website (http://www.ncsbn.org).

Wendt (2003, p. 277) states that the NCLEX test plan and practice analyses are not intended to serve as the primary source for nursing curriculum. As Wendt notes, however, these documents provide faculty with valuable data on entry-level nursing practice that can be used to update course content.

The activities identified in the practice analysis are incorporated in the test plan under the four categories of client needs. The client needs are the same for both the NCLEX-RN and the NCLEX-PN test (NCSBN, 2016c, 2017a):

1. Safe effective care environment
2. Health promotion and maintenance
3. Psychosocial integrity
4. Physiological integrity

Although the basic client needs are the same, the subcategories and weighting of the items differ. **Tables 15.1** and **15.2** illustrate the different subcategories and weighting of the exams. These tables also illustrate the range of items that an examinee would receive depending on the length of the test that the examinee receives. (The length of the exam is discussed later in this chapter.) Note that the difference in the client need subcategories reflects the difference in the activities of the two levels in nursing practice: For example, when compared with the RN exam, the PN exam does not include parenteral therapies, and coordinated care is identified instead of management of care.

Table 15.1 2016 NCLEX-RN Test Plan

NCLEX–RN BLUEPRINT April 2016 Pretest Items (Not scored) Scored Items		Minimum Exam 75 items 15 items 60 items	Maximum Exam 265 items 15 items 250 items
Safe effective care environment			
Management of care	17–23%	10–14	43–58
Safety and infection control	9–15%	6–10	23–38
Health promotion and maintenance	6–12%	4–8	15–30
Psychosocial integrity	6–12%	4–8	15–30
Physiological integrity			
Basic care and comfort	6–12%	4–8	15–30
Pharmacological and parenteral therapies	12–18%	8–12	30–45
Reduction of risk potential	9–15%	6–10	23–38
Physiological adaptation	11–17%	7–10	28–43

Data from National Council of State Boards of Nursing. (2016c). 2016 *NCLEX-RN detailed test plan*. Chicago, IL: Author.

Table 15.2 2017 NCLEX-PN Test Plan

NCLEX–PN BLUEPRINT April 2017 Pretest Items (Not scored) Scored Items		Minimum Exam 85 items 25 items 60 items	Maximum Exam 205 items 25 items 180 items
Safe effective care environment			
Coordinated care	18–24%	11–14	32–43
Safety and infection control	10–16%	6–10	18–29
Health promotion and maintenance	6–12%	4–8	11–22
Psychosocial integrity	9–15%	5–9	16–27
Physiological integrity			
Basic care and comfort	7–13%	4–8	13–23
Pharmacological therapies	10–16%	6–10	18–29
Reduction of risk potential	9–15%	5–9	16–27
Physiological adaptation	7–13%	4–8	13–23

Data from National Council of State Boards of Nursing. (2017). *2017 NCLEX–PN detailed test plan*. Chicago, IL: Author.

The percentages of items for each client need category also vary between the RN and PN test plans. These percentages determine the number of items each student receives in each category. Although the number of items administered varies among students, the percentage of items every student receives is consistent for each category. For example, an RN candidate who answers 75 items (the minimum number of items on the RN examination) would receive 60 scored items, with 4 to 7 items coming from the psychosocial category; while an RN candidate who answers 265 items (the maximum number of items on the RN examination) would receive 250 scored items, with 15 to 30 items from the psychosocial category. They each receive a different number of items, but they both receive 6% to 12% of the scored items from the psychosocial category (NCSBN, 2016c).

The NCLEX test plans are not two-way charts, as discussed in Chapter 4, "Implementing Systematic Test Development." The current NCLEX plans are one-way classification systems that assign a percentage of test items only to the categories and subcategories of the client needs.

The test plans also address several processes that are fundamental to the practice of nursing. These processes are not assigned a percentage of item representation in the test plan; rather, they are integrated in an unspecified manner throughout the four categories of client needs. These integrated processes include:

- Nursing process
- Caring
- Communication and documentation
- Teaching/learning (NCSBN, 2016c, 2017a)

The practice of having every item address both a nursing activity related to a client need and one or more integrated processes ensures that the items are relevant to nursing practice. You can be assured that you will not find any trivia on the NCLEX exams!

Characteristics of the NCLEX

Since 1994, the NCLEX examinations have used a computerized adaptive testing (CAT) format. The exams are administered on a computer by appointment at testing centers. The results, which reflect the minimum competency required for safe entry-level nursing practice, are used by the state boards of nursing to make decisions about licensure for nursing practice. Each examinee receives a unique test that is tailored to the individual's ability because the precise difficulty of every item is included in the computer program. While candidates answer different items, the test is fair to everyone because each student receives an exam that matches the test plan (NCSBN, 2016b, 2016h).

CAT Format

The NCLEX is administered on a computer using CAT. This method administers a unique exam to each candidate depending on the candidate's ability: The questions change depending on how well the candidate performs. The first item on the test has average difficulty. If the candidate answers the item correctly, the program presents a more difficult item; if the candidate answers incorrectly, the program presents an easier item. As the candidate progresses through the test, the computer program continuously estimates the candidate's ability based on the most recent response and all the previous responses. The items continue to become harder as the candidate answers them correctly, and they become easier as the candidate answers incorrectly (NCSBN, 2016b).

The NCLEX computer program does not allow candidates to return to previous items or progress to the next item until the item that is currently on the screen is answered. After the candidate responds to an item, the computer program searches the item bank to find an item that meets both the NCLEX test plan requirements and has a difficulty level based on the candidate's current ability. As the candidate continues to answer items, the estimate of the candidate's ability becomes more precise, until the candidate is correctly answering 50% of the items presented. This point is referred to as the candidate's ability estimate: the item difficulty level at which the candidate has a 50% chance of correctly answering an item (NCSBN, 2016b). This process produces a test that is targeted to each candidate.

Passing Standard

The state boards of nursing are charged by their states with regulating nursing practice to protect the public. The NCLEX exams are high-stakes examinations that must consider the welfare of the healthcare consumer as well as the future of the large number of graduate nurses who take the exam. In 2015, for example, more than 299,000 candidates took the NCLEX-RN and NCLEX-PN exams (NCSBN, 2016f). Therefore, it is important that the standard is set high enough to protect the public and low enough so that competent nurses who have completed an expensive and rigorous nursing program are not denied licensure (O'Neill, Marks, & Reynolds, 2005).

The minimum level of competency that a candidate must attain to pass the NCLEX is referred to as the passing standard. Although each member board of nursing is free to set whatever requirement it sees fit for licensing nurses, every board requires candidates to take the NCLEX, and all accept the passing standard that is set by the NCSBN. This allows for cost containment when developing the exam, and it also allows for portability of test results because the test offers the same content and passing standard across the country (O'Neill et al., 2005). In other words, candidates only have to pass the NCLEX test once, no matter how many states they apply to for licensure.

As Wendt and Kenny (2007) explain, establishing a cut score, or passing standard, is a critical element for ensuring the validity of an examination. The NCLEX passing standard reflects the nursing ability required to practice competently at the entry level. To ensure the accuracy of the passing standard, the NCSBN's board of directors evaluates the passing standard of the NCLEX every three years. When evaluating the passing standard, the board considers information from a variety of sources:

- Results of a standard setting exercise, which requires a panel of content experts to estimate the performance of minimally competent entry-level nurses on a representative sample of 180 individual items. In other words, the panel looks at each question and asks, "Should we expect a minimally competent nurse to answer this question correctly?"

- What the passing standard, the pass rates, and indicators of academic readiness have been historically.

- Results of the surveys of opinions of employers and educators related to competence of recent graduates.

- Information regarding the educational readiness of high school students who express interest in nursing.

Based on careful consideration of all this information, the NCSBN board of directors decided in December 2015 to keep the passing standard for the NCLEX-RN test at the level of 0.00 logits, which was instituted in April 2013. This passing standard will remain in effect through March 2019 (NCSBN, 2016g). The NCSBN board of directors decided in December of 2016 to keep the passing standard for the NCLEX-PN at −0.21 logits. This standard will remain in effect through March 2020 (NCSBN, 2016g, 2017b). You can track future changes in the passing standard on the NCSBN website (http://www.ncsbn.org).

Logits

Although many people understand what a percentage is, most do not understand what a logit is. Logit is an abbreviation for "log odd units," which is a unit of interval measurement. The logit is used on the NCLEX as a unit of measurement ability that predicts the probability of a candidate answering an item correctly (O'Neill, 2005; NCSBN, 2012).

The NCLEX-RN has 15 pretest items, or tryout items, and the NCLEX-PN has 25 pretest items; these are not scored. Refer again to Tables 15.1 and 15.2, which illustrate how the pretest items are included on the NCLEX test plan. Pretesting items allow the NCSBN to determine the precise difficulty of the items before they are used as scored items on a test. Each pretest item is given to thousands of candidates; the difficulty of these items is tracked, and the results are statistically analyzed. The precise difficulty level of the items, relative to each other (not relative to the candidates), is identified. Only when the precise difficulty level of a pretest item is established is it added to the NCLEX item pool for inclusion as a scored item on a future exam (NCSBN, 2016e).

Once a pretest item meets the rigorous statistical standards of the NCSBN and becomes a scored item, it is placed on a continuum, which includes all the scored items in a test pool. This continuum rank-orders the items from the least difficult to the most difficult. The examinee's ability level is described as the point on the item difficulty continuum where the candidate has a 50:50 chance of answering the item correctly. The current passing standard requires the examinees' ability level to be at the point on the item difficulty continuum that represents 0.00 logits or greater for the NCLEX-RN and −0.21 logits or greater for the NCLEX-PN (NCSBN, 2016g, 2017b).

The odds ratio on the NCLEX can be described as the chance of answering an item correctly relative to the chance of answering the item incorrectly. The logit represents a transformation of the odds ratio into a useful unit of probability. The NCLEX considers person ability, item difficulty, and the passing standard on a scale, which uses logits as the unit of measurement to identify whether a candidate is successful or unsuccessful on the NCLEX (O'Neill, 2005, p. 2). Refer to the NCSBN website for an explanation of how the logit is implemented in the NCLEX exams.

Examination Length

Both the NCLEX-RN and the NCLEX-PN are variable-length tests, although they have a minimum and a maximum number of items (NCSBN, 2016c, 2017a):

- The NCLEX-RN has 75–265 items, includes 15 pretest items, and has a 6-hour time limit. (Refer to Table 15.1 for a breakdown of the items according to the NCLEX-RN test plan.)

- The NCLEX-PN has 85–205 items, includes 25 pretest items, and has a 5-hour time limit. (Refer to Table 15.2 for a breakdown of the items according to the NCLEX-PN test plan.)

The actual length of an individual's exam is determined by the candidate's responses to the items. Once a candidate answers the minimum number of items, the computer program compares the candidate's ability level to the passing standard for the first time. At that point, if the computer program determines with 95% certainty that the candidate's ability is above or below the passing standard, the test ends. If the computer program cannot determine with 95% certainty that the candidate has passed or failed, the candidate continues to receive items. From that point on, the candidate's ability estimate is recalculated and compared with the passing standard after each item is answered. The exam ends once the candidate's ability level is clearly above or below the passing standard with a 95% certainty. Obviously, candidates who are above the passing standard pass and those who are below fail (O'Neill et al., 2005; NCSBN, 2016c, 2017a).

Only those candidates whose ability estimate continues to be minimally above or minimally below the passing standard such that it is too close for the computer program to determine pass or fail with 95% certainty receive the maximum number of items. The exam ends when the maximum time limit is met or the student has answered the maximum number of items (O'Neill et al., 2005; NCSBN, 2016c, 2017a).

Because the ability estimate for a candidate who answers the maximum number of items is very precise, the 95% certainty requirement is dropped and the computer program compares the candidate's ability estimate to the passing standard. This is referred to as the maximum item rule. If the ability estimate is above the passing standard, the candidate passes. If it is below or equal to the passing standard, the candidate fails (NCSBN, 2016c, 2017a).

As O'Neill et al. (2005, p. 150) explain, when a candidate runs out of time after answering the minimum number of items but before answering the maximum number of items, the pass/fail decision process is more complex. The candidate's ability estimate is compared with the passing standard for each of the last 60 items that the candidate answered. If the candidate's ability estimate is equal to or falls below the passing standard even once on the last 60 items, the candidate fails. To pass the examination, the candidate must have maintained an ability level above the passing standard when responding to every one of the last 60 items answered on the exam.

For example, suppose a candidate runs out of time after answering the 200th item. The computer program compares the examinee's ability estimate on the 200th item to the passing standard. If the ability estimate is at or below the passing standard, the examinee fails. If the ability estimate is above the passing standard, the computer program compares the examinee's ability estimate to the passing standard on the 199th item. If this is also above passing, the computer program compares the ability estimate to the passing standard after the response to the 198th item. This process continues through the last 60 items that the student responded to, in our case, back to the 141st item. The candidate does not need to have answered each of the last 60 items correctly. As long as the candidate has answered the minimum number of items and the ability estimate remains above the passing standard for every one of the last 60 responses, the candidate passes the test (O'Neill et al., 2005, p. 150; NCSBN, 2016c, 2017a).

This does not mean that the last 60 rule bases the pass/fail decision only on the candidate's responses to the last 60 items. Remember, the candidate's ability estimate at any point in the test is based on the responses to all items up to that point, so the candidate's ability estimate before the last 60 items influences the ability estimate of the last 60 items (O'Neill et al., 2005, p. 164). In the example above, the candidate's ability estimate on the 140th item is the basis for the ability estimate on each item up to the end of the test (the 200th item in this case). O'Neill and colleagues (2005, p. 164) maintain that the last 60 rule and the maximum item rule in effect offer a second chance to those examinees who were unsuccessful in demonstrating their competency at the 95% certainty level during the test.

The NCSBN does not release the results of the test to the candidates. The results are released only to the individual state boards of nursing, which sends the results to the individual candidates. Some states allow the students to obtain their results online two business days after they take the exam. Students should check with their state board of nursing to determine whether they can receive their results online.

NCLEX Item Development

The NCLEX is a high-stakes test. Decisions that can be life altering for nursing graduates are made based on the results of these examinations. The NCSBN takes its responsibility, to both the nursing graduates and the healthcare consumers, very seriously. Therefore, the NCLEX examinations are developed to meet exacting psychometric standards. As the previous discussion demonstrates, the development of the NCLEX test plans involves a painstaking process; the process for item development is painstaking as well.

No matter how well developed the test plan, the test will not measure what it claims to measure if the items do not address the test plan (see Chapter 5, "Selected-Response Format: Developing Multiple-Choice Items"). The NCSBN goes to great lengths to develop challenging items that address the test plan to obtain valid information on which to base the decision about whether a graduate will be allowed to practice nursing.

The NCSBN considers the Item Development Program to be essential for maintaining the quality of the NCLEX. For that reason, the Item Development Program is designed to create high-quality NCLEX test items. The NCSBN recruits currently licensed nurses to serve as volunteers on item development panels, which consist of item writers and item reviewers (NCSBN, 2016d). The volunteers are a diverse group, with backgrounds in all areas of nursing specialties and practice settings.

The Item Development brochure on the NCSBN website describes the roles and requirements for application to these panels. The item writers must be licensed to practice nursing and be currently teaching nursing students in a clinical setting or be employed in a clinical setting where they work directly with nurses who have been practicing for less than 1 year. Writers for the NCLEX-RN must also have a master's or higher degree in nursing. Item writers meet for 3- to 5-day sessions where they use a computer program to develop items that reflect the competencies of newly licensed nurses under the guidance of NCSBN test developers (NCSBN, 2016d).

Item reviewers evaluate the items after they are developed. The item reviewers are nurses who are currently practicing in a clinical setting where they work directly with nurses who have been practicing for less than 1 year. The panel of judges consists of one basic/undergraduate nursing faculty member and one newly licensed nurse, in addition to qualified item writers and reviewers (NCSBN, 2016d). Consult http://www.ncsbn.org for the latest information regarding the application process for the Item Development Program.

Characteristics of NCLEX Items

Because the purpose of the NCLEX is to measure the ability of nursing candidates to practice safely and effectively, the items must be developed to accurately assess those abilities. The items that are developed to address the activities of the practice analysis within the framework of client needs must require the students to use their knowledge in real-life situations to ensure competence and to safeguard the healthcare consumer.

Cognitive Levels

The practice of nursing requires problem solving and critical thinking; nurses have to be able to apply their knowledge. For that reason, NCLEX items are designed to measure higher-order thinking ability. The NCLEX item writers use Bloom's taxonomy as a guide to writing items that are at the application or higher levels of cognitive ability (NCSBN, 2016d). Refer to Chapter 5, "Selected-Response Format: Developing Multiple-Choice Items," and Chapter 6, "Writing Critical Thinking Multiple-Choice Items," for a variety of item examples that assess higher-order thinking ability.

Critical Thinking Ability

NCLEX item writers develop items that require students to apply problem solving and critical thinking ability to prioritize complex situations, make judgments based on criteria, or combine elements to make a decision (Wendt, 2003). Chapter 6, "Writing Critical Thinking Multiple-Choice Items," provides guidance for developing multiple-choice items that assess critical thinking on your classroom exams.

Alternate Formats

The NCSBN describes alternate items as those that use technology to present items other than the standard four-option multiple-choice item. Alternate items are subjected to the same rigorous quality control as the standard four-option multiple-choice items and are also scored as either correct or incorrect; there is no partial credit on the NCLEX (NCSBN, 2016h; Wendt, 2003). The alternate item types include:

- Fill in the blank
- Point and click
- Multiple response
- Chart/exhibit
- Drag and drop

Although the NCLEX examinations continue to contain predominantly four-option multiple-choice items, alternate items have been added to both the PN and RN test pools. Alternate items will not change test plans or lengthen the tests—they are simply being used as vehicles for assessing increased cognitive processing (Wendt, 2003). Refer to Chapter 5, "Selected-Response Format: Developing Multiple-Choice Items," and Chapter 6, "Writing Critical Thinking Multiple-Choice Items," for detailed discussions of alternate-format item development.

Preparing Nursing Students for the NCLEX

Student success on the NCLEX is a major concern for nursing faculty. Issues such as accreditation, student recruitment, and even the very existence of a program are greatly affected by student success or failure on this exam. Faculty members are therefore understandably concerned with identifying strategies to promote student success. Because specific content is not included in the test plan, it is not possible to teach to this test, nor should that be the case.

Curriculum Focus

The best preparation for the NCLEX that nurse educators can offer students is to follow the guidelines outlined in this text and thus offer students a sound educational experience. If you prepare your students to meet the objectives of your nursing program, they will pass NCLEX as a secondary gain. Of course, it is essential that you follow the process outlined thus far: identifying objectives and learning outcomes, providing teaching and learning strategies to facilitate the student attainment of the objectives, and assessing the students with tools that require higher-order thinking. Although there is incredible stress for both faculty and students surrounding the results of the NCLEX, the curriculum must focus on your program objectives or you will find yourself attempting to teach to the test rather than preparing your graduates to meet the objectives of your program.

NCLEX Test Plan Consideration

Two especially valuable publications, which are available for free on the NCSBN website, are the *Detailed Test Plan for the NCLEX-RN* and the *Detailed Test Plan for the NCLEX-PN*. These publications classify the activities that were identified in the practice analyses according to the four categories of client needs (NCSBN, 2016c, 2017a). In other words, both students and faculty can obtain the clearest picture for what is included on the NCLEX by reviewing the activities identified in the detailed test plans or by reading the practice analysis. These activities should be included somewhere in your curriculum not only because they are on the NCLEX but also because they identify the competencies that are required of your new graduates (Aucoin & Treas, 2005; Wendt et al., 2010).

Although it is wise to examine the NCLEX test plan carefully to be sure that your curriculum addresses the client care activities that are identified by the practice analysis, the NCLEX activities should be integrated into your curriculum, not act as the basis for it. For example, the RN test plan, as illustrated in Table 15.1, designates 6% to 12% of the NCLEX-RN test items as health promotion and maintenance. Would you limit health promotion and maintenance to 6% to 12% of your curriculum? Remember, the tests are based on the actual practice and opinions of new graduates. Stuart (2006) points out that new graduates are still attempting to master basic psychomotor skills and recommends that nursing education is based on evidence-based care needed by patients. While it is important to provide students with the opportunity to master the knowledge required for licensure, nurse educators must focus on curricula that goes beyond the confines of a minimal-competency examination (Giddens, 2009).

Historically, the education of nurses was referred to as training, a term that has, thankfully, become obsolete. The term *education* only gradually replaced *training* as nurses endeavored over decades to establish the professional status of their occupation. The current focus on the NCLEX pass rate could precipitate a crisis in nursing education: Teaching to a test can be equated to training. Do nurse educators really want to revert to training students to pass a test, or would they prefer to educate nurses to meet the objectives of a nursing program? One point cannot be ignored: The NCLEX should support nursing education, not orchestrate it.

Classroom Test Development

The NCLEX test development process is designed to ensure that the NCLEX exams are state-of-the-art tools for measuring the knowledge, skills, and abilities of entry-level nurses to ensure safe and effective practice (Wendt, 2003; Wendt et al., 2010). It is obvious that the process is an arduous one, as any designed to ensure the quality of the information on which high-stakes decisions are made would be. Although classroom tests cannot be subjected to the same developmental rigor as the NCLEX, the process sends a message to nurse educators: Trustworthy test results depend on careful test preparation. Careful development of classroom exams is crucial for two reasons:

1. Pass/fail decisions in nursing education are high-stakes, life-altering decisions.
2. Developing high-level, challenging exams that require students to think throughout the course of their nursing program prepares them for nursing practice as well as the NCLEX.

The suggestions offered in previous chapters help you to ensure the quality of your classroom exams. Also, the *Detailed Test Plan for the NCLEX-RN* and the *Detailed Test Plan for the NCLEX-PN* provide very useful guides for item development. These are the documents that the NCLEX item writers use as guides when developing test items for the NCLEX (NCSBN, 2016c, 2017a). These publications are valuable resources for faculty in several ways. For example, when developing a unit on pharmacological pain management, it would be very helpful to review the content listed for pharmacological pain management as a resource for both providing classroom instructional opportunities and developing exam items. These documents should be in every nurse educator's reference library.

Cross-Referencing the NCLEX Test Plans

Table 15.3 provides a worksheet for an NCLEX-RN exam-based cross-reference, and **Table 15.4** provides a worksheet for an NCLEX-PN exam-based cross-reference.

Table 15.3   An NCLEX-RN Cross-Reference Worksheet

Client Needs Content	1. Management of care (17%–23%)	2. Safety and infection control (9%–15%)	3. Health promotion and maintenance (6%–12%)	4. Psychosocial integrity (6%–12%)	5. Basic care and comfort (6%–12%)	6. Pharmacological and parenteral therapies (12%–18%)	7. Reduction of risk potential (9%–15%)	8. Physiological adaptation (11%–17%)
	1	2	3	4	5	6	7	8
I								
II								
III								
IV								
V								
VI								
VII								
VIII								

Data from National Council of State Boards of Nursing. (2016c). *2016 NCLEX-RN detailed test plan*. Chicago, IL: Author.

These charts offer a column to include content that creates a cross-reference for your classroom exams. They can be useful for evaluating exams that purport to be NCLEX preparation tests and are also useful as a cross-reference for evaluating if your classroom exams are addressing the activities that new nursing graduates are involved in, as identified in the practice analyses.

While cross-referencing for the NCLEX client's needs is helpful, it would be counterproductive to blueprint your classroom exams using this method. The only valid approach for developing a classroom test blueprint is to base it on the course content and your instructional objectives, as described in Chapter 4, "Implementing Systematic Test Development."

Table 15.4   An NCLEX-PN Cross-Reference Worksheet

	1. Coordinated care (18%–24%)	2. Safety and infection control (10%–16%)	3. Health promotion and maintenance (6%–12%)	4. Psychosocial integrity (9%–15%)	5. Basic care and comfort (7%–13%)	6. Pharmacological therapies (10%–16%)	7. Reduction of risk potential (9%–15%)	8. Physiological adaptation (7%–13%)
Objectives	1	2	3	4	5	6	7	8
Content								
I								
II								
III								
IV								
V								
VI								
VII								
VIII								

Data from National Council of State Boards of Nursing. (2017). *2017 NCLEX-PN detailed test plan*. Chicago, IL: Author.

Cross-Referencing for Integrated Processes

Just as the NCLEX test plans integrate several concepts and processes without specifically blueprinting them, you may also be interested in identifying constructs that are included in your exams but not specifically represented on your blueprints. The nursing process in particular is an area of interest for most faculty members. Nursing test items are most effective when written in terms of the nursing process (as Chapter 5, "Selected-Response Format: Developing Multiple-Choice Items," discusses). Appendix E, "Sample Item Stems for Phases of the Nursing Process," provides sample item stems for the five phases of the nursing process. You can use sample item stems as templates to assist you in developing nursing process multiple-choice items that reflect real-life clinical situations.

Tables 15.5, 15.6, and **15.7** provide cross-reference worksheets for the integrated processes of nursing process, cognitive levels, and communication/documentation, respectively.

Table 15.5   A Nursing Process Cross-Reference Worksheet

	Exam I	Exam II	Exam III	Final
Assessment				
Analysis				
Plan/implement				
Evaluate				
Total				

Table 15.6   A Cognitive Level Cross-Reference Worksheet

	Exam I	Exam II	Exam III	Final
Comprehensive				
Analysis				
Application				
Total				

Table 15.7   A Communication/Documentation Cross-Reference Worksheet

	Exam I	Exam II	Exam III	Final
Communication				
Documentation				
Total				

Although completing these worksheets will assist you with your test analysis, they can also be quite tedious to complete. However, as Chapter 14, "Instituting Item Banking and Test Development Software," discusses, test development software enables you to bypass tedious manual data entry and easily code and classify items so that completing grids such as these is simply a matter of clicking your mouse.

Standardized Examinations

Numerous commercial testing companies produce exams for student nurses. Entrance exams, course content exams, critical thinking exams, comprehensive exams, and exit exams are among the many types offered for assessing students all the way through their nursing programs. These assessment and remediation programs are costly, which is why there is big profit in providing testing services for nursing education. According to the NCSBN (2016f), 208,840 U.S.-educated candidates took the NCLEX-RN and NCLEX-PN for the first time in 2015. We can estimate that at least double that number is currently enrolled in schools of nursing across the country. Do the math: Commercial testing companies have the potential for making huge profits.

As Giddens (2009) notes, the cost of these programs poses the question: "Who is benefitting the most—the students or the testing companies?" You need to make sure that you clearly understand what you are buying and are not misled by marketing tactics.

Standardized examinations can be a valuable component of an assessment plan. When these exams are integrated throughout a nursing program, they provide valuable feedback for students and faculty. They provide helpful information for comparing your students to students in other nursing programs across the country. This information can assist you in identifying strengths and weaknesses in your program and, it is useful for evaluating and revising curriculum (National League for Nursing [NLN], 2012; Spector & Alexander, 2006).

Obviously, it is important to examine a test carefully before purchasing it for your program. Examine the test's psychometric parameters; they should be available from the vendor. Ask for a sample of the items and compare them with the criteria discussed previously to evaluate whether they are measuring higher-order thinking. If the items do not meet these standards, do not purchase the exam. If you are satisfied with the quality of the items, ask the following questions to determine whether the exam meets the criteria for a trustworthy standardized exam—in this case, one that has validity evidence related to your course content and objectives:

- What is the test blueprint or table of specifications?
- How was the test plan developed?
- What sample was the test normed on? Ask for the list of schools that participated in establishing the norms and the level of the students whose scores were used in the norming process.
- What is the reliability coefficient of the test?
- What specific content is covered in the test?
- Which schools currently use the test?
- How many items are on the exam?
- How much time is allowed to complete the exam?
- Which item formats are used on the test?

Although standardized exams are helpful tools, students can be negatively affected when the results of these tests are used for purposes other than those for which they were designed (NLN, 2012). For example, when you include the results of a standardized exam in a course grade, you must provide evidence that the test results are valid indicators of a student's mastery of the content and objectives of your course. When developing a test to inform decisions about student progression in a course of study, the content domain on the test must be limited to what the students have had the opportunity to learn during the course (American Educational Research Association [AERA], American Psychological Association, & National Council on Measurement in Education, 2014, p. 15). Discussions about validity establish that validity evidence is required for every interpretation of a test's results. If you do not have evidence that the standardized exam is measuring the content and objectives of your course, you cannot justify including the test results in the students' grades.

In fact, your students could require you to provide evidence of the legal defensibility of including a score from a standardized exam in their course grade. If you cannot demonstrate the relationship of the content on the test to the content taught in the classroom, the curriculum validity of the standardized exam could be questioned (Brookhart & Nitko, 2014). Even if the students do not challenge the legality of a test, professional ethics requires educators to establish validity evidence for every test result that is used to make decisions about students.

Progression Policies

Nursing programs are under so much pressure to have an above-average NCLEX first-time pass rate that one wonders whether the Lake Wobegon effect has taken hold in nursing education. The Lake Wobegon effect refers to an imaginary community where all children are above average (Lyman, 1998). This effect, applied to nursing, would mean that every state would report that all of their nursing graduates were above the national average for passing the NCLEX on their first attempt! Although these results are impossible, nurse educators across the country are expressing concern that they are being held to this standard. Giddens (2009) suggests that nurse educators should initiate discussion with the NCSBN to identify new mechanisms to validate entry-level competence.

Today, the pass rate for first-time U.S.-educated test takers continues to have a powerful hold on nursing programs. Schools that have first-time pass rates below their state's passing standard risk losing the approval of their state board of nursing (Spector & Alexander, 2006). Thus, it is understandable that nurse educators are implementing programs to maintain or increase the NCLEX first-time passing rate of their graduates.

Because of the increasing pressure for students to pass the NCLEX, schools across the country are implementing progression policies. A progression policy is a school policy that establishes the criteria that students must meet to progress through a nursing program. These policies, when carefully implemented throughout a nursing program, can help to maintain a level of quality in nursing education. The problem arises when schools use a single exam, such as an exit exam, as the sole criterion for graduation or permission to take the NCLEX (Spector & Alexander, 2006; Spurlock & Hunt, 2008). This approach is being implemented because nursing faculty are concerned that low-achieving students will fail the NCLEX and their program's pass rate will be unacceptable. Giddens (2009) asserts that this practice is unfair and borders on unethical educational practice. Spurlock (2013) notes that progression policies that prevent low-achieving students from taking the NCLEX only artificially increase licensure pass rates and do not improve the quality of the educational program. These policies are actually providing a disservice for the students who are at risk for failing the NCLEX because they divert attention from the real educational issues that are affecting the program.

NCLEX Predictor Exit Exams

NCLEX predictor exams or exit exams purport to predict which students will pass the NCLEX. Most also identify student weaknesses and offer remediation for the student to follow and thus improve their chances for passing NCLEX. An exit exam can be a very useful tool when it is used as part of an assessment program.

As with any standardized exam, it is important to review an exit exam carefully before purchasing it. If you are satisfied with the quality of the items, ask the following questions to determine whether the exam meets the criteria for a trustworthy standardized exam—in this case one that has established evidence of predictive validity as well as evidence based on the test content of the NCLEX:

- Which schools currently use the test?
- How many items are on the exam?
- How much time is allowed to complete the test?
- Are all items four-option multiple-choice?
- Is the exam based on the NCLEX test plan?
- Can I review a sample of how several items are coded related to the client needs?
- How are the nursing specialties (adult health, women's health, child health, and mental health) weighted in the exam?
- What is the cut score for predicting NCLEX passing? (The cut score is the minimum score that the student must attain to be predicted to pass the NCLEX.)
- What percentage of students who were predicted to fail (or not predicted to pass) actually passed the NCLEX last year?

The last two items are particularly important. The publishers of these exit exams usually advertise their high level of accuracy at predicting those who will pass the NCLEX exam; this predictive value is the test's negative predictive value score.

If a testing company sets its cut score for passing at a very high level, it is bound to identify accurately those who will pass NCLEX. For example, if you give students a test of 100 items and the cut score is 95, then the test will predict that those who score above 95% will pass NCLEX. Obviously, predicting that only a very few of the top students will pass NCLEX increases the chance that a high percentage of those who you predict to pass will pass. After all, 84.53% of the U.S.-educated first-time test takers passed NCLEX-RN, and 81.89% of the U.S.-educated first-time test takers passed the NCLEX-PN in 2015 (NCSBN, 2016f).

The most important indicator of a test's predictive ability is its positive predictive value scores. When students who are predicted to fail actually pass the test, the test has a low positive predictive value. A low positive predictive value has a negative impact on the students; it means that students who score low on an exit exam and are prohibited from graduating or taking the NCLEX actually would pass the NCLEX if they were allowed to take it (Spurlock & Hanks, 2004, pp. 542–543).

Table 15.8 illustrates a hypothetical example of predictive values for an exit exam. Suppose an exit exam of 100 items is given to 100 students. The cut score for the test is 90. Fifty students who obtain a score of 90 or above are predicted to pass the NCLEX. Therefore, 50% of the students who score below the cut score are not predicted to pass, which is the equivalent of predicting that those students will fail the NCLEX. All the students take the NCLEX. Forty-eight students who were predicted to pass actually pass the NCLEX, for a passing prediction of 96%. However, only 12 of 50 students who were not predicted to pass actually fail the NCLEX, for a failing prediction of 24%. In addition, the pass rate for the entire group is 86% as opposed to the 50% that was predicted by the test. The overall ability of the test to correctly classify students as predicted to pass or predicted to fail is only 60%.

Table 15.8   Illustration of Predictive Values Score Data

Students Predicted to Pass	Actual Pass	Actual Fail	Accurately Predicted	Predictive Value
50	48	2	48	96%

Students Predicted to Fail or Not Predicted to Pass	Actual Pass	Actual Fail	Accurately Predicted	Predictive Value
50	38	12	12	24%

Total Students	Predicted to Pass and Actually Passed	Predicted to Fail and Actually Failed	Accurately Predicted	Accuracy of Prediction	Predicted Pass Rate	Actual Pass Rate
100	48	12	60	60%	50%	86%

Testing companies want to show themselves in the best light, so they usually do not report their accuracy for correctly identifying those who will fail the NCLEX. In fact, most companies state that they do not predict failure at all. However, when students are prevented from taking the NCLEX because they did not attain a predetermined score on an exit exam, the effect is the same as predicting that they will fail (Spurlock, 2006; Spurlock & Hunt, 2008).

Testing companies often neglect to report NCLEX pass rates for students who do not achieve the benchmark score. Take, for example, Young and Wilson's (2012) validity study for predicting NCLEX-RN success based on the results on the HESI Exit Exam. In 2007, they conducted a survey that attempted to link obtaining the benchmark score on the HESI exam to passing the NCLEX-RN. The survey obtained responses from 72 nursing programs representing 4,383 nursing students. Of the 4,383 students, only 1,075 achieved the benchmark score or higher on their first attempt at taking the HESI exam. Out of these 1,075 who were predicted to pass NCLEX-RN on their first attempt, 1,066 actually passed. Based on these results, the HESI Company reported that their test has a predictive accuracy of 99%. Young and Wilson also reported that of the 730 who were required to take the HESI test a second time, 271 students achieved the benchmark score and 259 (95.57%) passed NCLEX-RN an their first attempt. An additional 367 students took the HESI test a third time; 148 of these scored at or above the benchmark and 138 (93.24%) went on to pass NCLEX-RN on their first attempt. Based on these findings, Young and Wilson claim that the HESI Exit Exam had a predictive accuracy of 97.93%, regardless of whether the student achieved the benchmark score on the first, second, or third attempt at taking the HESI test (p.12).

It is clear that this approach for evaluating predictive accuracy is very flawed. Yet many testing companies take a misleading approach when interpreting data in order to show themselves in the best light and increase the sales of their testing products. Young and Wilson (2012) are evaluating NCLEX success for 4,383 students, yet they only report the success rate for the 1,494 students who achieved the benchmark score on the HESI test. These 1,494 were predicted to pass NCLEX-RN on their first attempt; that means that 34% of the total group was predicted to pass. This is a very low prediction indeed, given that 84.53% of the first-time U.S.-educated examinees actually passed the NCLEX-RN on their first attempt in 2015 (NCSBN, 2016f).

This validity study is incomplete. What happened to the 2,889 students who were not predicted to pass? Did they all fail? What were the score intervals for all the students who took the HESI with their corresponding pass rates? How accurate is the HESI test for predicting failure on the NCLEX?

The actual objective of an exit exam should be to identify those who are at risk for failing and provide them with remediation so they can pass the NCLEX. Because exit exams target lower-performing students, the predictability of NCLEX pass rates at varying score points should be investigated and identified (Sosa & Sethares, 2015). Before you purchase an exit exam, particularly if you are including the results in your progression policy, find out how accurate it is at identifying student weaknesses and use the test results only as part of a comprehensive assessment of student abilities.

Spurlock (2006) identifies that an increasing number of nursing programs are implementing progression policies that prevent students from taking the NCLEX based on an unacceptable score on an exit exam. Young and Wilson (2012) state that 47% of the 45 schools that responded to their survey reported delaying or denying graduation to those students who failed to meet the benchmark score on the HESI Exit Exam.

What validity evidence is there for these policies? Is the exit exam blueprinted to provide evidence that the students have mastered the program objectives? If one of the objectives of the program is that the "students will pass an NCLEX predictor test," the decision may be justified, but how will the accrediting agencies view this objective? Consider the validity guidelines presented in the *Standards for Educational and Psychological Testing* (AERA et al., 2014, p. 15): "When student mastery of a delivered curriculum is tested for purposes of informing decisions about individual students, such as promotion or graduation, the framework elaborating a content domain is appropriately limited to what students have had an opportunity to learn from the curriculum as delivered."

Standardized exit exams can be useful tools as part of a school's assessment program; however, they cannot be used as the sole predictor for student success on the NCLEX. Morin (2006, p. 309) identifies that "there are several valid and reliable instruments available to help predict student success in the NCLEX-RN. None, however, should be used as the only predictor of success." It is inherently unfair to prevent a student from finishing a 2-, 3-, or 4-year program based on the results of one exam. Consider the time commitment and the financial obligation students have assumed. Students should not be promoted through a program of nursing study only to be turned away, often with substantial debt, because the program did not prepare them to take the licensure exam. It is true that the state boards of nursing are mandated to protect the public, but they are also concerned with fairness, attrition rates, and the quality of the education that nursing students receive.

The boards of nursing are responding to the increase in use of exit exams. Spector and Alexander (2006) reported the results of an informal survey of the 60 boards of nursing. Fifteen of the boards reported having concerns with the use of exit examinations, which they manage in various ways. One state requires that exit examinations alone not be used as a bar to graduation when all other program requirements have been met. Several states have investigated nursing programs for lack of fair and ethical practices when exit exams unfairly inhibited program completion. Many states have regulations requiring programs to have written policies stating the requirements for graduation. In these states, a program using an exit exam without a written policy would be in violation of state rules.

Even when a written policy includes an exit exam as a graduation requirement, this practice has ethical and legal implications. Standard 12.0 from the *Standards for Educational and Psychological Testing* (AERA et al., 2014, p. 198) clearly states, "In educational settings, a decision or characterization that will have a major impact on a student should take into consideration not just scores from a single test but other relevant information."

Spurlock and Hanks (2004, p. 544) point out that students who are prevented from graduating or taking the NCLEX based on an exam that has a low positive predictive value are being treated unjustly. If students who would have passed the NCLEX were prevented from taking the exam because they failed an exit exam that has a low ability to predict accurately failing the NCLEX, they would have a legitimate claim that they received unnecessary and injurious treatment.

Brookhart and Nitko (2014, p. 92) discuss the issue of due process when considering the legal defensibility of a high-stakes test. Previous discussion establishes that an exit exam is considered a high-stakes test when it is used to determine qualification for graduation or taking the NCLEX. Substantive due process is concerned with the appropriateness and the purpose of a requirement. Is it appropriate to deny graduation to a student who is predicted to fail the NCLEX based on the results of an exam that has a low ability to predict failure on NCLEX? Whether or not students seek legal redress related to a progression policy, educators have the professional responsibility to ensure that results of a standardized exam are valid for the intended interpretation and use (Brookhart & Nitko, 2014, p. 43).

Ask these two questions:

1. What is the predictive validity for accurately identifying those who will fail the NCLEX?
2. How can the results of one test be used to prevent students from taking the NCLEX?

Review Table 15.8 again for an example of how students could be affected by a progression policy that is based on the results of one exam. The hypothetical exit exam predicted that 50 students would fail the NCLEX. However, only 12 actually failed. In this case, if those 50 were prevented from taking the NCLEX, 38 students who would have passed would have been denied the opportunity to practice nursing. It is unlikely that a school would deny graduation to so many students, but even if the number was much smaller, the situation is still unfair. Only tests that are based on a program's curriculum should be used to permit or prohibit graduation.

Requiring students who obtain a low score on an exit exam to participate in a carefully structured remediation program is a reasonable policy. However, requiring students to retake an exam until they receive a passing score can be counterproductive. In fact, Spurlock and Hunt (2008) identified that only the first score on a popular national exit exam (HESI) was statistically significant for predicting NCLEX-RN outcomes. Young and Wilson (2012) also found that significantly more students who met the benchmark on their first attempt on the HESI Exit Exam passed NCLEX than those who met the benchmark on their second or third attempt. Their findings also indicated that 53% of the 45 schools surveyed required students who did not attain the benchmark to retake the HESI Exit Exam. Twenty percent of these schools required the students to retake the test more than four times! Faculty must consider that taking the test repeatedly results in a delay in taking the NCLEX that is associated with a decreased pass rate (NCSBN, 2002).

Before establishing a policy requiring students to retake a standardized test, ask yourself these questions:

- How many versions of the test are there?
- Have they been equated to ensure that they are parallel forms of the test?
- How many times can a student repeat the test?
- What does the student learn from repeatedly taking the same exam?
- What is the test really measuring after it is repeated several times?
- How long will the student be delayed in taking the NCLEX?

When deciding how to implement a standardized exam or what the "passing" or "cut" score will be, nursing faculty should be mindful of the exacting process that the NCSBN uses to determine where to set the passing standard for licensure. As O'Neill and colleagues (2005) point out, it is important to set the passing standard high enough to protect the public, but they also identify the importance of setting the standard low enough that competent nurses are not denied licensure. Nursing faculty have the responsibility to ensure that students are well prepared to succeed, not to prevent well-prepared students from succeeding.

Facilitating Student Success

If your students are not successful on a standardized exit exam, you must ask why this is so. Are your classroom exam items written at lower cognitive levels? Are the objectives and content of your courses appropriate? How can you justify preventing students from taking the NCLEX if they have successfully completed your program? Does the problem lie with your students or with the curriculum they have successfully completed? These are difficult questions to answer, but they are important ones that must be addressed in the interest of fairness.

Academic decisions cannot be based on the results of one test. Nurse educators must consider more of the evidence related to NCLEX success when developing progression policies. The literature documents that factors such as grade point average, nursing course grades, reading ability, and SAT scores are associated with NCLEX success more consistently than the results of an exit exam (Alameida, et al., 2011; Beeman & Waterhouse, 2001; Eddy & Epeneter, 2002; Haas, Nugent, & Rule, 2004; Higgins, 2005; Landry, Davis, Alameida, Prive, & Renwanz-Boyle, 2010; McGahee, Gramling, & Reid, 2010; Ostyre, 2001; Poorman, Mastorovich, Liberto, & Gerwick, 2010; Romeo, 2013; Schlairet, Green, & Benton, 2014; Seldomridge & DiBartolo, 2004; Thomas & Baker, 2011; Waterhouse & Beeman, 2003; Yellin & Geoffrion, 2001; Yin & Burger, 2003).

It is time to refocus from trying to predict NCLEX success to trying to facilitate student success. While there is an abundance of research related to predicting NCLEX success, the research related to examining instructional approaches that promote student achievement is limited (DiBartolo & Seldomridge, 2005). Griffiths, Papastrat, Czekanski, and Hagan (2004, p. 324) note that, while the factors that indicate student success on NCLEX have been extensively examined, the measures adopted to predict success are not absolutely reliable. It is essential for nursing faculty to consider strategies, such as curriculum revision or changes in instructional methods, to promote greater success for graduates and programs.

The basic premise applies: Prepare your students with a solid curriculum to meet your program objectives and they will also be prepared to pass the NCLEX (Koestler, 2015). Certainly, some of the students will not be successful, but it only makes sense to identify those individuals early in the program. Therefore, it is essential to challenge the students with exams that test their ability to think from the beginning of the program. You cannot expect students to be successful on the NCLEX, a test that includes only items that challenge students' thinking ability, when they have only been exposed to items that require memorization. In fact, graduates too often report that their nursing programs did not prepare them for the items on the NCLEX.

Johnson and Mighten's (2005, p. 321) study supports the assertion that is being voiced increasingly by nurse educators: Traditional lecture is not the most effective method for promoting the critical thinking skills that are necessary for completing a nursing program and passing the NCLEX. Numerous authors advocate alternative strategies for teaching that involve the student in active learning (Amerson, 2006; Bastable, 2007; Bellack, 2005; Bradshaw & Lowenstein, 2011; Candela, Dalley, & Benzel-Lindley, 2006; Clayton, 2006; Delpier, 2006; Diekelmann, 2002; Fay, Johnson, & Selz, 2006; Ferguson & Day, 2005; Hanna, Roberts, & Hurley, 2016; Herrman, 2008; Koestler, 2015; Mastrian, McGonigle, Mhan, & Bixler, 2011; Pugsley & Clayton, 2003; Valiga, 2003). Educators cannot expect students to think critically if they are not afforded the opportunity to develop critical thinking skills.

Ironside and Valiga (2006) believe that faculty across the country are moving toward excellence in nursing education, as evidenced by the increasing discussion and implementation of innovative strategies, beyond the traditional lecture, to promote student ability in both the classroom and practice arenas. Griffiths et al. (2004, p. 324) clearly summarize this situation: "The NCLEX experience is not an end-of-program experience, but rather a program-long opportunity to build the knowledge and skills that will ensure nursing program graduates demonstrate the quality of our academic efforts."

NCLEX Prep Courses

NCLEX prep courses are a good idea. Although they are no substitute for a solid nursing program, every student should be encouraged to take one. When these courses are well prepared, they help the graduates in several ways by:

- Decreasing test anxiety
- Consolidating a huge body of information
- Helping graduates to focus on important concepts
- Providing large numbers of practice items
- Offering the opportunity to discuss the rationales for test items
- Reinforcing what the graduate learned in the basic program

There is a prep course for every licensing and certification exam for every profession. That alone is a testimonial to their value. While every student should enroll in an NCLEX prep course, all courses are not alike. The key issue is the quality of the course. While 208,840 U.S.-educated candidates took the NCLEX-RN and the NCLEX-PN for the first time in 2015, more than 299,000 candidates in total took the NCLEX that same year (NCSBN, 2016f). Test prep is big business! Before recommending a course or providing a course on your campus for your students, you should examine the course materials and investigate several questions:

- What is the cost of the course?
- Are the faculty members experienced nurse educators?
- How long has the course been in operation?
- What is the NCLEX pass rate for students who complete the course?
- What additional help is offered for those who actually fail the NCLEX?
- Do the students have to listen to endless hours of content review that reiterates what they learned in their basic program?
- Are the students provided with lots of opportunity to practice and analyze items that require critical thinking?
- Who developed the items?
- What is the quality of the items?
- How much focus is placed on thinking through a problem as opposed to relying on test-taking tips?

Students make a significant financial commitment when taking an NCLEX test prep course, in addition to the $200 fee (NCSBN, 2016e) for taking the actual NCLEX. So it behooves them to shop carefully. A quality NCLEX review program does not rely on feeding students a lot of tips or rules they should follow steadfastly because the NCLEX developers know all the tips. A quality program reinforces what students have already learned and exposes them to new situations in which they must apply their knowledge. In other words, a quality program enhances the students' ability to apply the content that they have mastered in their basic nursing program.

In fact, students can be misled by some of the tips that are offered. With a linear test (one that presents the same items to all students), it can be beneficial to guess if you run out of time. Wild guessing will not help on the NCLEX CAT exam. In fact, it is likely to cause the candidate to fail because of the way the exam is scored. Yet some review courses encourage guessing. So be wary of a course that relies on tips. The students should go with what they know, even if they are violating a tip!

Here are several suggestions, both from my experience and the NCSBN publications (NCSBN, 2016d, 2016e), that you should share with your students:

- The NCSBN does not designate a preset number of students to fail the exam.
- The test is designed to measure entry-level practice, not advanced nursing practice.

- The exam tests important concepts, not trivia.
- When you read each item, ask yourself, "What is the problem or potential problem?" before you read the options.
- NCLEX tests your ability to think, not to memorize facts.
- Spend only 1 or 2 minutes on each item. Remember, some of the items included in the first 75 items for the NCLEX-RN test and 85 items for the NCLEX-PN test are pretest items and they do not count in your score, so move on.
- You have plenty of time, but pace yourself just in case you receive the maximum number of items. It is better to answer the maximum number of items than to run out of time.
- Stay calm. Do not worry if the items seem difficult; you can expect to miss 50% of the items.
- You cannot go back to review items or change your answers. You must answer before the computer gives you a new item. Make an intelligent guess and move on if an item seems too difficult for you.
- The number of items you receive does not determine whether you pass or fail.
- Schedule an appointment to take the exam as soon as possible after you graduate. Pass rates tend to decline for students who delay taking the exam.
- Take the exam seriously. The results have an important impact on the school's accreditation status.
- The NCLEX uses some terms that may not be familiar, such as prescriptions instead of doctor's orders.

Become familiar with the candidates section at http://www.ncsbn.org to review all the latest information on taking the NCLEX.

Summary

It is important for nurse educators to be familiar with the entire NCLEX process, as reviewed in detail in this chapter. The activities associated with the NCLEX, including subject areas and critical thinking skills, should be considered as an overlay to a sound curriculum. This chapter establishes the importance of being familiar with the issues surrounding NCLEX preparation. It behooves all nurse educators to carefully examine these issues to determine and implement fairly the policies and strategies that promote student success with NCLEX.

Henry Ford said, "Whether you believe that you can, or you believe that you cannot, you are correct." The best help that you can offer to your students for passing the NCLEX is to provide them with a solid curriculum, foster their critical thinking ability, challenge them with high-level exams, and encourage them to believe in themselves. If you establish your curriculum so that you have prepared your students to meet your program objectives, they will have the ability and the self-confidence that they need to pass NCLEX.

Learning Activities

1. Discuss the process for validating the results of the NCLEX-RN and NCLEX-PN exams. How is the validation process reflected in the test plans?

2. Describe the similarities and differences of the test plans for the NCLEX-RN and the NCLEX-PN tests. Discuss the rational for the differences in the test plans, including:
   - Subcategories of client needs
   - Percentages of items in each client needs category
   - Length and time allowed for each exam

3. Identify the range of items a student who answers 125 items on the NCLEX-RN exam would receive from each client needs category.

4. Develop an item from your area of expertise for each of the NCLEX alternative item formats, including:
   - Fill in the blank
   - Point and click
   - Multiple response
   - Chart/exhibit
   - Drag and drop

5. How would you explain the CAT format for the NCLEX to a student? Include:
   - The test plan
   - The maximum number of items on the test
   - The maximum length of time for the test
   - The meaning of pretest items
   - The ability estimate
   - The passing standard

6. Describe how the pass/fail decision is made for the NCLEX exam, including:
   - 95% certainty
   - Maximum number of items
   - Maximum time limit

7. How would you implement the use of a standardized exit exam in your nursing program?

8. What factors would you consider when recommending an NCLEX prep course?

9. What are the three most important recommendations you would you give a student who is preparing to take the NCLEX exam?

Web Links

American Association of Colleges of Nursing
http://www.aacn.org
National Council of State Boards of Nursing
http://www.ncsbn.org
National League for Nursing
http://www.nln.org

References

Alameida, M. D., Prince, A., Davis, H. C., Landry, L., Renwanz-Boyle, & Dunham, M. (2011). Predicting NCLEX-RN success in a diverse student population. *Journal of Nursing Education, 50*(5), 261–267.

American Educational Research Association, American Psychological Association, & National Council on Measurement in Education. (2014). *Standards for educational and psychological testing.* Washington, DC: American Educational Research Association.

Amerson, R. (2006). Energizing the nursing lecture: Application of the theory of multiple intelligence learning. *Nursing Education Perspectives, 27,* 194–196.

Aucoin, J. W., & Treas, L. (2005). Assumptions and realities of the NCLEX-RN. *Nursing Education Perspectives, 26,* 268–271.

Bastable, S. B. (2007). *Nurse as educator: Principles of teaching and learning for nursing practice* (3rd ed.). Sudbury, MA: Jones and Bartlett.

Beeman, P. B., & Waterhouse, J. K. (2001). NCLEX-RN performance: Predicting success on the computerized examination. *Journal of Professional Nursing, 17,* 158–165.

Bellack, J. P. (2005). Teaching for learning and improvement. *Journal of Nursing Education, 44,* 295–296.

Bradshaw, M. J., & Lowenstein, A. J. (2011). *Innovative teaching strategies in nursing and related health professions* (5th ed.). Sudbury, MA: Jones and Bartlett.

Brookhart, S. M., & Nitko, A. J. (2014). *Educational assessment of students* (7th ed.). Upper Saddle River, NJ: Pearson Education.

Candela, L., Dalley, K., & Benzel-Lindley, J. (2006). A case for learning-centered curricula. *Journal of Nursing Education, 45,* 59–65.

Chinn, R. N., & Hertz, N. R. (2010). *Job analysis: A guide for credentialing organizations.* Lexington, KY: Council of Licensure, Enforcement and Regulation.

Clayton, L. H. (2006). Concept mapping: An effective, active teaching-learning model. *Nursing Education Perspectives, 27,* 197–203.

Delpier, T. (2006). Cases 101: Learning to teach with cases. *Nursing Education Perspectives, 27,* 203–209.

DiBartolo, M. C., & Seldomridge, L. A. (2005). A review of intervention studies to promote NCLEX-RN success of baccalaureate students. *Nurse Educator, 30,* 166–171.

Diekelmann, N. (2002). "Too much content . . .": Epistemologies' grasp and nursing education. *Journal of Nursing Education, 41,* 469–470.

Eddy, L. L., & Epeneter, B. J. (2002). The NCLEX-RN experience: Qualitative interviews with graduates of a baccalaureate nursing program. *Journal of Nursing Education, 41,* 273–278.

Fay, V. P., Johnson, J., & Selz, N. (2006). Active learning in nursing. *Nurse Educator, 31,* 65–68.

Ferguson, L., & Day, R. A. (2005). Evidence-based nursing education: Myth or reality? *Journal of Nursing Education, 44,* 107–115.

Giddens, J. F. (2009). Changing paradigms and challenging assumptions: Redefining quality and NCLEX-RN pass rates. *Journal of Nursing Education, 48,* 123–124.

Griffiths, M. J., Papastrat, K., Czekanski, K., & Hagan, K. (2004). Research briefs: The lived experience of NCLEX failure. *Journal of Nursing Education, 43,* 322–325.

Haas, R. E., Nugent, K. E., & Rule, R. A. (2004). The use of discriminant function analysis to predict student success on the NCLEX-RN. *Journal of Nursing Education, 43,* 440–446.

Hanna, K., Roberts, T, & Hurley, S. (2016). Collaborative testing as NCLEX enrichment. *Nurse Educator, 31*(4), 171–174.

Herrman, J. W. (2008). *Creative teaching strategies for the nurse educator.* Philadelphia, PA: F. A. Davis.

Higgins, B. (2005). Strategies for lowering attrition rates and raising NCLEX-RN pass rates. *Journal of Nursing Education, 44,* 541–547.

Ironside, P. M., & Valiga, T. M. (2006). Creating a vision for the future of nursing education. *Nursing Education Perspectives, 27,* 120–121.

Johnson, J. P., & Mighten, A. (2005). A comparison of teaching strategies: Lecture notes combined with structured group discussion versus lecture only. *Journal of Nursing Education, 44,* 319–322.

Koestler, D. L. (2015). Improving NCLEX-RN first-time pass rates with a balanced curriculum. *Nursing Education Perspectives, 36,* 55–57.

Landry, L. G., Davis, H., Alameida, M. D., Prive, A., & Renwanz-Boyle, A. (2010). Predictors of NCLEX-RN success across 3 prelicensure program types. *Nurse Educator, 35,* 259–263.

Lyman, H. L. (1998). *Test scores and what they mean* (6th ed.). Boston, MA: Allyn and Bacon.

Mastrian, K. G., McGonigle, D., Mhan, W. L., & Bixler, B. (2011). *Integrating technology in nursing education.* Sudbury, MA: Jones and Bartlett.

McGahee, T. W., Gramling, L., & Reid, T. R. (2010). NCLEX-RN success: Are there predictors? *Southern Online Journal of Nursing Research, 10*(4). Retrieved from http://www.resourcenter.net/images/SNRS/Files/SOJNR_articles2/Vol10Num04 Main.html

Morin, K. H. (2006). Commentary: Use of the HESI Exit Examination in schools of nursing. *Journal of Nursing Education, 45*(8), 308–310.

National Council of State Boards of Nursing. (2002). *The NCLEX delay pass rate study.* Chicago, IL: Author.

National Council of State Boards of Nursing. (2012). What is a logit? Retrieved from https://www.ncsbn.org/What_is_a_logit/pdf

National Council of State Boards of Nursing. (2013). *2012 LPN/VN practice analysis: Linking the NCLEX-PN examination to practice.* Chicago, IL: Author.

National Council of State Boards of Nursing. (2014). *NCSBN news release: NCSBN opens registration for NCLEX in Canada.* Retrieved from www.nanb.nb.ca/media /news/NCSBN_News_Release_10-22-2014-E.pdf

National Council of State Boards of Nursing. (2015). *2014 RN practice analysis: Linking the NCLEX-RN examination to practice.* Chicago, IL: Author.

National Council of State Boards of Nursing. (2016a). *2015 LPN/VN practice analysis: Linking the NCLEX-PN examination to practice.* Chicago, IL: Author.

National Council of State Boards of Nursing. (2016b). *Computerized adaptive testing (CAT).* Retrieved from https://ncsbn.org/1216.htm

National Council of State Boards of Nursing. (2016c). *Detailed test plan for the National Council licensure examination for registered nurses.* Chicago, IL: Author.

National Council of State Boards of Nursing. (2016d). *Item development brochure*. Retrieved from https://www.ncsbn.org/item_Development_Brochure.pdf

National Council of State Boards of Nursing. (2016e). *NCLEX examination candidate bulletin*. Chicago, IL: Author.

National Council of State Boards of Nursing. (2016f). *NCLEX pass rates 2015*. Retrieved from https://www.ncsbn.org/7285.htm

National Council of State Boards of Nursing. (2016g). *Setting the NCLEX passing standard*. Retrieved from https://www.ncsbn.org/2630.htm

National Council of State Boards of Nursing. (2016h). *What the exam looks like*. Retrieved from https://www.ncsbn.org/2334.htm

National Council of State Boards of Nursing. (2017a). *2017 detailed test plan for the National Council licensure examination for licensed practical/vocational nurses*. Chicago, IL: Author.

National Council of State Boards of Nursing. (2017b). *NCSBN board of directors upholds current passing standard for NCLEX-PN examination*. Retrieved from https://ncsbn,org/10107.htm

National League for Nursing. (2012). *The fair testing imperative in nursing education*. Retrieved from http://www.nln.org/facultyprograms/facultyresources/fair_testing_guidelines.htm

O'Neill, T. R. (2005). Definition of a logit. *NCLEX Psychometric Technical Brief, 2*(2), 1–3.

O'Neill, T. R., Marks, C. M., & Reynolds, M. (2005). Re-evaluating the NCLEX-RN passing standard. *Journal of Nursing Measurement, 13,* 147–165.

Ostyre, M. E. (2001). Predicting NCLEX-PN performance for practical nursing students. *Nurse Educator, 26,* 170–174.

Poorman, S. G., Mastorovich, M. L., Liberto, T. L., & Gerwick, M. (2010). A cognitive behaviorial approach for at-risk senior nursing students preparing to take the NCLEX. *Nurse Educator, 35,* 172–175.

Pugsley, K. E., & Clayton, L. H. (2003). Traditional lecture or experiential learning: Changing student attitudes. *Journal of Nursing Education, 42,* 520–523.

Romeo, E. M. (2013). The predictive ability of critical thinking, nursing GPA, and SAT scores on first-time NCLEX-RN performance. *Nursing Education Perspectives, 55,* 248–253.

Schlairet, M. C., Green, R., & Benton, M. J. (2014). The flipped classroom: Strategies for an undergraduate nursing course. *Nurse Educator, 39*(6), 321–325.

Seldomridge, L. A., & DiBartolo, M. C. (2004). Can success and failure be predicted for baccalaureate graduates on the computerized NCLEX-RN? *Journal of Professional Nursing, 20,* 361–368.

Smith, J. E., & Crawford, L. H. (2002). The link between entry-level RN practice and the NCLEX-RN examination. *Nurse Educator, 27,* 109–112.

Sosa, M., & Sethares, K. (2015). An integrative review of the use and outcomes of HESI testing in baccalaureate nursing programs. *Nursing Education Perspectives, 36*(4), 237–243.

Spector, N., & Alexander, M. (2006). Exit exams from a regulatory perspective. *Journal of Nursing Education, 45,* 291–292.

Spurlock, D. (2006). Do no harm: Progression policies and high-stakes testing in nursing education. *Journal of Nursing Education, 45,* 297–302.

Spurlock, D. (2013). The promise and peril of high-stakes testing in nursing education. *Journal of Nursing Regulation, 4*(1), 4–8.

Spurlock, D. R., & Hanks, C. (2004). Establishing progression policies with the HESI exit examination: A review of the evidence. *Journal of Nursing Education, 43,* 539–545.

Spurlock, D. R., & Hunt, L. A. (2008). A study of the usefulness of the HESI exit exam in predicting NCLEX failure. *Journal of Nursing Education, 47,* 157–166.

Stuart, G. W. (2006). Guest editorial: What is the NCLEX really testing? *Nursing Outlook, 54,* 1–2.

Thomas, M. H., & Baker, S. S. (2011). NCLEX-RN success: Evidenced based strategies. *Nurse Educator, 36,* 246–249.

Valiga, T. M. (2003). Teaching thinking: Is it worth the effort? *Journal of Nursing Education, 42,* 479–480.

Waterhouse, J. K., & Beeman, P. B. (2003). Predicting NCLEX-RN success: Can it be simplified? *Nursing Education Perspectives, 24,* 35–39.

Wendt, A. (2003). The NCLEX-RN examination: Charting the course of nursing practice. *Nurse Educator, 28,* 276–280.

Wendt, A., & Kenny, L. (2007). Setting the passing standard for the National Council Licensure Examination for Registered Nurses. *Nurse Educator, 32,* 104–108.

Wendt, A., Kenny, L., & Brown, K. (2010). Keeping the NCLEX-RN current. *Nurse Educator, 35,* 1–3.

Yellin, E., & Geoffrion, A. (2001). Associate degree nurse success in NCLEX-RN, predictors and implications. *Nurse Educator, 26,* 208–211.

Yin, T., & Burger, C. (2003). Predictors of NCLEX-RN success of associate degree nursing graduates. *Nurse Educator, 28,* 232–236.

Young, A., & Wilson, P. (2012). Predicting NCLEX-RN success: The seventh validity study HESI Exit Exam. *Computers, Informatics, Nursing, 30*(1), 55–60.

Appendix A

Steps for Implementing a Systematic Assessment Plan

1. Define the constructs to be introduced in the course.
2. Develop instructional objectives.
3. Write learning outcomes for each objective.
4. Outline the course content/concepts.
5. Schedule exams and due dates for other assignments.
6. Develop a grading plan based on the guidelines.
7. Identify teaching/learning activities to address course content, concepts, and objectives.
8. Determine assessment tasks that are appropriate to measure the achievement of course content, concepts, and objectives.
9. Determine what content, concepts, and course objectives to include on each assessment task.
10. Blueprint exams and assignments to address course content, concepts, and objectives only.
11. Include all the above information in the course syllabus.
12. Discuss all the above information with students.
13. Write exam items to address the blueprint.
14. Assemble the exams based on the blueprint specifications.
15. Review exams to verify that they meet the blueprint specifications.
16. Administer and score the exams based on the guidelines.
17. Analyze the results of the exams.
18. Conduct student exam review.
19. Assign scores to the exams.
20. Provide students with feedback regarding their achievement.

© Anteromite/Shutterstock

21. Offer remediation to students as needed.
22. Use item analyses to improve and bank items with their data.
23. Assign grades at the end of the semester based on the predefined grading plan that was shared with students.
24. Confidentially communicate the grades to students.

Appendix B

Basic Test Statistics

Measures of central tendency: Measures designed to provide a single value that best represents the typical score in a distribution. These measures illustrate how scores in a distribution are concentrated.

Mean: The score that represents the arithmetic average of all the scores on a test. Obtained by dividing the sum of a set of scores by the number of scores.

Median: The middle score in a set of ranked scores that divides the group into two equal halves (the 50th percentile).

Mode: The score that occurs most frequently in a set of scores. It is the score that is obtained by the largest number of test takers.

Measures of dispersion: These measures describe the variability of a set of scores or how scores are spread out in a distribution.

Range: The distance between the lowest and highest scores. The range is distorted by extreme scores.

Variance (SD^2) and standard deviation (SD): Measures of the dispersion of scores around the mean of a distribution. The more the scores cluster around the mean, the smaller the variance; the smaller the variance, the greater the similarity of the group. SD is the square root of the variance. Large values of these indices indicate that the scores are spread out away from the mean.

Percentile rank: A score that indicates the percentage of lower scores in the norm group. If a score of 54 on a test is equal to the 40th percentile, it indicates that 40% of the students in the group achieved a score equal to or lower than 54, while 60% of those in the group received scores higher than 54. A percentile rank does not show what percentage of questions the examinee answered correctly on the test.

Correlation coefficient: An index that indicates the relationship between two sets of measures. This index ranges from -1.0, which indicates a perfect negative relationship, to $+1.0$, which indicates a perfect positive relationship. A value of 0.0 indicates no relationship between the two measures.

Reliability coefficient: An index of the consistency of test scores. This index ranges from 1.0, which is perfect consistency, to 0.0, which indicates the absence of reliability.

Standard error of measurement (SEM): An estimate of the possible amount by which a score (or group of scores) can differ from the true score, based on errors in measurement. The higher the SEM, the lower the score reliability.

© Anteromite/Shutterstock

Difficulty index (p value): The percentage of correct responses to an item. This value is obtained by dividing the sum of those who answered the item correctly by the total number who took the test. This index ranges from 0.0 to +1.0, with 0.0 indicating that no one answered correctly and +1.0 indicating that all test takers answered the item correctly.

Discrimination index (D value) or point biserial index (PBI): Indicates the quality of a test item by identifying the capability of the item to differentiate between high scorers and low scorers on a test. The higher the D value or PBI, the better the test item. The index ranges between −1.0 and +1.0. A positive discrimination index occurs when more students in the highest scoring group answered the item correctly than those in the lowest scoring group. A negative index means that more students in the lowest scoring group answered the item correctly than those in the highest scoring group.

Suggested Range for PBI Values on a Classroom Exam

>0.40	Very good
0.30 to 0.39	Good; examine stem and options for clarity
0.20 to 0.29	Marginal; identify problems with stem and/or options
0.10 to 0.19	Weak; revise stem and/or options before banking the item
0.00 to 0.09	Very weak; consider rejecting or accepting multiple answers for the item
<0.00	Unacceptable; reject or accept multiple answers for the item

Appendix C

Basic Style Guide

This appendix presents an outline of the guidelines that are suggested for item writing. The rules of grammar and punctuation are very complex, so you should have at least one good style reference if you write at all. Each of the references cited at the end of this appendix is worth owning. Remember, no document is read more carefully than your tests are by the students who take them.

While it is important to observe the rules of grammar and punctuation, keep in mind that the rules may not always apply in item writing. Developing a style and being consistent are the key elements for professional-looking classroom exams.

- Write all items in the present tense. Keeping all sentences in the present tense avoids confusion concerning the time of different actions and makes the problem in the question seem to be occurring as the student is attempting to solve it.

    A nurse is assessing a client (present tense)

    NOT

    A nurse assessed a client (past tense)

    EVEN WORSE

    A client has been assessed (passive voice)

- Avoid using the passive voice. The active voice means that the subject of the sentence is the doer; in the passive, the subject is acted upon. The active voice is more direct and concise than the passive voice. Past events that have an impact on the actions of the nurse should be included, but the problem should be occurring now. Misuse of voice does not constitute a grammatical error, but it does affect the readability of the items, particularly for English language learners (ELLs).

    A nurse is assessing a client (present tense) who had surgery 4 hours ago.

    NOT

    A client who had surgery is being assessed by a nurse. (passive voice)

- End a stem that presents a question with a question mark, followed by options that begin with an uppercase letter. To maintain consistency, because some of the options will be fragments, do not use periods at the end of the options unless you are quoting someone.

Which of these actions should a nurse take?

A. Obtain the client's blood pressure
B. Elevate the head of the client's bed
C. Give the client the prescribed sedative
D. Instruct the client to cough and breathe deeply

Which of these instructions should a nurse give to a client who has had stable angina for several years?

A. "Wear a scarf across your face if you have to go outside when the weather is very cold."
B. "Take your prescribed nitroglycerin every evening when you are going to bed."
C. "Restrict the amount of water you drink every day to 500 milliliters."
D. "Participate in vigorous aerobic exercise three times a week."

- Do not use any punctuation at the end of a stem that is an incomplete statement. Begin each option that is completing the stem with a lowercase letter and end the option with a period.

A nurse should assess the client for

A. hyperthermia.
B. rusty sputum.
C. chest pain.
D. hypotension.

- Use the word *nurse* instead of *you* as the subject of the question. We want to know what a nurse should do. You might do anything!

Which of these questions should a nurse ask?

NOT

Which of these questions should you ask?

- Use *should* instead of *would* when referring to a nurse's actions. *Should* denotes obligation or necessity, while *would* suggests what might happen. Items should focus on what should occur, not on what an individual nurse might do. Technically, because anything might happen, every option that follows the word *would* might be correct.

Which of these measures should a nurse include in the client's care plan?

NOT

Which of these measures would a nurse include in the client's care plan?

- Be consistent with terms. Decide on terms such as *client* or *patient*, *physician* or *primary care provider*, and use them consistently. *Client* is the preferred term in most textbooks and on the licensure and certification exams.

Which of these instructions should a nurse give to a client?

- Be careful with the use of the words *signs* and *symptoms*. A *sign* is an objective finding that is observed by an examiner. A *symptom* is a subjective indication as perceived by the client. A *manifestation* is a perceptible indication of a disease. If *sign* is used in the stem, every option that follows must be a sign; if *symptom* is used, every option that follows must be a symptom. Use *manifestation* if the options include both signs and symptoms. In fact, use *manifestation* or *manifestations* in all cases. This will decrease the introduction of error into your test items.

A nurse should observe the client for which of these manifestations?

- *A* is the indefinite article that refers to a person who is not previously specified. *A* refers to any member in the category. *A* nurse refers to any or every nurse. *The* is a definitive article. It is used before a person who has already been mentioned; that is, you are referring to a specific nurse or client who was previously mentioned. The first time you refer to a nurse or a client, use *a*. The second time, use *the*.

A nurse is teaching a client who has congestive heart failure and is on a low sodium diet. Which of these instructions should *the* nurse include?

- Avoid ambiguities by specifying who is saying or doing what to whom in the stem. Do not leave anything to the imagination of the examinees.

Which of these statements, if made by a client who is on a low sodium diet, should indicate to a nurse that the client is adhering to the diet prescription?

NOT

Which of these statements should indicate to a nurse that a client understands how to follow a low sodium diet? (It is unclear who is making the statement.)

- Avoid using descriptors for clients or nurses. Gender, names, ages, marital status, and occupation are all extraneous information that could introduce bias into your test items unless these descriptors pertain to the problem that is being posed.

A nurse is caring for a client who had an appendectomy. . . .

NOT

A nurse is caring for Mrs. Bock, a 45-year-old woman who had an appendectomy. . . .

- Health problems are very unflattering adjectives.

  A client who has hypertension

  NOT

  A hypertensive client

- Use the term *medication* for all legal medications. Save the term *drug* for reference to illegal substances.

  A client is taking all these medications.

  NOT

  A client is taking all these drugs.

- Refer to all medications using only the generic names. The NCLEX has decided to use only the generic names so it makes sense to accustom students to this format.

  A client is taking furosemide. Which of these side effects of furosemide should a nurse caution the client about?

- The first time a phrase that is commonly referred to as an abbreviation is used, spell out the phrase and put the abbreviation in parentheses (no matter how common you think the abbreviation is). Use only the abbreviation once it is introduced.

  A client is scheduled to have a nasogastric tube (NGT) inserted. Which of these explanations should a nurse offer the client about the purpose of the NGT?

  Do not include the abbreviation if it is not used again in the question.

  Which of these measures should a nurse include in the care plan for a client who has a nasogastric tube?

- Label all laboratory values and vital signs.

  A client has a blood pressure of 110/82 mmHg and serum potassium of 3.8 mEq/L.

  NOT

  A client has a blood pressure of 110/82 and serum potassium of 3.8.

- Use both Fahrenheit and Centigrade when reporting temperature.

  A client has a temperature of 100.4°F (38°C).

  NOT

  A client has a temperature of 100.4°F.

  EVEN WORSE

  A client has a temperature of 100.4°.

- Clarify all abbreviations (for example, decide whether to use mL or ml) and use them consistently. Periods are not necessary after an abbreviation. Use abbreviations only after a number

  How many milliliters should the client receive?

  NOT

  How many mL should the client receive?

  Do not label the options when a unit of measurement is spelled out in the stem.

  How many milliliters should the client receive?

  A. 5
  B. 7
  C. 9
  D. 10

  How many tablets should the client receive?

  A. 0.5
  B. 1.0
  C. 1.5
  D. 2.0

  A complaining client has a very negative connotation. Use reports instead.

  A client reports having abdominal pain.

  NOT

  A client complains of abdominal pain.

- Avoid referring to a client as being "with a health problem." *With* is a preposition that means "in the company of" or "having as a possession, attribute, or feature." A client is not accompanied by a health problem and certainly would not consider a health problem to be an attribute or a characteristic. *Has* is the third-person present singular of the verb *to have*. One meaning of *to have* is to be affected by something, particularly something of a medical nature. Use a client who *has* a health problem.

A client who has colon cancer. . . .

NOT

A client with colon cancer. . . .

- It is inappropriate to use contractions in formal writing, and a test should be considered formal. However, it is preferred to use contractions when you are quoting someone. The goal is to make the situation seem realistic.

A nurse who cannot understand what a client is saying says to the client, "Could you repeat what you just said? I didn't understand you."

NOT

A nurse who can't understand what a client is saying says to the client, "I didn't understand you. Could you repeat what you just said?"

- Avoid using brand names that might be unfamiliar to some students.

A new mother says to a nurse, "My baby just finished drinking the infant formula."

NOT

A new mother says to a nurse, "My baby just finished drinking the Enfamil."

- A measure is an activity that is a means to an end. The activities related to the planning phase of the nursing process are an ongoing series of actions that are designed to achieve a planned outcome. The use of a verb here would connote that the action will occur only once instead of continuing until the outcome is achieved. Express measures that connote ongoing activities as gerunds. A gerund is a verb plus *-ing* and acts as a noun.

Which of these measures should a nurse include in the care plan for a client who has a nursing diagnosis of fluid volume deficit?

A. Monitoring. . .
B. Observing. . .
C. Measuring. . .
D. Providing. . .

NOT

A. Monitor. . .
B. Observe. . .
C. Measure. . .
D. Provide. . .

- Use a verb for an activity that occurs as a one-time action. These actions relate to the implementation phase of the nursing process.

  Which of these actions should a nurse take when a client develops dyspnea?

  A. Stop. . .
  B. Elevate. . .
  C. Report. . .
  D. Administer. . .

  NOT

  A. Stopping. . .
  B. Elevating. . .
  C. Reporting. . .
  D. Administering. . .

- Spell out numbers one through nine; write numbers 10 and higher as numerals. This rule does not apply to ages, figures containing decimals, percentages, temperature, dates, math calculations, or times of day.

  A client who has performed eight repetitions. . .

  A 6-year-old child. . .

  A client who was hospitalized for 16 days. . .

- Arrange numbers in options in sequence, usually from smallest to largest. Scrambled values require students to hunt for the answer.

  A. 11
  B. 16
  C. 32
  D. 46

  NOT

  A. 32
  B. 46
  C. 11
  D. 16

- Terms should also be arranged in sequence.

  A nurse should identify the client's anxiety level as

  A. mild.
  B. moderate.
  C. severe.
  D. panic.

  NOT

  A nurse should identify the client's anxiety level as

  A. severe.
  B. panic.
  C. mild.
  D. moderate.

- Make the style agree in a series that includes numbers that would ordinarily be spelled out and numbers that would ordinarily be given as numerals.

  A. 2
  B. 6
  C. 14
  D. 19

  NOT

  A. Two
  B. Six
  C. 14
  D. 19

- Spell out a number that begins a sentence.

  Twenty minutes after taking a medication. . . .

  NOT

  20 minutes after taking a medication. . . .

- Omit the period after a number in an option. It could be misconstrued as a decimal point and could cause confusion.

A. 9
B. 12
C. 16
D. 22

NOT

A. 9.
B. 16.
C. 22.
D. 12.

- Negative stems are discouraged, but if you choose to use a word that reverses the meaning of the question, such as "The client needs ***FURTHER*** instructions," the font for the negative word should be bold, italic, and caps to draw attention to the reversal. Highlight only words that reverse the meaning of the stem. Once you start to highlight adjectives and adverbs, such as *first*, *last*, *most*, *least*, and *priority*, the impact of highlighting diminishes. Students are more likely to overlook the emphasis placed on the word.

    Which of these statements, if made by the client, should indicate to a nurse that the client needs ***FURTHER*** instruction?

    NOT

    Which of these statements, if made by the client, should indicate to a nurse that the client needs further instruction?

- Use hyphens when two or more adjectives are placed together to modify a noun.

    A 2-year-old child. . . .

    A nurse uses a 1-inch needle. . . .

    A well-known celebrity is admitted. . . .

    Remember, the key word in the phrase *style guide* is "guide." All these suggestions are guidelines. Some of the guidelines are designed to raise a red flag—to alert you to a potential problem with an item and to caution you to examine the language you have used closely. When considering these guidelines, keep in mind that these style guides are associated with items that work successfully on multiple-choice exams. In the end, however, you are the final judge of the appropriateness of an item.

Suggested Reading

Stilman, A. (2010). *Grammatically correct: An essential guide to punctuation, style, usage, and more* (2nd ed.). Cincinnati, OH: F & W Media.

Strunk, W., & Strunk, W., Jr. (2011). 2011 revised edition: The elements of style. Cambridge, UK: The Elements of Style Press.

Targeting Cognitive Levels for Multiple-Choice Item Writing

Knowledge: Recalling material that was previously learned. Refers to the simple remembering of a fact, concept, theory, or principle.

The learner is expected to recall information exactly as presented in a textbook or from a classroom lecture and then select the correct answer from the choices presented. Knowledge questions do not require understanding or judgment. Knowledge questions test students' ability to remember previously learned facts, to recall information, and to recognize the correct choice.

Knowledge verbs:

define	recognize
identify	relate
know	reproduce
label	select
list	state
name	tabulate
quote	tell
recall	write

Sample knowledge item:

A nurse should explain to a client who has hypothyroidism that the purpose of levothyroxine is to

    A. replace thyroid hormone.*

    B. stimulate the action of the thyroid gland.

    C. provide thyroid-stimulating hormone.

    D. block the stimulation of the thyroid gland.

Comprehension: The ability to grasp the meaning of material, which is demonstrated by translating material from one form to another.

Comprehension questions test the student's ability to understand information, translate facts, explain the importance of the information, take in information and give it back another way, and make predictions based on understanding.

Comprehension verbs:

change	interpret
compare	outline
convert	predict
describe	rank
differentiate	rearrange
discuss	reorder
distinguish	rephrase
estimate	reword
explain	summarize
extrapolate	transform
illustrate	translate
infer	

Sample comprehension item:

A nurse should explain to a client who is taking warfarin sodium that it is important to regulate the intake of which of these foods?

    A. Liver

    B. Spinach*

    C. Whole milk

    D. Grapefruit

Application: The ability to use learned material in new and concrete situations.

Application questions test the student's ability to apply concepts, laws, methods, phenomena, principles, procedures, rules, and theories to solve problems in unique, real-life situations.

Application verbs:

accelerate	identify
apply	illustrate
arrange	initiate
ascertain	instruct
ask	limit
assist	locate
associate	measure
avoid	minimize
balance	modify
calculate	motivate
change	observe
check	obtain
classify	offer
compose	operate
compute	prepare
construct	prevent
control	promote
demonstrate	relate
design	remove
determine	restrict
develop	revise
discourage	schedule
elevate	show
employ	solve
encourage	stop
enhance	suppress
ensure	teach
examine	test
formulate	transfer
generalize	use
guide	utilize

Sample application item:

A client who took NPH insulin at 8 a.m. this morning reports feeling weak and tremulous at 4 p.m. Which of these actions should a nurse take?

    A. Take the client's blood pressure

    B. Give the client's PRN dose of insulin

    C. Check the client's capillary blood sugar*

    D. Advise the client to lie down with legs elevated

Analysis: The ability to break down material into its component parts so that its organizational structure can be understood.

    Analysis questions test the student's ability to break down information, see a relationship among the parts, recognize the effects, identify patterns, and understand the meaning of information.

Analysis verbs:

analyze	differentiate
arrange	distinguish
associate	divide
categorize	estimate
classify	examine
compare	infer
connect	investigate
contrast	look for trends
correlate	order
debate	question
deduce	recognize error
delineate	separate
detect	solve
determine	subdivide
diagram	verify

Sample analysis item:

Which of these manifestations, if identified in a client during the immediate postoperative period, should a nurse associate with the development of hypovolemic shock?

    A. Hypertension

    B. Increased pulse*

    C. Hyperthermia

    D. Rapid capillary refill

Appendix E

Sample Item Stems for Phases of the Nursing Process

I. Assessment

Process of collecting, verifying, and communicating relevant client data

Which of these (manifestations, side effects) should a nurse investigate first when assessing a client who has (undergone a dx test, nursing dx, medical dx, medication prescription)?

A nurse assesses that a client who has (dx) has (manifestations, vital signs). What additional data should the nurse collect to establish a nursing diagnosis of (. . .)? What (information, data) should the nurse obtain next? Select all that apply.

When assessing a client who has (dx), a nurse should determine whether the client has which of these (signs, symptoms, clinical manifestations, laboratory values)? Select all that apply.

Which of these questions is the most important one for a nurse to ask when assessing a client who has (dx, manifestations)?

To identify whether a client is developing a (side effect of medication, complication of a procedure, progression of a disease), which of these questions should a nurse ask the client?

Which of these questions should a nurse ask a client to assist in establishing a nursing diagnosis of (. . .)? Select all that apply.

Which of these data are most important for a nurse to obtain when assessing a client who has (manifestation, dx)?

A nurse assesses that a client has (manifestation). What further information should the nurse obtain? Which of these questions is the most important for the nurse to ask the client?

When a client develops (manifestations, vital signs), what additional data should a nurse obtain? (insert chart with client manifestations)

A nurse assesses that a client has (several manifestations, vital signs). (insert chart with client manifestations) Which of these additional assessments should the nurse make?

II. Analysis

Process of interpreting assessment data to identify actual or potential client health problems

A nurse identifies that a client who has (dx) demonstrates (manifestations, laboratory values). This finding would help substantiate a nursing diagnosis of. . . .

A client who has (dx) says to a nurse, ". . . ." A nurse should recognize this statement as indicative of. . . .

When assessing a client who has (dx), which of these findings would indicate (complication, advanced disease progress)?

Which of these factors in a client's history is most likely related to the development of (dx)? (insert chart with history findings)

A nurse assesses that a client that has all of these nursing diagnoses. Which one should receive priority for this client?

A nurse assesses that a client who has (dx) has a (laboratory test, dx test) that reveals (. . .). Which of these nursing diagnoses is appropriate for this client? Select all that apply.

Which of these findings, if identified in a client who (has dx, had procedure, is taking medication), should a nurse report to a physician immediately?

A nurse assesses a client who (has dx/is taking medication). Which of these client findings requires immediate follow-up by the nurse? (insert chart with client findings)

A nurse obtains a health history from a client who (has dx/is taking medication). Which of these client findings should the nurse follow-up immediately?

Which of these findings, if identified in a client who (has dx, is receiving Rx), indicates that the client is at risk for developing (complication)?

A nurse should recognize that a client who (has dx/is taking medication) is at risk for developing (complication, side effect) if the client. . . .

A client who has (dx, been in an accident, sustained an injury) is admitted to the emergency department with manifestations indicated in the chart below. Which of the injuries should be treated first? (insert chart with client manifestations)

III. Planning

Process of establishing desired client outcomes and designing strategies to achieve those outcomes

Which of these outcomes should a nurse to establish with a client who has (manifestations, nursing dx, medical dx) of. . . ?

A nurse is developing a plan of care with a client who has (manifestations, nursing dx, medical dx). Which of these outcomes should receive priority in the plan?

Which of these measures should (be included/receive priority) in the care plan for a client who has (manifestations, nursing dx, medical dx)?

When a client (has nursing dx, has medical dx, has a manifestation of/is receiving medication), which of these (pieces of equipment, medications) should a nurse have available?

A nurse should include which of these teaching strategies when planning care for a client who has (nursing dx, medical dx, developmental level)?

Which of these measures, if included in the care plan for a client who has (dx), is the most effective one to (reduce, relieve) (clinical manifestation)?

The teaching plan for a client who is taking (medication or class of medication) should include which of these instructions? Select all that apply.

When planning home care for a client who has (dx), which of these (measures) should a nurse assist the client and family to identify as the priority? Which of these referrals should a nurse make?

Which of these outcomes is most appropriate to establish for a client who has (nursing dx)? Select all that apply.

A nurse is planning staff assignments. Which of these tasks should the nurse assign to a nursing assistant?

A nurse should assign which of these staff members to care for (a client who has dx, an elderly client, an anxious client)?

Which of these laboratory results is most important for a nurse to monitor for a client who has (dx)?

Which of these nursing measures most effective in assisting a client who has (nursing dx, medical dx) in order to achieve the outcome of . . . ?

IV. Implementation

Process of initiating and completing nursing actions to accomplish the defined outcomes

A nurse should instruct a client who (has dx, is at risk for. . .) to make which of these lifestyle modifications? Select all that apply.

A client is scheduled to start taking (medication). A nurse should teach the client to observe for side effects, which include. . . . Select all that apply.

The parents of a (. . .)-year-old child express concern to a nurse about (child's behavior). Which of these explanations (related to age/developmental level) is most appropriate for the nurse to give the parents?

A client who has (dx) has prescriptions for all the medications listed in the table below. Which one should the nurse administer when the client reports . . . ?(insert chart with client medications)

Before administering (medication, treatment) to a client, which of these (laboratory values, vital signs) should a nurse check? Select all that apply.

When a client who has (dx, surgical procedure) develops (manifestation, laboratory value), which of these actions should a nurse take (first, initially)?

Which of these assessments of a client who has (dx) requires immediate nursing intervention?

Which of these approaches is most appropriate for a nurse to take when (performing a procedure) on a (age/developmental level) child?

Which of these explanations should a nurse give to a client who is scheduled to have (surgery, procedure)?

A client (states, acts, experiences an unusual event) or a nurse (performs a procedure, witnesses an accident). Which of these statements should the nurse record in the client's medical record?

A client who is scheduled for (surgery, procedure, treatment) says to a nurse, ". . . ." Which of these responses should the nurse make?

A nurse observes a (colleague, nursing assistant) including all these measures when (performing a procedure). Which one requires the nurse to intervene? Which of these actions is most appropriate for the nurse to take?

V. Evaluation

Process of measuring the client's response to treatments, medications, and nursing actions and progress toward achieving defined outcomes

A nurse instructs a client about (treatment, procedure, medication). Which of these statements, if made by the client indicates that the client (has the correct understanding of the instruction/needs *FURTHER* instruction)?

A client who has (dx) is (taking medication, receiving treatment). Which of these statements, if made by the client, indicates that the (medication, treatment) is having (an *UNTOWARD*, the desired) effect?

When a client who has a (dx) is being treated with (medication, treatment), which of these (manifestations, laboratory data) indicates that the client's condition is (improving, *WORSENING*)? Select all that apply.

A client who has (dx) is receiving (medication, treatment). Which of these responses should a nurse expect the client to have if the (medication, treatment) is achieving the desired therapeutic effect?

A client is on a (diet). Which of these meals, if selected by the client, indicates that the client has the correct understanding of the diet plan?

A client who has (dx) is receiving (medication, treatment). Which of these (laboratory, assessment) findings should a nurse recognize as indicating that the treatment is having (the desired effect) (an *UNTOWARD* effect)?

An outcome for a client who has a (dx) of (. . .) is. . . . Which of these client (statements, behaviors, findings) indicates that the interventions to meet this outcome have been (successful, *UNSUCCESSFUL*)?

Which of these client observations is the most reliable indicator that a client has the correct understanding of how to (give injection, follow diet, avoid side effects)?

Which of these statements is the most accurate recording of a client's response to a (medication, treatment, procedure)?

Which of these (actions, statements) of a client who has (dx) is the best indicator of the client's acceptance of (dx, diet, death, body image change)?

Sample Item Stems for Client Needs Using the Nursing Process Format

I. Management of Care

Assess

A nurse receives a change-of-shift report for all these clients. Which client should the nurse assess first?

Which of these assessments should a nurse make to determine the equipment needs for a client who has (dx, nursing dx) and is being discharged home? Select all that apply.

Which of these questions should a nurse ask to assess if a client understands (advanced directives, legal rights, informed consent)?

Which of these assessments of a client who has (nursing dx, medical dx) should a nurse include to determine if the client is correctly following the (instructions, treatment plan)?

A nurse is completing an admission assessment for a client who is scheduled to have (surgery, procedure). To assess if the client's care is compliant with the Patients' Bill of Rights, which of these questions should the nurse ask?

Analyze

A client who has (dx, been in an accident, sustained an injury) is admitted to an emergency department with (several manifestations). Which of these nursing interventions is the priority?

A nurse identifies these findings when assessing the following clients. Which one should the nurse report to the primary care provider?

A home care nurse receives the following voice mails from several clients. Which one should the nurse call back first?

A nurse identifies all of these findings when assessing a client who has (dx) (insert a chart with client findings). Which finding should the nurse report to the primary care provider immediately?

A nurse assesses a client who has (dx) and determines that the client has all of these nursing diagnoses. Which one is the priority?

Which of these nurses is acting in the role of client advocate?

Which of these interdisciplinary situations represents (case management, collaboration, cooperation, collegiality)?

A nurse is triaging clients who are admitted to an emergency department after being in a (multi-vehicle automobile accident, house fire, landslide). Which one should be treated first?

Plan

After receiving a report for a client at the beginning of a shift (insert a chart with client manifestations) which of these actions should a nurse take first?

A home care nurse is planning to visit all these clients today. Which one should the nurse visit first? In which order should the nurse see the clients?

Which of these measures (instructions) should a nurse include in the care plan (discharge plan) for a (age) client who has (dx, self-care deficit, medication prescription)?

A nurse receives a change-of-shift report for these clients. In which order should the nurse assess the clients?

A hospitalized client who has (dx) says to a nurse, "I'm going to sign myself out and I want to have a copy of my chart." Which of these responses should the nurse offer?

When caring for a client who has (dx, nursing dx), a nurse plans interdisciplinary interventions. Which of these activities represents (case management, collaboration, etc.)?

Implement

A client who has (dx) has all these prescriptions. Which one should the nurse implement when the client develops (manifestations)?

A nurse observes a (colleague, nursing assistant, student nurse) including all these measures when (performing a procedure). Which one would require the nurse to intervene?

A nurse observes a (colleague, nursing assistant, student nurse) including all these measures when (performing a procedure). Which of these actions should the nurse take?

A client who has a terminal illness says to a nurse, "I don't want any heroic measures when I die, but I don't know how to tell my son. What should I do?" How should the nurse assist the client to approach this discussion?

Which of these tasks would be appropriate for a nurse to assign to an unlicensed nursing assistant?

A client who is being treated for (chronic illness, life-threatening injury) says to a nurse, "I really am unhappy with my doctor. I need to find someone who I can relate to." Which of these responses should the nurse offer?

A student nurse is assigned to take care of a client who has (dx, manifestation). The student refuses to enter the client's room and says to the instructor, "I would like a different client assignment?" Which of these responses should the instructor make?

Which of these situations represents a breach of private healthcare information?

Which of these instructions should a nurse include when preparing a client who has (dx, injury) for discharge to (home, hospice, nursing home)?

A client who has (dx) says to a nurse, "I have decided to stop treatment." Which of these responses should the nurse offer?

The spouse of client who is hospitalized for treatment of (dx) asks a nurse, ("How is my wife responding to the chemotherapy?" "What is the medication that my wife is receiving?") Which of these responses should the nurse offer?

A nurse enters the room of a client who has a terminal illness and has an advance directive that specifies comfort care only. The nurse finds the client unresponsive. (The family is in the room.) Which of these actions should the nurse take?

A staff nurse approaches a charge nurse and says, "I cannot remember my password (for the computer, medication cart). Can I use yours for today?" Which of these responses should the charge nurse make?

Evaluate

Which of these questions should a nurse include to determine if a client comprehends and consents to having (surgery, invasive procedure)?

Which of these statements, if made by a client who is scheduled to have (surgery, treatment, dx procedure), would indicate that the client (has the correct understanding, needs ***FURTHER*** instruction)?

A nurse delegates (task) to a nursing assistant. Which of these observations would indicate that the nursing assistant has completed the task successfully?

Which of these observations would indicate that a nursing assistant needs guidance for (managing time effectively, setting priorities, recognizing when to report client findings)?

A nurse manager institutes a new teaching plan to introduce staff nurses to the new (electronic medication record, electronic client chart, etc.). Which of these findings would best indicate that the teaching plan is successful?

A charge nurse implements a plan to teach staff members to (respond to a code, implement disaster plan, use new technology). Which of these methods is the best method to evaluate the staff members' understanding of the instruction?

II. Safety and Infection Control

Assess

Which of these questions should a nurse ask a client regarding (identity, health history, allergies, etc.) before (admission to outpatient performing physical assessment)?

When assessing a client for (risk for falls, skin integrity, etc.), which of these (observations, questions, etc.) should a nurse include?

Which of these assessments should a nurse make of a client who is scheduled to have an (MRI, CT scan, etc.)?

Which of these assessments should a nurse make before administering (medication, treatment)?

Which of these (questions, observation) should a nurse (ask, make) to determine if a (client, nursing assistant) is (using equipment correctly, employing ergonomic principles, implementing asepsis techniques) correctly?

Analyze

A nurse assesses that a client has (describe manifestations of a visual, hearing, sensory impairment). Which of these safety measures should a nurse discuss with the (client, daughter, etc.)?

A nurse observes the results of a client's (Mantoux test, sputum test, CBC, INR, etc.). Which of these findings indicates that the client needs (instruction, room assignment, treatment, etc.)?

A client who has a medical diagnosis of (stroke, dementia, etc.) has all these nursing diagnoses. Which one is the priority?

All these findings are identified in a client's assessment. Which one puts the client at highest risk for (falls, infection, etc.)?

A nurse establishes all these nursing diagnoses after assessing a client. Which one is the priority?

Plan

Which of these safety measures should a nurse include in the care plan for a client who has (nursing dx, visual impairment, restraints)?

A nurse is planning care for a client who has (type of infection) and is on (type of precautions). Which personal protective equipment should the nurse put on before entering the room?

A nurse is teaching a client who has (infectious disease, newly implanted device) for discharge home. Which of these instructions should the nurse include?

A nurse is preparing to administer (blood transfusion, initial insulin injection, chemotherapy) to a client. Which of these measures should the nurse include in the client's care plan?

Which of these clients should a nurse recommend for discharge when preparing the hospital for an impending (hurricane, tornado, etc.)?

Implement

A nurse observes a colleague (mishandling hazardous waste, contaminating sterile field, etc.). Which of these actions should a nurse take?

Which of these instructions should a nurse give to a (nursing assistant, client) to ensure safe use of (equipment)? Select all that apply.

Which of these questions (related to allergies, identification) should a nurse ask before (nutritional instruction, treatment, procedure)?

Which of these instructions should a nurse give to (client's family, nursing assistant) regarding the use of (type of equipment, restraints)?

Which of these suggestions should a nurse give to a homebound client who has (infection, ataxia, confusion, vertigo, etc.)? Select all that apply.

Which of these infection control precautions should a nurse implement for a client who has (nursing dx, medical dx, manifestations)?

Evaluate

Which of these statements, if made by a client who has (dx) indicates that the client correctly understands infection control precautions?

Which of these statements, if made by the daughter of a client who has (dx) is being discharged to (home, daughter's home, assisted living) indicates that the (client, daughter) understands (safety precautions)?

A nurse manager develops and initiates a new plan to decrease the incidence of (urinary tract infections, pressure ulcers, etc.). Which of these findings would be the best evidence that the plan is successful?

Which of these actions, if implemented by a nursing assistant would indicate that the assistant needs **FURTHER** instruction (related to infection control, safe equipment use, use of restraints, security precautions, handling infectious waste, etc.)?

A nurse prepares a client who has (AIDS, pneumonia, wound infection, TB, etc.) for hospital discharge. Which of these statements, if made by the client, indicates that the client needs **FURTHER** instruction?

III. Health Promotion and Maintenance

Assess

Which of these questions should a nurse ask to determine if a client uses culturally preferred therapies for treatment of (nursing dx, medical dx)?

Which of these assessments should a nurse make to determine the developmental level of a(n) (XX)-year-old child?

Which of these (observations, questions) should a nurse (include, ask) when assessing the (self-care ability, developmental stage, disease prevention ability) of a client? Select all that apply.

Which of these (observations, questions) should a nurse (include, ask) when assessing the (nutritional status, lifestyle choices, immunization status) of a client?

Which of these approaches is the most effective approach for assessing a client's (nutritional status, lifestyle choices, learning style, etc.)?

Analyze

A nurse assesses that a(n) (XX)-year-old child exhibits (behavior). Which of these toys should the nurse select for the child?

A nurse identifies all these findings when assessing a newborn. (insert chart describing findings) Which of these Apgar scores should the nurse assign to the infant?

Which of these findings, if identified when examining (an infant, a toddler, a preschooler, etc.) should a nurse refer to the client's primary healthcare provider?

A nurse assesses a client's (family systems, lifestyle choices, etc.) and identifies all these nursing diagnoses. Which one is the priority?

A nurse identifies that a client has (cholesterol level, CBC, etc.). The client has all of these nursing diagnoses. Which one is the priority?

Plan

Which of these activities should a nurse plan for a(n) (XX)-year-old child who is hospitalized and on (bed rest, infection control precautions, activity restriction)?

Which of these instructions should a nurse include when discussing the (aging process, ante/intra/postpartum care, newborn care, family planning, health screening, immunizations, growth and development) with (client, parents)?

Which of these instructions should a nurse include in a plan for teaching a group of (senior citizens, parents) about (health screening, lifestyle changes, developmental stages, etc.)?

Which of these approaches would be most effective when discussing (health promotion programs, disease prevention, human sexuality, high-risk behaviors) with a group of (adolescents, teenagers, retired adults, etc.)?

When teaching a group of parents of toddlers about (preventing accidental poisoning, normal growth and development, etc.), which of these instructions should a nurse include? Select all that apply.

Implement

Which of these instructions should a nurse give to a (male client, female client) about a self-administered (testicular exam, breast exam, disease prevention, specific high-risk behaviors)?

Which of these instructions should a nurse include when discussing growth and development with the parents of a(n) (XX)-year-old child who is demonstrating (behavior)?

Which of these instructions should a nurse give to the caretaker of a(n) (XX)-year-old client who has (dementia, poor mobility, etc.).

Which of these measures should a nurse include when completing a physical assessment of a client's (lower extremities, abdomen, etc.)?

Which of these immunizations should a(n) (XX) year-old child receive?

Which of these health screenings should a nurse recommend for a(n) (XX)-year-old (male, female)?

Evaluate

A nurse instructs a client regarding (growth and development, prevention of specific disease, family planning, childhood immunizations, self-care for specific disease). Which of these (responses, statements, actions) by the client should a nurse interpret as indicating that the client (has the correct understanding of the instructions, needs **FURTHER** instruction)?

Which of these statements, if made by a client, indicates that the client understands the (precautions for preventing disease, newborn care, etc.)? Select all that apply.

Which of these statements, if made by a client, indicates that the client understands (strategies to achieve optimal health, effect of the aging process, benefits of health screening)?

Which of these actions, if demonstrated by a client who has (HIV, an STD, etc.) indicates that the client (has the correct understanding of the instructions, needs **FURTHER** instruction)?

Which of these statements, if made by the parents of a(n) (XX)-year-old child indicates that the parents understand (developmental stages, immunizations schedules, etc.)? Select all that apply.

IV. Psychosocial Integrity

Assess

Which of these assessments should a nurse make to determine a client's (coping mechanisms, stress management, support systems, etc.)?

A client says, "(. . .)" to a nurse. (Which of these responses should the nurse make? Which of these responses would be most effective?)

Which of these approaches is the best one to determine a client's (religious or spiritual influences on health, coping mechanisms, support systems, chemical dependency, etc.)?

Which of these is the best approach to assessing a client's (sensory/perceptual alterations, stress management, spiritual influences, coping mechanisms)?

Which of these assessments of a(n) (child, elderly client) should a nurse report as suspected abuse?

A nurse identifies all these findings when assessing a client who (has psychopathology, has chemical dependency, is receiving end-of-life care, etc.). Which of these additional assessments should the nurse make?

Analyze

Which of these assessment findings of a client who has (nursing dx, medical dx) should a nurse follow up immediately?

A nurse assesses a client and identifies all the findings in the table below. (insert chart with findings)

Which of these nursing diagnoses should the nurse include for the client? Select all that apply.

A nurse identifies that a client has all these nursing diagnoses. (insert chart with list of diagnoses) Which one is the priority?

A nurse identifies all these findings when assessing a client. (insert chart with findings). Which of these therapeutic communication techniques should the nurse use?

A client who has (medical dx, nursing dx) has all the prescriptions (not medications) listed in the table below. Which one should the nurse implement when the client (develops manifestations, exhibits behavior)?

A client who is admitted to the hospital for detoxification has all these manifestations. (insert chart with manifestations) Which one should the nurse follow up first?

Plan

A nurse identifies all these findings when assessing a client. (insert chart with findings). Which of these measures should the nurse include in the client's care plan? Select all that apply.

In which of these situations should a nurse employ crisis intervention? Select all that apply.

A nurse identifies that a client's (religious beliefs, culture, sensory/perceptual alteration, coping mechanism) is interfering with the client's acceptance of the treatment plan. Which of these measures should the nurse include in the client's care plan? Select all that apply.

Which of these measures should a nurse include when planning end-of-life care for a client (who is in denial, whose family is in denial)?

Which of these measures should a nurse include in the care plan for a hospitalized client who has (sensory/perceptual alteration)?

Which of these measures should a nurse include in the care plan for a client who is (addicted to cocaine, an alcoholic) who is hospitalized for detoxification? Select all that apply.

Implement

A client who is scheduled to have (surgery, procedure, treatment) says to a nurse, "(. . .)." Which of these responses should the nurse offer?

A client who has (psychopathology, chemical dependency, sensory/perceptual alteration) is experiencing (grief and loss, body image change) demonstrates (behavior). Which of these interventions should a nurse initiate?

The daughter of a client who (is receiving end-of-life care, has specific pathophysiology, has sensory/perceptual alteration) says to a nurse, ". . . ." Which of these (responses, instructions) should the nurse offer?

A client refuses lifesaving (treatment, procedure) based on religious beliefs. Which of these actions should a nurse take?

A nurse identifies that a(n) (elderly client, 2-year-old child, etc.) has (several bruises, difficulty managing stress). Which of these actions should a nurse take? Select all that apply.

A client who had (disfiguring surgery) says to a nurse, "(I . . .)." Which of these responses should a nurse offer?

Evaluate

A client who has (terminal illness, coronary artery disease, etc.) plans to use (guided imagery, relaxation, etc.) to manage stress. Which of these client statements indicates the correct understanding of (guided imagery, relaxation, etc.)?

A nurse reviews stress management techniques with a group of parents of pre-school-age, school-age (children). Which of these statements, if made by a parent, indicates the correct understanding of the stress management techniques.

Which of these observations of a client indicates that the client correctly understands the instructions related to (stress management, coping mechanisms)? Select all that apply.

Which of these statements, if made by a client, indicates that the client has the correct understanding of (stress management, end-of-life care)?

Which of these client behaviors should a nurse recognize as evidence that the nursing interventions to improve the client's (stress management, coping mechanism, etc.) are successful?

V. Basic Care and Comfort

Assess

Which of these assessments should a nurse include when assessing a client who has a history of (vertigo, tinnitus, dizziness)?

Which of these questions should a nurse include when assessing a client's (nutrition, elimination, personal care, rest and sleep pattern)? Select all that apply.

A nurse assesses a client's (mobility, nutritional, elimination, etc.) status and identifies (manifestations). Which of these further assessments should the nurse make?

When assessing a client's understanding of (alternative therapies, nonpharmacologic comfort interventions, nutrition, etc.) the client says to a nurse, ". . . ." Which of these further assessments should the nurse make?

Which of these assessments should a nurse include when assessing a client's (nutritional status, mobility status, rest and sleep pattern, etc.)? Select all that apply.

A nurse should include which of these observations when assessing a client's (nutritional status, hydration status, elimination status, mobility status, skin integrity, etc.)? Select all that apply.

Analyze

Which of these assessment findings indicates that a client needs assistance with (assistive devices, personal care, nutrition, etc.)?

A nurse assesses a client's (mobility, nutritional status, etc.) and identifies the findings indicated in the table below. Which of these nursing diagnoses should the nurse identify? Select all that apply.

A nurse assesses a client's (mobility, nutritional status, etc.) and identifies all these nursing diagnoses. Which one is the priority?

A nurse identifies all these findings as identified in the table below when assessing a client's (nutrition, hydration, mobility, personal hygiene, rest and sleep, etc.) status. (insert chart with findings) Which finding requires immediate follow up?

Which of these assessment findings of a client who has a (medical dx, nursing dx) of (dx related to nutrition, elimination, fluids, etc.) should a nurse report immediately to the primary care provider?

Plan

Which of these measures should a nurse include in the care plan for a client who has (manifestation related to difficulty eating or drinking, BMI of . . ., nasogastric tube feeding, gastrostomy tube feeding, increased blood glucose level, increased urine specific gravity)?

Which of these measures should a nurse include when (performing postmortem care, irrigating a client's bladder, inserting a nasogastric or urethral catheter, etc.)? Select all that apply.

Which of these measures should a nurse include when providing (alternative or complimentary) therapy? Select all that apply.

Which of these (therapies, interventions) should a nurse include when planning interventions for a client who (is subject to skin breakdown, requires TPN, requires tube feeding, etc.)?

Which of these measures should a nurse include in the care plan for a client who has findings (related to nutrition, fluid retention, pain, immobility, etc.) identified in the chart below? (insert chart with client findings)

Implement

A nurse should include which of these instructions when teaching a client to use (assistive device, alternative therapy, alternative methods to promote voiding, orthopedic devices, nonpharmacological pain management, etc.)?

Which of these actions should a nurse take when a client has symptoms of (dehydration, nutritional deficit, elimination difficulty, etc.)?

Which of these instructions should a nurse include when teaching a (client, client's family) to (prevent complications of immobility, use nonpharmacological comfort measures, follow prescribed diet)?

A nurse is educating the family of a client who has (medical dx) about (palliative care, assisting with personal hygiene, providing adequate nutrition, etc.). Which of these instructions should the nurse include? Select all that apply.

Which of these suggestions should a nurse offer to a client who reports having (insomnia, difficulty following diet, pain, incontinence, etc.)?

Evaluate

Which of these observations indicates that a client's use of (alternative therapy) is having the desired effect?

A nurse initiates all of these actions (insert chart with list of actions) to assist a client who has (assistive device, sensory impairment, altered nutrition, etc.). Which of these observations indicates that the interventions are successful?

Which of these findings, if identified in a client who uses (assistive device, non-pharmacological interventions for pain management, etc.) indicates that the client is using the (. . .) correctly?

A nurse teaches a client who has (medical dx) about (using assistive device, using complimentary or nonpharmacological therapy practices, following special diet, using orthopedic device, obtaining adequate rest.) Which of these statements by the client is the best evidence that the teaching was effective?

Which of these client observations is the most reliable indicator that the client has the correct understanding about (using assistive device, following prescribed diet, etc.)?

VI. Pharmacological and Parenteral Therapies

Assess

Which of these assessments should a nurse make before administering a dose of (medication) to a client?

Which of these assessments should a nurse make when a client is taking (identify two medications)?

A nurse assesses that a client who is (taking medication, having an intravenous transfusion, having a blood transfusion) has (vital signs, manifestations). Which additional assessment should the nurse make? Select all that apply.

Which of these questions is most important to ask when assessing a client who has (medical dx) and is taking (medication)?

Which of these questions should a nurse ask to identify if a client who has (medical dx) is developing a side effect of (medication)?

Analyze

Which of these assessment findings, if identified in a client who is taking (medication), should a nurse follow up?

Which of these nursing diagnoses should a nurse identify for a client who is taking (medication) and has all of the assessment findings identified in the chart below? (insert chart with assessment findings)

A client who has (medical dx, nursing dx) has all the medication prescriptions listed in the table below. Which one should the nurse implement when the client (develops manifestations, exhibits behavior)?

Which of these findings, if identified when assessing a client, is a contraindication for (medication)?

A client who has (type blood) needs a transfusion. In an emergency situation, which of these blood types is safe for the client to receive?

A nurse identifies that a client who has (medical dx) is taking all the medications. Listed in the chart below (insert chart with medications). Which combination of medications should the nurse recognize as incompatible?

Plan

Which of these instructions should a nurse plan to include when teaching a client who is scheduled to start taking (medication)?

Which of these measures should a nurse include when planning care for a client who is receiving (medication, TPN, blood transfusion, etc.)? Select all that apply.

Which of these measures should a nurse include when planning care for a client who (has an ostomy, is on a ventilator, has an arterial line, etc.)?

Which of these measures should receive priority when monitoring a client who is receiving (medication, a transfusion, intravenous infusion, etc.)?

Which of these laboratory test results would be most important for a nurse to monitor for a client who has (medical dx) and is taking (medication)?

A nurse should include which of these teaching strategies when planning care for a client who is taking (injectable medication, pain medication, controlled substance, PCA, etc.).

Implement

After administering a dose of intravenous (medication), a client (exhibits manifestations). Which of these actions should the nurse take?

A client who is receiving (a transfusion, TPN) develops (manifestations). Which of these actions should a nurse take?

Which of these measures should a nurse include when administering a blood transfusion to a client? Select all that apply.

A nurse is preparing to administer (medication dose). The medication is available as (dose per tablet or ml). How (many milliliters, tablets) should the nurse administer?

A nurse is preparing to administer (dose) intravenously over (time). The medication is provided from the pharmacy as (dose per ml). The nurse should regulate the intravenous infusion to run at how many milliliters per hour?

A client is scheduled to receive an intravenous infusion of (ml) over (number of) hours. A nurse should regulate the intravenous infusion to run at how many milliliters per hour?

Evaluate

Which of these client manifestations should a nurse recognize as an adverse effect to (medication)?

Which of these client statements indicates that the client has the (correct, *INCORRECT*) understanding of how to take (medication)?

A client who has (medical dx) is taking (medication). Which of these client findings indicates that the medication is having the (desired, an *UNTOWARD*) effect?

A nurse instructs a client to self-administer (insulin, heparin, etc.). Which of these client observations is the best indicator that the client correctly understands the instructions?

When a client who has (medical dx) is being treated with (medication), which of these (manifestations, vital signs, laboratory data) indicates that the (medication) is (*WORSENING*, improving)?

VII. Reduction of Risk Potential

Assess

Which of these assessments should a nurse make before sending a client for (MRI, CT scan, bronchoscopy, etc.)?

Which of these questions should a nurse ask a client who is scheduled to have (MRI, CT scan, bronchoscopy, etc.)?

Which of these additional assessments should a nurse make when a client has lab result indicated in the chart below? (insert chart with lab results)

When a client who has (medical dx) develops (vital signs, lab results), which of these additional assessments should the nurse make?

To identify if a client is developing a complication of a (diagnostic test, treatment, procedure), which of these assessments should a nurse include?

Which of these assessments should a nurse make after a client has (procedure, treatment)? Select all that apply.

Analyze

Which of these findings, if identified when assessing a client who is scheduled to have (bronchoscopy, MRI, angiogram, etc.), should a nurse report to the physician?

Which of these findings, if identified when assessing a client, would be a contraindication for (procedure)?

Which of these (vital signs, lab values) would indicate that a client is having an untoward reaction to (a procedure)? Select all that apply.

Which of these findings, if identified in a client's history, indicates that the client is at risk for developing a complication of (dx test, surgical procedure, etc.)?

Which of these findings, if identified when completing a (gastrointestinal, respiratory, cardiovascular, etc.) focused assessment, should a nurse follow up immediately? Select all that apply.

Plan

Which of these measures should a nurse include in the care plan for a client who is scheduled to have (MRI, PET scan, CT scan, etc.)? Select all that apply.

Which of these laboratory values is most important for a nurse to monitor for a client who has (medical dx)?

A nurse should plan to include which of these instructions when teaching a client who is scheduled to have (ECT, cardiac catheterization, NGT inserted, surgery, procedure, etc.)?

The care plan for a client who had (cast applied, surgical procedure, chest tube inserted, etc.) should include which of these measures?

Which of these measures should a nurse include when planning care for a client who is (on prolonged bed rest, receiving nasogastric tube feedings, at risk for falling, etc.)? Select all that apply.

Implement

Which of these precautions should a nurse take before sending a client for an (MRI, arteriogram, bronchoscopy, endoscopy, etc.)?

A nurse identifies (redness, swelling, pain, etc.) at a client's (intravenous insertion site, femoral artery insertion site, surgical incision, etc.). Which of these actions should the nurse take?

Which of these instructions should a nurse include when teaching a client who is scheduled to have (an MRI, conscious sedation, an electrocardiogram, surgery, a laboratory test, etc.)? Select all that apply.

Which of these actions should a nurse include when (obtaining an arterial blood specimen, performing an EKG, performing fetal heart monitoring, performing diagnostic testing, etc.)?

Which of these actions should a nurse include when completing a focused assessment of a client's (gastrointestinal, respiratory, circulatory, etc.) system?

Evaluate

Which of these laboratory values, if identified in a client who is receiving (treatment), indicates that the treatment is (successful, unsuccessful)? (insert chart with lab values)

Which of these findings, if identified in a client who has a(n) (chest tube, tracheostomy, continuous bladder drainage, etc.) indicates that the treatment is effective?

A client has (vital signs, lab values, manifestations) before (procedure, surgery, etc.). Which of these findings, if identified after the (procedure, surgery, etc.) would indicate that the treatment was (successful, unsuccessful)?

A nurse identifies that a client's (chest tube, telemetry monitor, drainage tube, etc.) is (describe functioning). Which finding indicates that the treatment is functioning correctly?

A client has (procedure, surgery, treatment). Which of these statements, if entered in the client's medical record, documents that the (procedure, surgery, treatment) was (successful, unsuccessful)?

VIII. Physiological Adaptation

Assess

Which of these assessments should a nurse include when assessing a client who has (F&E imbalance, infectious disease, specific illness, etc.)?

Which of these assessments should a nurse make before (suctioning, performing dialysis, administering oxygen, administering TPN, etc.)?

A nurse assesses a client who has (dx) and identifies all of these findings. (insert chart with findings) Which of these further assessments should the nurse make?

Which of these observations, if made when assessing a client who has (a wound, ostomy, tracheostomy, etc.), requires further assessment?

When assessing a client who (has an infectious disease, is receiving chemo or radiation therapy, etc.), which of these findings indicates the need for further assessment?

Analyze

A nurse identifies all of these findings when assessing a client who has (medical dx, receiving therapy, F&E imbalance, etc.). (insert chart with findings) Which of the findings is the priority for follow up?

A nurse identifies all these nursing diagnoses for a client who (is receiving dialysis, on telemetry, has a pacemaker, etc.). Which one is the priority?

Which of these findings, if identified when assessing a client (who has medical dx) (should be followed up, is a contraindication for a medication)?

Which of these findings, if identified in a client who is (receiving treatment), indicates that the client may be developing complication of the (medication)?

A nurse assesses a client who has (dx) and identifies all these findings. (insert chart with findings) Which finding should be reported to the primary care provider immediately?

A nurse assesses a client who is (receiving chemotherapy, radiation, etc.) and identifies all of these findings. (insert chart with findings) Which finding should be reported to the primary care provider?

Plan

Which of these instructions should a nurse plan to include when teaching a client who is scheduled to (start peritoneal dialysis, have an implanted pacemaker, etc.)?

Which of these measures should a nurse include when planning care for a client who is scheduled to have (surgery, dialysis, an arterial line, etc.)? Select all that apply.

When teaching a client about (ostomy care, incentive spirometry, a pacing device, etc.) which of these instructions should a nurse plan to include? Select all that apply.

Which of these measures should a nurse include when preparing to (suction, provide wound care, etc.) for a client?

Which of these outcomes should a nurse establish with a client who has a(n) (alteration in body system, F&E imbalance, etc.)

Implement

Which of these actions should a nurse take when a client who has (acute or chronic condition) develops (manifestation)?

Which of these actions should a nurse include when caring for a client who has a(n) (telemetry, pacemaker, arterial line, etc.) develops (complication)?

Which of these interventions should a nurse include when (changing an arterial line dressing, caring for a client on mechanical ventilation, providing pulmonary hygiene, etc.)?

A nurse identifies that a client who has (medical dx) is experiencing (complications). Which of these actions should the nurse take?

A client who is (receiving therapy) develops (untoward reaction). Which of these actions should a nurse take?

A client who has (medical dx) says to a nurse, ". . . ." Which of these responses should the nurse offer?

Which of these instructions is the priority when teaching a client who has (medical dx) to manage self-care?

Evaluate

A nurse instructs a client who has a(n) (ostomy, pacemaker, wound, etc.). Which of these behaviors, if identified when observing the client, indicates that the client correctly understands the instructions.

A client who has (medical dx) has all these treatments prescribed. (insert chart with prescribed treatments) Which of these findings, if identified when observing a client, indicates that the client is following the prescribed treatment regimen?

Which of these observations is most indicative that a client who has (medical dx) correctly understands the instructions related to (procedure)?

A nurse establishes the outcome of (. . .) with a client who has (. . .). Which of these client (behaviors, responses, findings) is the best indication that the outcome is attained?

Which of these client findings, if identified in a client who (was treated for an infectious disease, received oxygen therapy, received illness management activities, etc.), indicates that the interventions were successful?

Which of these findings, if identified in a client who is receiving (chemotherapy, radiation, hemodialysis, etc.), would indicate that the treatment is (successful, unsuccessful)?

Index

Page numbers followed by *f*, *t*, *b*, and *e* indicate figures, tables, boxes, and exhibits, respectively.

A

AACN. *See* American Association of Colleges of Nursing
abbreviations, style guide for test items, 380–381
ability estimates, NCLEX passing standard and, 350
academic dishonesty, 216–220
    academic integrity policy, 221
    cheating, 215, 216–217
    deterring, 218–220
    plagiarism, 220–221
    strategies to prevent, 217–218
academic integrity policy, 221
achievement, student. *See also* grades, assigning; mastery (performance) learning
    assessing, 2–3, 12, 13, 17–21, 119
    of course objectives, 16, 33, 58–59, 79, 365
achievement test, 17, 23, 68, 83–84, 240, 245, 258. *See also* tests
action in the stem, 113–117*e*
action verbs, 36
active learning, 119, 295
active voice, style guide for test items, 377
Adams, John, 11
adequate information, 185, 185*e*
adjectives, 385
administration of tests, 212
    reliability and, 232
AERA. *See* American Educational Research Association
affective learning domain, 7, 51
    Bloom's taxonomy of, 46–48, 47*t*, 296, 352
    in clinical/laboratory experience, 297–298
AFT. *See* American Federation of Teachers
Alexander, M., 362
all of the above, avoiding use of, 110, 110*e*
alphabetizing, options, 103
alternative formats, NCLEX examinations, 352–353
ambiguities, avoidance of, 379
ambiguous statements, 166–167*e*
American Association of Colleges of Nursing (AACN), 4–5
American Educational Research Association (AERA), 23. *See also Standards for Educational and Psychological Testing*
American Federation of Teachers (AFT), 6

American Nurses Association, *Code of Ethics*, 295
American Psychological Association, 6, 23. *See also Standards for Educational and Psychological Testing*
analysis
    cognitive level of, 43, 46
        test items written at, 66, 68, 125, 134–136, 146, 148, 193
    item stems for, 392
analytic scoring rubric, 195, 197*t*
anchor papers, scoring essay items and, 192
Anderson, L. W., 83, 84
    taxonomy, 46–48, 47*t*
Anderson, V. J., 319
Anna, D. J., 213
answer options, equal representation of, in item bank, 203
answer selection, on tests, 91
anxiety, test
    humor-induced, 22, 118
    reducing, 69–70, 84, 92, 203–204, 208, 215–216
application, cognitive level of
    generally, 43, 47
    test items written at, 66, 68, 125, 134, 139, 146, 193
application question, 135–136*e*
appropriate objective, 51–52
articles, indefinite, 379
ascending order, for item options, 95
assessment. *See also* evaluation; measurement
  data collection for, 12
  format, appropriate, 61–62
  instructional role of, 1–10
    assessment and self-efficacy, 3–4
    assessment competency standards, 6, 6*b*
    assessment inadequacies, 4–5
    assessment instruments, 7
    in educational instruction, 2
    ethical responsibilities, 3
    learning activities, 8
    need for systematic approach to assessment, 7
    process of assessment, 1–3, 2*f*
  item stems for, 391
  language of, 11–29
    basic test statistics, 27–28
    evaluation, 13–15
    grade, 21
    instructional objectives, 15–16

411